Post-traumatic Stress Disorder

World Psychiatric Association *Evidence and Experience in Psychiatry* Series

Series Editor: Helen Herrman, WPA Secretary for Publications, University of Melbourne, Australia

Depressive Disorders, 3e
Edited by Helen Herrman, Mario Maj and Norman Sartorius
ISBN: 9780470987209

Substance Abuse Disorders
Edited by Hamid Ghodse, Helen Herrman, Mario Maj and Norman Sartorius
ISBN: 9780470745106

Schizophrenia 2e
Edited by Mario Maj, Norman Sartorius
ISBN: 9780470849644

Dementia 2e
Edited by Mario Maj, Norman Sartorius
ISBN: 9780470849637

Obsessive-Compulsive Disorders 2e
Edited by Mario Maj, Norman Sartorius, Ahmed Okasha, Joseph Zohar
ISBN: 9780470849668

Bipolar Disorders
Edited by Mario Maj, Hagop S Akiskal, Juan José López-Ibor, Norman Sartorius
ISBN: 9780471560371

Eating Disorders
Edited by Mario Maj, Kathrine Halmi, Juan José López-Ibor, Norman Sartorius
ISBN: 9780470848654

Phobias
Edited by Mario Maj, Hagop S Akiskal, Juan José López-Ibor, Ahmed Okasha
ISBN: 9780470858332

Personality Disorders
Edited by Mario Maj, Hagop S Akiskal, Juan E Mezzich
ISBN: 9780470090367

Somatoform Disorders
Edited by Mario Maj, Hagop S Akiskal, Juan E Mezzich, Ahmed Okasha
ISBN: 9780470016121

Current Science and Clinical Practice Series

Schizophrenia
Edited by Wolfgang Gaebel
ISBN: 9780470710548

Obsessive Compulsive Disorder
Edited by Joseph Zohar
ISBN: 9780470711255

Other recent World Psychiatric Association titles

Special Populations

The Mental Health of Children and Adolescents: an area of global neglect
Edited by Helmut Remschmidt, Barry Nurcombe, Myron L. Belfer, Norman Sartorius and Ahmed Okasha
ISBN: 9780470512456

Contemporary Topics in Women's Mental Health: global perspectives in a changing society
Edited by Prabha S. Chandra, Helen Herrman, Marianne Kastrup, Marta Rondon, Unaiza Niaz, Ahmed Okasha, Jane Fisher
ISBN: 9780470754115

Approaches to Practice and Research

Religion and Psychiatry: beyond boundaries
Edited by Peter J Verhagen, Herman M van Praag, Juan José López-Ibor, John Cox, Driss Moussaoui
ISBN: 9780470694718

Psychiatric Diagnosis: challenges and prospects
Edited by Ihsan M. Salloum and Juan E. Mezzich
ISBN: 9780470725696

Recovery in Mental Health: reshaping scientific and clinical responsibilities
By Michaela Amering and Margit Schmolke
ISBN: 9780470997963

Handbook of Service User Involvement in Mental Health Research
Edited by Jan Wallcraft, Beate Schrank and Michaela Amering
ISBN: 9780470997956

Psychiatrists and Traditional Healers: unwitting partners in global mental health
Edited by Mario Incayawar, Ronald Wintrob and Lise Bouchard,
ISBN: 9780470516836

Depression and Comorbidity

Depression and Diabetes
Edited by Wayne Katon, Mario Maj and Norman Sartorius
ISBN: 9780470688380

Depression and Heart Disease
Edited by Alexander Glassman, Mario Maj and Norman Sartorius
ISBN: 9780470710579

Depression and Cancer
Edited by David W. Kissane, Mario Maj and Norman Sartorius
ISBN: 9780470689660

Post-traumatic Stress Disorder

Editors

Dan J. Stein, MD, PhD
Professor and Chair
Department of Psychiatry
University of Cape Town
Cape Town, South Africa;
Visiting Professor
Mount Sinai School of Medicine
New York, NY, USA

Matthew J. Friedman, MD
Professor of Psychiatry and of Pharmacology & Toxicology
Dartmouth Medical School;
Executive Director
National Center for Posttraumatic Stress Disorder
US Department of Veterans Affairs
Hanover, NH, USA

Carlos Blanco, MD, PhD
Professor of Psychiatry
Department of Psychiatry
Columbia University
New York, NY, USA

WILEY-BLACKWELL
A John Wiley & Sons, Ltd., Publication

This edition first published 2011

Wiley-Blackwell is an imprint of John Wiley & Sons, formed by the merger of Wiley's global Scientific, Technical and Medical business with Blackwell Publishing.

Registered office: John Wiley & Sons, Ltd, The Atrium, Southern Gate, Chichester, West Sussex, PO19 8SQ, UK

Editorial offices:
9600 Garsington Road, Oxford, OX4 2DQ, UK
The Atrium, Southern Gate, Chichester, West Sussex, PO19 8SQ, UK
111 River Street, Hoboken, NJ 07030-5774, USA

For details of our global editorial offices, for customer services and for information about how to apply for permission to reuse the copyright material in this book please see our website at www.wiley.com/wiley-blackwell.

Library of Congress Cataloging-in-Publication Data

Post-traumatic stress disorder / [edited by] Dan Stein, Matthew Friedman, and Carlos Blanco.
p. ; cm.
Includes bibliographical references and index.
ISBN 978-0-470-68897-7 (cloth)
1. Post-traumatic stress disorder. I. Stein, Dan J. II. Friedman, Matthew J. III. Blanco, Carlos, 1962-
[DNLM: 1. Stress Disorders, Post-Traumatic. WM 172]
RC552.P67P6616 2011
616.85′21–dc23

2011014924

A catalogue record for this book is available from the British Library.

This book is published in the following electronic format: ePDF 9781119998488; Wiley Online Library: 9781119998471; ePub 9781119971481; Mobi 9781119971498

Typeset in 11/13pt Times Roman by Laserwords Private Limited, Chennai, India

First Impression 2011

Contents

Preface **xi**

List of Contributors **xv**

1 PTSD and Related Disorders **1**
Matthew J. Friedman

Commentaries

1.1 Walking the Line in Defining PTSD: Comprehensiveness Versus Core Features 35
Chris R. Brewin

1.2 Trauma-Related Disorders in the Clinical and Legal Settings 38
Elie G. Karam

1.3 Redefining PTSD in DSM-5: Conundrums and Potentially Unintended Risks 42
Alexander C. McFarlane

2 Epidemiology of PTSD **49**
Carlos Blanco

Commentaries

2.1 Challenges and Future Horizons in Epidemiological Research into PTSD 75
Abdulrahman M. El-Sayed and Sandro Galea

2.2 Preventing Mental Ill-Health Following Trauma 79
Helen Herrman

2.3 PTSD Epidemiology with Particular Reference to Gender 82
Marianne Kastrup

3 Neurobiology of PTSD **89**
Arieh Y. Shalev, Asaf Gilboa and Ann M. Rasmusson

Commentaries

3.1 Translational Theory-Driven Hypotheses and Testing Are Enhancing Our Understanding of PTSD and its Treatment 139
Brian H. Harvey

3.2 Precipitating and design approaches to PTSD 142
Eric Vermetten

4 Pharmacotherapy of PTSD 149
Dan J. Stein and Jonathan C. Ipser

Commentaries
4.1 Critical View of the Pharmacological Treatment of Trauma 163
Marcelo F. Mello
4.2 Shortcomings and Future Directions of the Pharmacotherapy of PTSD 164
Michael Van Ameringen and Beth Patterson
4.3 Dire Need for New PTSD Pharmacotherapeutics 167
Murray B. Stein

5 Psychological Interventions for Trauma Exposure and PTSD 171
Richard A. Bryant

Commentaries
5.1 Psychological Interventions for PTSD in Children 203
Lucy Berliner
5.2 Challenges in the Dissemination and Implementation of Exposure-Based CBT for the Treatment of Hispanics with PTSD 205
Rafael Kichic, Mildred Vera, and María L. Reyes-Rabanillo
5.3 What Else Do We Need to Know about Evidence-Based Psychological Interventions for PTSD? 208
Karina Lovell
5.4 Another Perspective on Exposure Therapy for PTSD 211
Barbara Olasov Rothbaum

6 (Disaster) Public Mental Health 217
Joop de Jong

Commentaries
6.1 An Excellent Model for Low- and Middle-Income Countries 263
Dean Ajdukovic
6.2 Disaster Mental Health and Public Health: An Integrative Approach to Recovery 266
Suresh Bada Math, Channaveerachari Naveen Kumar and Maria Christine Nirmala
6.3 Transcultural Aspects of Response to Disasters 272
Tarek A. Okasha

6.4 Disaster Public Health: Health Needs, Psychological First Aid and Cultural Awareness 275
Robert J. Ursano, Matthew N. Goldenberg, Derrick Hamaoka and David M. Benedek

Index **281**

Preface

Post-traumatic stress disorder (PTSD) is arguably the most controversial of all the psychiatric diagnoses. There are disagreements about the qualifying events that count as sufficiently traumatic to precipitate PTSD, disagreements about the nature of the typical symptoms that follow exposure to trauma, disagreements about how best to prevent and treat PTSD, and disagreements about what kind of compensation is owed to people with PTSD by society.

At the same time, there have been major advances in our understanding of many aspects of PTSD. The diagnostic classifications of both the World Health Organization (WHO) and the American Psychiatric Association (APA) include the same broad symptom categories (e.g. re-experiencing, avoidance/numbing and arousal) and emphasise that exposure to extremely stressful events can produce profound alterations in cognitions, emotions and behaviour that may persist for decades or a lifetime.

There is also a growing appreciation of the public health burden of PTSD. Trauma continues to be a pervasive aspect of life in the 21st century, in high-, middle- and low-income countries [1]. Furthermore, PTSD and other trauma-related disorders are highly prevalent and disabling, are often associated with other psychiatric and medical disorders, and lead to significant costs for society [2, 3].

We are gradually advancing our scientific understanding of how exposure to traumatic events can produce neurobiological and psychological alterations which, if untreated, may persist indefinitely [4]. Furthermore, although there is not complete consensus across different clinical guidelines [5], there is general agreement that cognitive behaviour therapy and certain medications are the most effective clinical approaches for PTSD.

Many challenges remain. Fundamental information on the psychobiology of PTSD must be translated into effective, evidence-based clinical interventions. The development and testing of additional evidence-based treatments, especially treatments that are culturally sensitive and effective in more traditional ethnocultural settings, is required [6]. A further challenge is to move beyond the traditional clinic to the public health arena, where the focus must shift to resilience, prevention and selective interventions for populations at risk following disasters or mass violence [7].

The World Psychiatric Association (WPA) Evidence & Experience series provides a useful opportunity to work towards an evidence-based and integrative approach to different psychiatric conditions. In this volume, expert clinicians and researchers from around the world rigorously synthesise the data on PTSD, and provide balanced and judicious approaches to the controversies and challenges noted above. The chapters cover many aspects of PTSD, ranging from work on epidemiology and nosology, through research on psychobiology, to work on pharmacotherapy, psychotherapy and community approaches to intervention. Commentaries on each chapter, again from authors around the globe, provide additional depth.

Taken together, this work documents the many advances in empirical work on PTSD, negotiates a middle path through the theoretical controversies and provides clinicians and policy-makers with a practical approach to clinical and community interventions. Given that the field has learned much in recent decades about the kinds of trauma that are typically associated with PTSD, about the natural course of symptoms in response to such traumas, about optimal ways to evaluate and measure such symptoms, and about the best pharmacotherapeutic, psychotherapeutic and community approaches to the prevention and management of PTSD, we believe that this volume is timely. We hope that it will be useful to a broad range of readers.

We thank the many individuals who contributed to this volume, particularly the chapter authors. We also thank Joan Marsh of Wiley-Blackwell, Helen Herrman and Mario Maj of the WPA, and Marianne Kastrup, for their guidance and support; their vision and enthusiasm were pivotal in ensuring the initiation and progress of the volume. We wish to dedicate it to those individuals who have shared their symptoms and histories with us, teaching us the clinical aspects of PTSD and providing inspiring models of courage and resilience in the face of immense adversity.

Dan J. Stein, Carlos Blanco, Matthew J. Friedman

REFERENCES

1. Green, B.L., Friedman, M.J., de Jong, J. *et al.* (2003) *Trauma Interventions in War and Peace: Prevention, Practice, and Policy*, Kluwer Academic/Plenum, Amsterdam.
2. Watson, P.J., Gibson, L. and Ruzek, J.I. (2007) Public health interventions following disasters and mass violence, in *Handbook of PTSD: Science and Practice* (eds M.J. Friedman, T.M. Keane and P.A. Resick), Guilford Press, New York, pp. 521–539.
3. Blumenfield, M. and Ursano, R.J. (2008) *Intervention and Resilience after Mass Trauma*, Cambridge University Press, Cambridge, UK.
4. Friedman, M.J., Keane, T.M. and Resick, P.A. (2007) *Handbook of PTSD: Science and Practice*, Guilford Press, New York.

5. Forbes, D., Creamer, M.C., Bisson, J.I. *et al.* (2010) A guide to guidelines for the treatment of PTSD and related conditions. *Journal of Traumatic Stress*, **23**, 537–552.
6. Marsella, A.J, Johnson, J.L., Watson, P. and Gryczynski, J. (2008) *Ethnocultural Perspectives on Disaster and Trauma: Foundations, Issues and Applications*, Springer, New York.
7. Friedman, M.J. (2005). Every crisis is an opportunity. *CNS Spectrums*, **10**, 96–98.

List of Contributors

Dean Ajdukovic
Department of Psychology, University of Zagreb, Zagreb, Croatia

David M. Benedek
Department of Psychiatry and Neuroscience; Department of Psychiatry; Center for the Study of Traumatic Stress, Uniformed Services University of the Health Sciences, Bethesda, MD, USA

Lucy Berliner
Harborview Center for Sexual Assault & Traumatic Stress, School of Social Work, University of Washington, Seattle, WA, USA

Carlos Blanco
Department of Psychiatry, Columbia University, New York, NY, USA

Chris R. Brewin
Clinical Educational and Health Psychology, University College London, London, UK

Richard A. Bryant
University of New South Wales, Sydney, Australia

Abdulrahman M. El-Sayed
Department of Epidemiology, Mailman School of Public Health, Columbia University, New York, NY, USA

Matthew J. Friedman
Department of Psychiatry and of Pharmacology & Toxicology, Dartmouth Medical School; National Center for Posttraumatic Stress Disorder, US Department of Veterans Affairs, Hanover, NH, USA

Sandro Galea
Department of Epidemiology, Mailman School of Public Health, Columbia University, New York, NY, USA

Asaf Gilboa
The Rotman Research Institute, Baycrest Centre, Toronto, ON, Canada

Matthew N. Goldenberg
Department of Psychiatry; Center for the Study of Traumatic Stress, Uniformed Services University of the Health Sciences, Bethesda, MD, USA

Derrick Hamaoka
Department of Psychiatry; Center for the Study of Traumatic Stress, Uniformed Services University of the Health Sciences, Bethesda, MD, USA

Brian H. Harvey
Division of Pharmacology, Unit for Drug Research and Development, School of Pharmacy, North-West University (Potchefstroom campus), Potchefstroom, South Africa

Helen Herrman
Centre for Youth Mental Health, University of Melbourne, Victoria, Australia

Jonathan C. Ipser
Department of Psychiatry, University of Cape Town, Cape Town, South Africa

Joop de Jong
Department of Psychiatry, VU University Amsterdam, The Netherlands; Boston University, USA; Rhodes University, South Africa

Elie G. Karam
Department of Psychiatry and Clinical Psychology; Balamand University Medical School and St Georges Hospital University Medical Center; Institute for Development Research Advocacy and Applied Care (IDRAAC); Medical Institute for Neuropsychological Disorders (MIND), Beirut, Lebanon

Marianne Kastrup
Videnscenter for Transkulturel Psykiatri, Psykiatrisk Center København, Strandboulevarden, Denmark

Rafael Kichic
Anxiety Clinic, Institute of Cognitive Neurology (INECO) and Institute of Neurosciences, Favaloro University, Buenos Aires, Argentina

Channaveerachari Naveen Kumar
Department of Psychiatry, National Institute of Mental Health and Neurosciences (NIMHANS), Bangalore, India

Karina Lovell
The School of Nursing, Midwifery and Social Work, The University of Manchester, Manchester, UK

Suresh Bada Math
Department of Psychiatry, National Institute of Mental Health and Neurosciences (NIMHANS), Bangalore, India

Alexander C. McFarlane
Department of Psychiatry, University of Adelaide Node, Centre for Military and Veterans' Health, University of Adelaide, Adelaide, Australia

Marcelo F. Mello
Department of Psychiatry, Universidade Federal de São Paulo, São Paulo, Brazil

Maria Christine Nirmala
Lead Knowledge Management, Private Multinational Company, Bangalore, India

Tarek A. Okasha
Department of Psychiatry, Institute of Psychiatry, Faculty of Medicine, Ain Shams University, Cairo, Egypt

Beth Patterson
Department of Psychiatry and Behavioural Neurosciences, McMaster University, Hamilton, Ontario, Canada

Ann M. Rasmusson
Women's Health Sciences Division, National Center for PTSD, VA Boston Healthcare System; Boston University School of Medicine, Boston, MA, USA

María L. Reyes-Rabanillo
Psychiatry Service, Veterans Affairs Caribbean Healthcare System, San Juan, Puerto Rico

Barbara Olasov Rothbaum
Department of Psychiatry, Trauma and Anxiety Recovery Program, Emory University School of Medicine, Atlanta, GA, USA

Arieh Y. Shalev
Department of Psychiatry, Hadassah University Hospital, Jerusalem, Israel

Dan J. Stein
Department of Psychiatry, University of Cape Town, Cape Town, South Africa; Mount Sinai School of Medicine, New York, NY, USA

Murray B. Stein
Department of Psychiatry and Family and Preventive Medicine, University of California San Diego, CA, USA

Robert J. Ursano
Department of Psychiatry and Neuroscience; Department of Psychiatry; Center for the Study of Traumatic Stress, Uniformed Services University of the Health Sciences, Bethesda, MD, USA

Michael Van Ameringen
Department of Psychiatry and Behavioural Neurosciences, McMaster University, Hamilton, Ontario, Canada

Mildred Vera
Department of Health Services Administration, Medical Sciences Campus, University of Puerto Rico, San Juan, Puerto Rico

Eric Vermetten
Military Mental Health, Department of Defence; Department of Psychiatry, University Medical Center, Utrecht, The Netherlands

CHAPTER 1

PTSD and Related Disorders

Matthew J. Friedman
Department of Psychiatry and of Pharmacology & Toxicology, Dartmouth Medical School; National Center for Posttraumatic Stress Disorder, US Department of Veterans Affairs, Hanover, NH, USA

INTRODUCTION

Of the many diagnoses in the Diagnostic and Statistical Manual IV-TR (DSM-IV-TR) [1], very few invoke an aetiology in their diagnostic criteria: (i) organic mental disorders (e.g. caused by a neurological abnormality); (ii) substance-use disorders (e.g. caused by psychoactive chemical agents); (iii) post-traumatic stress disorder (PTSD); (iv) acute stress disorder (ASD); and (v) adjustment disorders (ADs) [2] – the latter three are all caused by exposure to a stressful environmental event that exceeds the coping capacity of the affected individual. The presumed causal relationship between the stressor and PTSD, ASD and AD is complicated and controversial, as will be discussed below. Controversy notwithstanding, acceptance of this causal relationship, initially in the DSM-III [3], has equipped practitioners and scientists with a conceptual tool that has profoundly influenced clinical practice over the past 30 years.

PTSD is primarily a disorder of reactivity rather than of an altered baseline state as in major depressive disorder or general anxiety disorder. Its psychopathology is characteristically expressed during interactions with the interpersonal or physical environment. People with PTSD are consumed by concerns about personal safety. They persistently scan the environment for threatening stimuli. When in doubt, they are more likely to assume that danger is present and will react accordingly. The avoidance and hyperarousal symptoms described below can be understood within this context. The primacy of traumatic over other memories (e.g. the reexperiencing symptoms) can also be understood as a pathological exaggeration of an adaptive human response to remember as much as possible about dangerous encounters in order to avoid similar threats in the future.

The sustained anxiety about potential threats to life and limb, pervasive and uncontrollable sense of danger, and maladaptive preoccupation with concerns

Post-traumatic Stress Disorder, First Edition. Edited by Dan Stein, Matthew Friedman, and Carlos Blanco.

about personal safety and the safety of one's family can be explicated in terms of psychological models such as classic Pavlovian fear conditioning, two-factor theory or emotional processing theory [4–6]. The traumatic (unconditioned) stimulus (the rape, assault, disaster, etc.) automatically evokes the post-traumatic (unconditioned) emotional response (fear, helplessness and/or horror). The intensity of this emotional reaction provokes avoidance or protective behaviours that reduce the emotional impact of the stimulus. Conditioned stimuli, reminders of such traumatic events (e.g. seeing someone who resembles the original assailant, confronting war-zone reminders, exposure to high winds or torrential downpours reminiscent of a hurricane, etc.), evoke similar conditioned responses manifested as fear-induced avoidance and protective behaviours.

Such psychological models can also be explicated within the context of neurocircuitry that mediates the processing of threatening or fearful stimuli. In short, traumatic stimuli activate the amygdala, which in turn produces outputs to the hippocampus, medial prefrontal cortex, locus coeruleus, thalamus, hypothalamus, insula and dorsal/ventral striatum [7–9]. In PTSD, the normal restraint on the amygdala exerted by the medial prefrontal cortex – especially the anterior cingulate gyrus and orbitofrontal cortex – is severely disrupted. Such disinhibition of the amygdala creates an abnormal psychobiological state of hypervigilance in which innocuous or ambiguous stimuli are more likely to be misinterpreted as threatening. To be hypervigilant in a dangerous situation is adaptive. To remain so after the danger has passed is not.

Fear-conditioning models help to explain many PTSD symptoms such as intrusive recollections (e.g. nightmares and psychological/physiological reactions to traumatic reminders), avoidance behaviours and hyperarousal symptoms such as hypervigilence. Emotional numbing, another important manifestation of PTSD, has been explicated in terms of stress-induced analgesia [10]. Such emotional anaesthesia is potentially even more disruptive and disturbing to the affected individual and loved ones than other symptoms because it may produce an insurmountable emotional barrier between the PTSD patient and his or her family. Such individuals are unable to experience loving feelings or to reciprocate those of partners and children. As a result, they isolate themselves and become emotionally inaccessible to loved ones to whom they had previously been very close. They also cut themselves off from friends. Finally, there are PTSD symptoms that jeopardise the capacity to function effectively at work, such as diminished ability to concentrate, irritability and loss of interest in work or school. In short, there is a perceived discontinuity between the pre- and post-traumatic self. People with PTSD see themselves as altered by their traumatic experience. They feel as if they have been drastically and irrevocably changed by this encounter. Others have described this discontinuity as a 'broken connection' with the past [11]; or as 'shattered assumptions' about oneself and one's world [12].

HISTORICAL ANTECEDENTS

Before the mid-nineteenth century, the psychological impact of exposure to traumatic stress was recorded by poets, dramatists and novelists. Trimble [13], Shay [14] and others have pointed out that Homer, Shakespeare and Dickens (to name only a few) had sophisticated understanding of the profound impact of traumatic stressors on cognitions, feelings and behaviour. Medicalisation of such invisible wounds, usually (but not always) received in combat, occurred on both sides of the Atlantic during the mid-nineteenth century. Explanatory models pointed to the heart (e.g. soldier's heart, Da Costa's syndrome and neurocirculatory asthenia), the nervous system (e.g. railway spine, shell shock) and the psyche (e.g. nostalgia, traumatic neurosis) as the (invisibly) affected system.

In the 1970s, spurred on by social movements in the USA and around the world, what had previously been contextualised primarily as a problem among military personnel and veterans was broadened to include victims of domestic violence, rape and child abuse. The women's movement emphasised sexual and physical assault on women while child advocacy groups emphasised physical and sexual abuse in children. Thus, new clinical entities took their places alongside combat-related syndromes. These included: rape trauma syndrome, battered woman syndrome, child abuse syndrome and others [15–17].

In other words, by the late 1970s clinicians had a wide variety of post-traumatic diagnostic options from which to choose, although none were recognised in the DSM-II [18]. Indeed, from a PTSD perspective, DSM-II was a step backwards, since DSM-I [19] contained the ill-defined 'gross stress reaction', which provided a useful, but temporary, diagnostic niche for military veterans, ex-prisoners of war, rape victims and Nazi Holocaust survivors. (If 'gross stress reaction' persisted, the diagnosis had to be changed to 'neurotic reaction'.) In DSM-II, however, even this diagnostic option was eliminated, so that 'situational reaction' was the only available diagnosis for people who exhibited clinically significant reactions to catastrophic experiences. Besides trivialising post-traumatic reactions (since this category included any unpleasant experience), 'situational reactions' were also considered temporary.

The DSM-III [3] process recognised that these differently labelled syndromes (e.g. rape trauma, post-Vietnam, war sailor, concentration camp syndromes, etc.) were all characterised by a very similar pattern of symptoms that became embodied within the PTSD diagnostic criteria. Hence, the emphasis shifted from the specific traumatic stressor to the relatively similar pattern of clinical expression that could be observed among survivors of a growing list of different severe stressful experiences. The various stressors were aggregated into Criterion A, while the clinical presentation was explicated by the PTSD symptoms themselves (Criteria B–D).

There have been some alterations of the original DSM-III PTSD criteria. The number of possible symptoms has increased from 12 to 17. The original three symptom clusters (reexperiencing, numbing and miscellaneous) have been rearranged into the present triad of reexperiencing, avoidance/numbing and hyperarousal. Criterion E (duration of symptoms must exceed one month) was included in the DSM-III-R in 1987 and Criterion F (that the symptoms must cause clinically significant distress or functional impairment) was added in the DSM-IV in 1994. Most importantly, the fundamental concept that exposure to overwhelming stress may precede the onset of clinically significant and persistent alterations in cognitions, feelings and behaviour has endured. Epidemiological studies have confirmed the DSM-III perspective and shown that exposure to extreme stress sometimes precedes severe and long-lasting psychopathology [20–24]. Such research has also shown, unfortunately, that exposure to traumatic stress is all too common across the population and that the prevalence of rape, domestic violence, child abuse and so on is unacceptably high. Thus, when it was time for the next revision of the diagnostic criteria for DSM-IV [25] it was clear that it was incorrect to characterise Criterion A, exposure to a traumatic event, as an event that 'is generally outside the range of usual human experience'.

PTSD: DSM-IV-TR DIAGNOSTIC CRITERIA

Criterion A1

The DSM-IV Criterion A was divided into objective (A1) and subjective (A2) components. Criterion A1 resembled the DSM-III-R [26] Criterion A, except that a greater number of events were included as stressor events. These included: being diagnosed with a life-threatening illness, child sexual abuse (without threatened or actual violence), learning about the sudden unexpected death of a family member or close friend, and learning that one's child has a life-threatening illness. The 'learning about' traumatic exposure (injury or death) of a loved one has proven to be one of the most controversial changes to Criterion A (see below). In DSM-IV, however, in addition to exposure to an A1 event, it was necessary that exposed individuals experience an intense (fear-conditioned) emotional reaction (Criterion A2) characterised as 'fear, helplessness or horror'. Although this had been foreshadowed in DSM-III-R's text description, the subjective response was now made an explicit (A2) criterion [27]. It is also worth noting that the timing of A2 was unclear and later subject to different interpretations, with some saying it might happen some time after the event rather than being strictly peritraumatic.

As we consider DSM-IV Criterion A1, there are several questions that must be addressed: (i) Should exposure to a potentially traumatic event be considered aetiologically or temporally significant with regard to the later development of PTSD? (ii) Can we really distinguish 'traumatic' from 'nontraumatic' stressors? (iii) Should Criterion A1 be eliminated from DSM-5?

Does traumatic exposure 'cause' PTSD?

DSM-III and DSM-IV are unclear about the aetiological significance of the Criterion A event [27, 28]. On the one hand, they both suggest that traumatic exposure 'causes' PTSD (e.g. 'evokes' the characteristic PTSD symptoms). On the other, they both suggest that the traumatic event constitutes a watershed experience that temporally precedes the expression of PTSD symptoms.

We have learned a number of things since 1980 that have a direct bearing on this question. First, we know that people differ with regard to resilience and vulnerability, so that most people exposed to traumatic events do not develop PTSD. Epidemiological research has identified a number of risk and protective factors that differentially affect the susceptibility of different individuals to develop PTSD following exposure. Resilience is a complicated attribute that includes genetic, psychobiological, cognitive, emotional, behavioural, cultural and social components [7, 29]. Second, we must also recognise that events differ with regard to the conditional probability that PTSD will follow exposure. For example, the conditional probability of PTSD following rape is much higher than that for exposure to natural disasters. In other words, there is a complex interaction between individual susceptibility and the toxicity of a given stressful event. Therefore, while we acknowledge that no event in and of itself can cause PTSD, we must also recognise that some events are much more likely to precede PTSD onset than others. It is more appropriate to consider the stressor as a powerful temporal antecedent with a variable conditional probability of preceding the development of PTSD than as an event that 'causes' PTSD. Such a conceptualisation tempers the attribution of causality and makes it possible to incorporate our growing understanding of how clinical outcomes are influenced by risk/protective factors and gene × environment interactions. In short, exposure to an A1 event is a necessary but not a sufficient condition for the subsequent development of PTSD. With this understanding, however, it must be understood that exposure to the traumatic event is absolutely critical, genetic loading notwithstanding [30]. As noted by Kilpatrick *et al.* [31] when summarising findings from the DSM-IV Field Trials, the argument over how best to operationalise Criterion A boils down to a debate over how broad versus how narrow Criterion A should be. A broad definition of Criterion A would include any event that can produce PTSD symptoms. In contrast, advocates for a more restrictive definition fear that broadening the criterion would trivialise the PTSD diagnosis and defeat the purpose of the original DSM-III PTSD construct by permitting people exposed to less stressful events to meet Criterion A. The DSM-IV Field Trials appeared to allay this concern as few people developed PTSD unless they experienced extremely stressful life events. Kilpatrick *et al.* [32] have recently replicated this Field Trial finding in two independent cohorts, the Florida Hurricane Study (FHS) and the National Survey of Adolescents (NSA). They found that among FHS study participants, 96.6% of those meeting PTSD Criteria B–F had previously been exposed to an A1 event. In the NSA study, 95.5% of those meeting Criteria B–F had been exposed to an A1 traumatic stressor. In other words, they found that very few people meet full PTSD diagnostic criteria without prior exposure to a recognisable traumatic event, as stipulated in DSM-IV.

Others, less comfortable with the greater number of qualifying A1 events in DSM-IV than in DSM-III, have objected that expansion of qualifying A1 events has diluted the basic PTSD construct. They have argued that under DSM-IV people who have received the PTSD diagnosis for less threatening events should really be diagnosed with an adjustment or anxiety disorder not otherwise specified (NOS) [32]. The major sticking point has been the DSM-IV addition of being 'confronted with' (or learning about) traumatic experiences of family members or close friends. This expansion has been called 'bracket creep' [30] or 'criterion creep' [33] and is presumed to have a particularly adverse impact in forensic settings or disability evaluations, where it has been blamed for frivolous tort or compensation claims.

Breslau and Kessler [34] tested the implications of the broad DSM-IV Criterion A1 verus DSM-III. Among a representative sample of over 2000 individuals, lifetime exposure to traumatic events defined by a narrow set of qualifying A1 events was compared to prevalence of exposure to a broad set of events. The narrow set included seven events of 'assaultive violence' (e.g. combat, rape, assault, etc.) and seven 'other injury events' (e.g. serious accident, natural disaster, witnessing death/serious injury, etc.). The broad set further included five events from the category 'learning about' traumatic events affecting close relatives (e.g. rape, assault, accident, etc.). Narrow-set exposure was 68.1% compared to broad-set exposure of 89.6%. Thus, there was a 59.2% increase in lifetime exposure to a traumatic event due to the expanded Criterion A1. More importantly, A1 events included within the expanded Criterion A1 contributed 38% of total PTSD cases. Although the wide discrepancy between the Kilpatrick *et al.* [31] and Breslau and Kessler [34] studies may have more to do with methodology than with Criterion A1 itself, [27] this finding has fuelled the controversy about how best to operationalise Criterion A1.

Kilpatrick *et al.* [32] have disputed the 'bracket/criterion creep' arguments. They point out that the DSM-IV Field Trials, as well as the aforementioned FHS and NSA data, indicate that very few individuals meet PTSD Criteria B–F without prior exposure to an A1 event. Brewin *et al.* [35] make a similar argument (see below). The non-A1 events most likely to precede the onset of PTSD B–F symptoms were sudden death of close relatives, serious illness and having a child with a potentially terminal illness [31, 32, 34]. One might ask whether these current non-A1 events should be redesignated as A1 events and if so, whether that would dilute the PTSD construct.

Dohrenwend [36] has suggested a different and very thoughtful approach to this issue. He has proposed that prototypical major negative events be rated objectively along six dimensions: valence (negative), source (external, uncontrollable, 'fateful'), unpredictable, central (life-threatening, deprivation of basic needs and goals), magnitude (likelihood of causing great negative changes) and likelihood to exhaust the individual. He further proposes that research be done to empirically derive A1 events by detecting which of these six dimensions reliably predict PTSD B–F symptoms. Events characterised by such dimensions would be designated A1 events while others would not. Dohrenwend has also argued that such a dimensional approach would obviate the need for a subjective Criterion A2 (see below). Research on this approach would be extremely useful. It would also be important to address the question of clinical feasibility by determining how well busy clinicians could utilise Dohrenwend's approach in clinical practice.

It seems that major questions regarding Criterion A1 can only be addressed through more research. The basic investigative approach would require the development of a comprehensive menu of prototypical major negative events in order to find out which reliably precede the onset of PTSD B–F symptoms and which do not. In order to ensure generalisability, both clinical and population samples that included sufficient diversity to address related questions regarding trauma type (e.g. sexual, military, disaster), gender, ethnicity, age, cultural and other factors would be needed. Dohrenwend's dimensional proposal could also be investigated in such a design. A longitudinal approach to this question would be best (ideally starting before traumatic exposure, but at the very least beginning immediately after such exposure).

Should Criterion A1 be eliminated?

It has been suggested that PTSD caseness and prevalence would change very little if Criterion A1 were completely eliminated. The DSM-IV PTSD Work Group also considered complete elimination of Criterion A but rejected this option because of concerns that 'the loosening of Criterion A may lead to widespread and frivolous use of the concept' [37]. Although several articles suggest that the full PTSD syndrome might be expressed following nontraumatic events (thereby fortifying 'bracket/criterion creep' arguments [30, 33]), most of these reports have been dismissed as methodologically flawed because proper clinical interviews are not utilised and because the data merely show an increase in PTSD symptoms, but not the full diagnosis. Indeed, when assessed by a structured clinical interview, there are actually very few examples of individuals who do not meet Criterion A who do meet full PTSD diagnostic criteria [35]. Furthermore, it is unclear in most of these reports whether the non-A1 event actually served as a reminder or trigger for a previously experienced traumatic event and therefore precipitated a PTSD relapse, rather than new-onset PTSD.

Arguments for eliminating Criterion A are: (i) traumatic exposure may sometimes precede onset of other diagnoses (e.g. depression, substance-use disorder) rather than PTSD; (ii) non-A1 events sometimes do appear to precede onset of PTSD B–F symptoms; (iii) it would bring PTSD more in line with other anxiety and affective disorders which do not require that symptom onset be preceded by a specific event; and (iv) lack of utility of Criterion A2 [35]. Most PTSD experts, responding to an unpublished survey undertaken by APA as part of the DSM-5 process, strongly supported retaining Criterion A1 but generally agreed that it needed to be modified to address the issues discussed in this review. Suggested modifications included: emphasising the temporal rather than the aetiological relationship between A1 and B–F symptoms, narrowing the criterion to eliminate second-hand exposure (e.g. the 'confronted by' criteria) and incorporating Dohrenwend's dimensional approach. All agreed that any final decisions should be informed by empirical evidence.

Criterion A2

As noted above, the DSM-IV Work Group stipulated that in addition to exposure to an A1 event, individuals thus exposed must also experience an intense subjective reaction characterised as 'fear, helplessness or horror'. It was expected that imposition of Criterion A2 would ensure that the only people eligible for the PTSD diagnosis would be those who had reacted strongly to the threatening event. It was also expected that imposition of this new Criterion A2 would function as a 'gatekeeper' and keep out any 'frivolous' PTSD diagnoses due to broadening of Criterion A1. The expectation, based on data from the DSM-IV Field Trials [31], was that few people exposed to low-magnitude (nontraumatic) events would meet Criterion A2 and therefore that most would not be eligible for the PTSD diagnosis.

Research indicates that DSM-IV's expectations regarding A2 have not been realised. As a result, the utility of Criterion A2 has been seriously questioned. Three negative studies found no effect of A2 on PTSD prevalence: in a community sample from Michigan; in a sample of older male military veterans; and in the World Health Organization's World Mental Health Survey, which included almost 103 000 respondents [34, 38, 39].

People whose occupation requires frequent traumatic exposure, such as military, police and emergency medical personnel, may not experience fear, helplessness or horror during or immediately following a trauma exposure because of their training. Other studies show that a substantial minority of individuals within community samples (e.g. ~20%) may meet all PTSD A1, B–F Criteria without meeting A2. Except for the absence of A2, there were no differences with regard to severity or impairment between A2 positive and A2 negative cohorts [40, 41]. Similar results have been found with recent female rape or assault victims [42]. Furthermore, people can develop PTSD following mild traumatic brain injury (TBI), in which case they may be unaware of any peritraumatic emotional response because of a loss of consciousness [43, 44]. These examples all indicate that some people can develop PTSD without an A2 response.

Another problem with A2 concerns the timeframe in which it is assessed. Since most PTSD cases are evaluated months or years after a traumatic event, and since assessment of A2 requires a retrospective recall of how the person responded during or shortly after the event, there is concern that subsequent recall of acute responses to trauma is unreliable and is influenced by mood biases associated with PTSD levels (or other factors) at the time of recall [45]. Therefore, questions about the accuracy of retrospective A2 reports obtained at varying intervals between trauma exposure and assessment have raised additional concerns about the usefulness of A2.

Based on all of this information, a number of investigators have called for the elimination of Criterion A2. Not only has it failed to predict the likelihood of PTSD, but it has also failed to realise the expectations of DSM-IV that it would serve as a 'gatekeeper' to offset any increased prevalence of PTSD caused by the expansion of qualifying A1 events [40]. McNally [30] has argued that we should eliminate A2 because 'in the language of behaviourism, it confounds the response with the stimulus. In the language of medicine, it confounds the host with the pathogen' (page 598).

On the other hand, there is consistent evidence that the absence of A2 strongly predicts A1-exposed people who will not develop PTSD [31, 34, 38, 39, 46]. Schnurr *et al*. [38] suggest that A2 may be most useful during the immediate aftermath of a traumatic event, by identifying individuals unlikely to develop PTSD. While this may be extremely useful in a war zone or disaster triage site, it does not appear to have a major bearing on improving diagnostic accuracy.

Finally, A2's 'fear, helplessness and horror' are all predicated on a fear-conditioning model of PTSD. This has been challenged as too narrow. There is now considerable data showing that other strong peritraumatic emotions are also associated with PTSD, such as: sadness, grief, anger, guilt, shame and disgust [31, 46–48].

Summarising Criteria A1 and A2

As DSM-5 moves forward, a major priority will be to address the aforementioned concerns regarding Criterion A. For A1, it will have to reduce the ambiguity about what is and what is not a traumatic event. For A2, it will have to consider the utility of this criterion in making the PTSD diagnosis and whether 'fear, helplessness or horror' should be expanded to include both peritraumatic dissociation and other intense peritraumatic emotions such as guilt, shame and anger. Given that peritraumatic emotions are likely to endure among those who do not recover from traumatic events and are eventually diagnosed with PTSD, it seems appropriate to include non-fear-based post-traumatic symptoms in DSM-5 [28].

Kilpatrick *et al*. [32] suggest that a key question about Criterion A is whether it should be designed to maximise sensitivity (thereby including all events that are capable of producing PTSD) or whether it should maximise specificity (thereby limiting qualifying events to those most likely to precede PTSD). A broad, less restricted definition would ensure that all individuals meeting other PTSD criteria would be eligible for treatment or other services. A more restricted definition would resolve current ambiguities in tort or compensation cases. Kilpatrick *et al*. maintain that until consensus has been achieved regarding sensitivity versus specificity, it will be impossible to define Criterion A.

The proposed DSM-5 criteria for PTSD [28] have retained Criterion A. It is expected that in the narrative description its temporal rather than aetiological significance will be emphasised. The major reason proposed for retaining Criterion A is that PTSD does not develop unless an individual is exposed to an event that is intensely stressful. Such individuals are keenly aware of a significant discontinuity in their lives because of subsequent preoccupation with memories, feelings and behaviours that are associated with that event. This is consistent with recommendations from other investigators. For example, McNally [30] has argued that the memory of the trauma is the 'heart of the diagnosis' and the organising core around which the B–F symptoms can be understood as a coherent syndrome.

Proposed DSM-5 diagnostic criteria for PTSD [28] indicate that Criterion A1 will probably not change substantially because there is insufficient data to address the concerns outlined in this review. It has retained DSM-IV language emphasising that qualifying events must involve direct exposure to actual or threatened death, serious injury or a threat to the physical integrity of others. With regard to the most controversial aspect of DSM-IV Criterion A1, being 'confronted by' traumatic events, the proposal for DSM-5 limits such 'confrontation' to learning about the traumatic exposure of a close friend or loved one or learning about aversive details of unnatural deaths, serious injuries or serious assaults to others. This includes learning about the homicide of a family member, learning about a gruesome death or learning the grotesque details of rape, genocide or other abusive violence to others. It also applies to work-related exposure to gruesome and horrific evidence of traumatic events, as with police personnel, firefighters, graves registration workers and emergency medical technicians. Finally, the revised Criterion A explicitly excludes witnessing traumatic events through electronic media, television, video games, movies or pictures.

Because of aforementioned concerns about differences in resilience and gene × environment interactions, there is legitimate concern that vulnerable individuals might develop bonafide B–F symptoms following events not generally considered 'traumatic'. The proposed DSM-5 solution to this diagnostic issue is the addition of an ASD/PTSD subtype of AD. Such an approach would provide a diagnostic niche for vulnerable individuals who express PTSD B–F symptoms following exposure to a nontraumatic event [2].

As for Criterion A2, the current proposal is to eliminate it in DSM-5 for all the reasons cited above [28].

Factor structure of PTSD

The DSM-IV PTSD construct consists of three symptom clusters: B, reexperiencing; C, avoidance/numbing; and D, hyperarousal. Many studies have utilised confirmatory factor analysis to test whether the three symptom clusters of DSM-IV provide the best model for the latent structure of PTSD. A thorough review of this extensive literature can be found elsewhere [49]. In short, the vast majority of studies support a four-factor model. Five support a two-factor solution. Of the four studies supporting a three-factor model, only one mirrors the three factors found in the DSM-IV PTSD diagnostic criteria [50].

Among the four-factor models, reexperiencing, avoidance and arousal have emerged as distinct clusters in all studies. There has been disagreement, however, about the fourth factor. In many studies, 'numbing' has been identified, while a 'dysphoria' factor has emerged elsewhere [28]. What is most noteworthy, from a DSM-IV perspective, is that none of these studies support a single avoidance/numbing cluster. The general dysphoria factor might be considered to be related to the negative emotional state frequently observed among individuals with PTSD [47]. It also supports arguments that PTSD should be considered an internalising disorder within the dysthymic/anxious misery subcategory along with major depression, dysthymia and general anxiety disorder [51, 52].

In summary, most confirmatory factor analyses support a four-, rather than a three-factor DSM-IV model. The majority of studies indicate that serious consideration should be given to including a separate fourth, 'numbing', symptom cluster in DSM-5. Finally, there is virtually no evidence in support of DSM-IV's Criterion C (avoidance/numbing) since avoidance and numbing are consistently distinct from one another in both the four- and two-factor solutions.

Based on these findings, the proposed DSM-5 criteria for PTSD [28] are nested within a four-factor model. The reexperiencing, avoidance and arousal (now renamed 'arousal and reactivity') clusters have remained. The fourth factor, 'negative alterations in cognitions and mood' replaces the DSM-IV numbing cluster. Most DSM-IV symptoms have been retained, although some have been redefined, while three new symptoms have been introduced (see below).

Can the B–D symptom clusters be improved?[1]

In addition to the fear-based anxiety symptoms, which provide the context for the current DSM-IV PTSD diagnostic criteria, the empirical literature strongly suggests that, as noted earlier in this review, traumatic exposure may be followed

[1] The proposed revision of B–D symptoms reviewed in this section is based on the work of the DSM-5 Trauma, PTSD and Dissociative Disorders Sub-Work Group of the Anxiety Disorders Work Group. In addition to the author, Patricia Resick, Chris Brewin, Richard Bryant, Dean Kilpatrick, Roberto Lewis-Fernandez, Katherine Phillips, Terry Keane, David Spiegel, Robert Ursano, Robert Pynoos and Eric Vermetten participated in this process. The official review of that work can be found in Friedman *et al*. [28].

by a variety of non-fear-based anxiety symptoms such as dysphoric anhedonic symptoms, aggressive/externalising symptoms, guilt/shame symptoms, dissociative symptoms and negative appraisals about oneself and the world [28, 47]. Such findings suggest that the DSM-IV PTSD diagnostic criteria should be revised to incorporate such symptoms in order to provide a better characterisation of the spectrum of post-traumatic symptomatology encountered by clinicians on a regular basis.

Criterion B

Traumatic nightmares (B2) and dissociative flashbacks (B3) rank among the most recognisable and distinctive symptoms of PTSD. Indeed, some have suggested that only these two symptoms should be retained in the B cluster symptoms and that others be eliminated because they overlap with symptoms seen in other disorders [53]. Specifically, they argue that intrusive recollections (B1) be eliminated because it is too similar to rumination seen in depression, while emotional and physiological arousal following exposure to traumatic reminders (B4 and B5) are too similar to symptoms found in specific and social phobia disorders. Despite such concerns, the current proposed DSM-5 criteria [28] have retained all three (B1, B4 and B5) controversial symptoms but have modified them to address these concerns.

The concern about B1 is that DSM-III/IV 'recurrent intrusive recollections' includes both intrusive images and thoughts, as discussed in more detail elsewhere [28]. There is a growing body of evidence to show that intrusive imagery and recurrent thought processes such as ruminations are quite distinct [54], with the former occurring uniquely in PTSD and the latter also found in other disorders such as depression. The intrusive images in PTSD are sensory memories of short duration, have a here-and-now quality and lack context, while ruminative thoughts in depression are evaluative and longer lasting. In addition, rumination appears to function as a cognitive avoidance strategy [35, 55–57]. Therefore, the proposed DSM-5 Criterion B1 was revised to eliminate thoughts/ruminations and to restrict this criterion to involuntary and intrusive distressing memories that usually include sensory, emotional, physiological or behavioural (but not cognitive) components.

B4 and B5 are triggered intrusive emotional and physiological experiences, respectively. The B4 and B5 criteria have been retained because it appears that elicitation of emotional and physiological reactivity to trauma-related stimuli is a key characteristic of PTSD. It is consistent with major fear-conditioning models of the disorder. It is the guiding rationale for critical laboratory paradigms in which distinctive alterations in psychological and neurobiological reactivity among PTSD participants can be reliably detected after exposure to trauma-related stimuli [58]. Furthermore, it is a principle that has informed our most effective cognitive behaviour therapies (CBTs), where emotions and cognitions elicited by traumatic reminders are processed therapeutically. B4 is intense emotional distress, which may be the only kind of recollection possible in individuals who sustained a TBI and have no conscious memories of the traumatic event. Indeed, it has been shown that trauma survivors with severe TBI and with no memory of the event can still meet PTSD criteria because they satisfy B4 or B5 in response to traumatic reminders [44]. In other words, these symptoms are conditioned responses in fear-conditioning models.

Criterion C

In accordance with the confirmatory factor analysis results reviewed above, DSM-IV's avoidance/numbing criterion will be split into C (avoidance) and D (negative alterations in cognitions and mood clusters). As stated previously, the proposed DSM-5 criteria now reflect the true latent structure of PTSD, which consists of four, rather than three factors.

The avoidance (C1 and C2) symptoms are completely consistent with a fear-conditioning model of PTSD. Indeed, Brewin *et al*. [35] have proposed that these are the only C-cluster symptoms uniquely associated with PTSD. C1 consits of efforts to avoid internal reminders associated with the traumatic events (e.g. thoughts, feelings or physical sensations) while C2 consists of efforts to avoid external reminders of the traumatic event (e.g. people, places, conversations, activities, objects or situations). These avoidance symptoms have been preserved in the proposed criteria for DSM-5.

Perhaps the most noticeable change in the DSM-5 proposal is the new D cluster, which encompasses, redefines and recontextualises the DSM-IV C3–C7 'numbing' symptoms. Some have proposed complete elimination of those symptoms because of their nonspecific overlap with general dysphoric symptoms present in other disorders [35, 59] and with the anhedonia found in depression [60], while others have argued strongly for expanding this cluster beyond a fear-conditioning context [28, 47]. As noted earlier, there are a number of negative appraisals and mood states associated with PTSD which have not been clearly explicated or included in DSM-III/IV. Some have been vaguely embedded within C3–C7 while others have not been included at all. According to the proposed criteria for DSM-5, they are now included in a unique cluster of symptoms which are distinct from reexperiencing, avoidance and arousal/reactivity symptoms.

There is very strong evidence that catastrophic or maladaptive appraisals are characteristic of traumatic stress responses that are associated with disorder or impairment [61]. Erroneous cognitions about the causes or consequences of the traumatic event, which lead individuals with PTSD to blame themselves or others, are major therapeutic targets in CBT. They are frequently found among survivors of childhood sexual abuse, rape/assault survivors and military personnel. Indeed, specific and effective strategies to address such self-blame is a consistent component of CBT for PTSD patients [61–63]. Sometimes, such self-blame is due to perceived personal failings, inadequacies or weakness [64, 65]. Therefore, given the prominence of self-blame among individuals with PTSD, it has been proposed as a new symptom for DSM-5.

Another maladaptive appraisal is DSM-IV symptom C7, a sense of foreshortened future, which has often been interpreted too narrowly in DSM-IV as the 'belief that one's life will be shorter or changed'. The empirical literature supports the observations of CBT therapists that individuals with PTSD have persistent negative expectations about themselves, others, or their future (e.g. 'I am a bad person; nothing good can happen to me; I can never trust again'). They do not expect to have a career, marriage, children or a normal life span [64, 66–70]. This has been retained in DSM-5 with the explicit stipulation that it concerns persistent negative expectations regarding many important aspects of life and not just a negative expectation about one's life span.

In addition to the negative appraisals about past, present and future included in the proposed DSM-5 Criterion D, people with PTSD have a wide variety of negative emotional states besides fear, helplessness and horror. Indeed, one of the arguments for moving PTSD out of the Anxiety Disorders category is the presence of many other negative mood states [71]. These include anger [69, 72–75], guilt [76–78] and shame [72, 79, 80]. This is the rationale for proposing a pervasive negative emotional state 'as a new symptom for DSM-5'.

There is abundant evidence for retaining other symptoms currently included in the DSM-IV numbing (C3–C7) cluster. These include dissociative amnesia [81, 82], diminished interest in significant activities, feeling detached or estranged from others and psychic numbing: persistent inability to experience positive emotions. These are all consistently endorsed by individuals with PTSD, as shown in the many confirmatory factor analysis studies reviewed above.

To summarise, it is proposed that the DSM-IV avoidance/numbing cluster be divided into two separate clusters: Criterion C, 'Persistent Avoidance of Stimuli Associated with the Trauma' and Criterion D, 'Negative Alterations in Cognitions and Mood Associated with the Trauma'. The dissociative aspects of amnesia are emphasised. The expectation of a foreshortened future has been explicitly expanded to include negative expectations about one's self, others, or one's future. Other DSM-5 symptoms that have been retained unchanged are: diminished interest in significant activities, feeling detached or estranged from others and psychic numbing. Finally, the empirical literature indicates that two new symptoms should be added: pervasive negative emotional state (e.g. fear, horror, anger, guilt or shame) and persistent distorted blame of self or others about the cause or consequences of the traumatic event.

Criterion D

Four of the five DSM-IV Criterion D symptoms are endorsed frequently by individuals with PTSD and are retained, unchanged, in the proposed DSM-5 criteria. These are insomnia, problems in concentration, hypervigilence and startle reactions. A review of the literature suggests, however, that this symptom cluster encompasses more than hyperarousal and should also include alterations in reactivity that are associated with the traumatic event. Such a reframing of this symptom cluster makes it possible to include behavioural as well as emotional indicators of such post-traumatic alterations. Therefore, it has been proposed that two new symptoms be added to this cluster: aggressive behaviour and reckless behaviour [28].

There is growing evidence, especially among military veterans, that PTSD is associated with more than an irritable mood state (DSM-IV's C2). Indeed, it appears that PTSD predicts aggressive behaviour and violence among military or veteran cohorts following deployment to a war zone [83–86]. Aggressive behaviour has also been observed among female flood survivors with PTSD [87]. Sometimes the aggressive behaviour, rather than other PTSD symptoms, becomes the major clinical focus. Such evidence prompted the DSM-5 proposal to include new-onset post-traumatic aggressive behaviour.

There is also growing evidence that PTSD is associated with reckless and self-destructive behaviour. This has been reported among Israeli adolescents, especially boys, exposed to recurrent terrorism, who exhibited marked increases in risk-taking behaviour [88]. Reckless driving has been observed among individuals with PTSD [89–91]. Finally, risky sexual behavior, sometimes associated with HIV risk, has been reported among college women, female prisoners and adult male survivors of childhood sexual abuse [92, 93]. Based on this evidence, it has been proposed that post-traumatic reckless behaviour be included as a new symptom in DSM-5.

Duration – Criterion E

A month must elapse between traumatic exposure and eligibility for a PTSD diagnosis. The DSM-III/IV rational for this stipulation is to set aside a window in which normal recovery can take place. Since most people exhibit distress during the acute aftermath of traumatic exposure, this one-month window provides an interval for normal post-traumatic recovery without pathologising normal distress exhibited during this period. Individuals who exhibit clinically significant distress or functional impairment during this initial month may qualify for either an ASD or an AD diagnosis (see below). The DSM-5 PTSD proposal preserves this one-month interval. It should be noted that because Criteria B–D in DSM-IV have been expanded to Criteria B–E in DSM-5, Criterion E in DSM-IV will become Criterion F in DSM-5.

'Delayed-onset' PTSD is also preserved in the DSM-5 proposal. This is an important consideration with regard to disability claims as well as forensic psychiatry. It appears that when delayed onset of the full PTSD syndrome occurs, it is preceded by the presence of subsyndromal PTSD symptoms that have increased to exceed the diagnostic threshold. It is very rare for people to suddenly develop PTSD months or years after the trauma when they had been completely asymptomatic during this prodromal period. Indeed, delayed onsets of PTSD, which generally represent exacerbations or reactivations of prior symptoms, have been estimated to account for 38.2 and 15.3% of military and civilian cases of PTSD, respectively [94]. It is no longer controversial, however, that delayed-onset PTSD does actually occur [95–97], although it appears to be very uncommon after natural disasters [98]. Based on the current literature, it has been suggested that this delayed clinical trajectory might be better described as delayed-'development' PTSD rather than 'onset', since PTSD symptoms are usually present well before the traumatised individual meets full PTSD diagnostic criteria.

The final DSM-5 proposal concerning duration is to eliminate the current three-month demarcation point between acute and chronic PTSD. This DSM-IV distinction is based on longitudinal studies of rape victims [99] and motor-vehicle accident survivors [100], which indicate that initially high PTSD rates tend to decline steeply and approach an asymptote at three months. Given a paucity of research on this subject as well as questions about the utility of such a distinction, it has been proposed that the distinction between acute and chronic PTSD be eliminated in DSM-5.

Functional impairment – Criterion F

DSM-IV added a 'significant distress or functional impairment' (F) criterion for PTSD and a number of other disorders. This means that a person who meets the requisite Criteria A–E would not receive a PTSD diagnosis unless he or she also exhibited clinically significant distress or functional impairment. Some regard this question as somewhat redundant since 'significant distress' is implicit in many PTSD symptoms. Because Criterion F is not unique to PTSD, DSM-5 is considering this in a much wider context. There are two distinct issues that must be addressed. First, should 'significant distress' be linked to 'functional impairment' or should both be assessed independently, and if so, how? Second, should significant distress and/or functional impairment remain a diagnostic criterion? If not, how should such information be incorporated into a diagnostic assessment? However Criterion F is defined for DSM-5, it will become Criterion G, because Criteria B–D have expanded to Criteria B–E.

Summary: proposed PTSD diagnostic criteria for DSM-5

The proposed revisions incorporate the following evidence: (i) There is ambiguity in the wording of Criterion A1; (ii) Criterion A2 has no utility in predicting onset of PTSD; and (iii) Criterion C appears to encompass two distinct clusters of symptoms, avoidance and numbing. The proposed diagnostic criteria represent a relatively conservative revision of DSM-IV with four clusters: reexperiencing symptoms, avoidance behaviour, negative alterations in cognitions and mood, and alterations in arousal and reactivity. Finally, in DSM-IV, only B1–5 and C1–2 are specifically anchored to the traumatic event. In these proposed criteria, it is stipulated that all B–G symptoms 'began or worsened after the traumatic event'.

ACUTE STRESS DISORDER

ASD was introduced in DSM-IV to provide a diagnostic niche for acutely traumatised individuals with clinically significant post-traumatic symptoms within the first month following exposure to a traumatic event. Whereas PTSD cannot be diagnosed before one month has elapsed, ASD cannot be diagnosed after one month has elapsed. Since most people exhibit significant distress during the immediate aftermath of traumatic exposure, ASD cannot be diagnosed until at least two days have elapsed following the event. In military or post-disaster parlance, extreme distress during the first 48 hours is called an 'acute stress reaction' or 'combat stress reaction', a normal response to extreme stress from which normal recovery is expected. Finally, since most distressed acutely traumatised individuals will recover during the first month, most CBT therapists delay formal treatment until 10–14 days have passed since the traumatic event, to make sure that recovery is unlikely without psychotherapy.

Another important difference between ASD and PTSD is the greater emphasis on dissociative symptoms in the former diagnosis. In DSM-IV, an individual must exhibit at least three (out of five possible) dissociative symptoms to meet ASD diagnostic criteria, whereas none are required for PTSD. The five dissociative symptoms are: reduction in awareness, derealisation, depersonalisation, numbing and amnesia. Otherwise, an individual must only exhibit one symptom out of each of three PTSD symptom clusters: reexperiencing, avoidance and arousal.

As reviewed by Bryant *et al*. [101], there were two reasons for introducing ASD into DSM-IV: to describe clinically significant post-traumatic reactions during the first month and to predict survivors at high risk of developing subsequent PTSD [102, 103]. A systematic literature review assessed the prevalence and predictive capacity of ASD [104]. It also reviewed the predictive capacity of subsyndromal ASD (defined as meeting three of the four ASD symptom criteria, usually lacking the three-symptom dissociative requirement). The rates of full ASD range from 7 to 28% with a mean of 13%, whereas the prevalence of subsyndromal ASD has ranged from 10 to 32%, with a mean rate of 23%. The higher prevalence for subsyndromal PTSD is because a significant number of severely distressed people meet all ASD criteria except for dissociative symptoms during the first months after traumatic exposure.

Although people who meet ASD criteria are at higher risk for developing PTSD, the majority of people who develop PTSD have never met ASD criteria [105]. Predictability is considerably better for subsyndromal PTSD (when the requirement for three dissociative symptoms is eliminated). Bryant *et al.* [101] suggest that this may be at least partially explained by the fact that the reexperiencing, avoidance and arousal ASD symptom clusters are very similar to the same clusters in PTSD, while most ASD dissociative symptoms are not found in PTSD.

DSM-IV's great emphasis on dissociation as a predictor of PTSD was based on evidence suggesting that peritraumatic dissociation was a risk factor for PTSD. Subsequent research has indicated that peritraumatic dissociation is not an independent predictor of PTSD [101]. Indeed, maintaining a requirement for these dissociative symptoms to meet ASD criteria has eliminated many high-risk, acutely traumatised individuals from consideration. Furthermore, persistent, rather than peritraumatic, dissociation appears to be more predictive of ASD and subsequent PTSD [106].

The proposed criteria for DSM-5 are predicated on the following: (i) clinically significant post-traumatic distress during the first month may take variable forms; (ii) dissociative symptoms may or may not be present during this period among people at high risk of developing PTSD; (iii) people who exhibit persistent distress during the first month following trauma exposure are at a higher risk of developing PTSD subsequently; and (iv) it is important to identify such individuals during this period so that they may receive effective CBT treatment in order to prevent the later development of PTSD [101]. As a result, the stipulation that acutely traumatised individuals meet ASD diagnostic criteria in each of four (dissociative, reexperiencing, avoidance and arousal) symptom categories has been eliminated in the proposed ASD criteria for DSM-5.

The proposed ASD Criterion A for DSM-5 is the same as that for PTSD, with clarification of Criterion A1 and elimination of A2 as discussed above. Individuals must exhibit eight out of the proposed fourteen symptoms, irrespective of the symptom category in which these symptoms reside. Proposed ASD symptoms for DSM-5 include: four reexperiencing symptoms (e.g. intrusive memories, traumatic nightmares, flashbacks and distress in response to traumatic reminders); three dissociative symptoms (e.g. emotional numbing, depersonalisation/derealisation and amnesia); two avoidance symptoms (e.g. avoidance of internal reminders and avoidance of external reminders); and five arousal symptoms (e.g. insomnia, hypervigilence, irritability, exaggerated startle response and agitation or restlessness). The proposed threshold of eight out of these fourteen symptoms is based on a recent analysis of three large datasets from Israel, the UK and Australia [101]. Future prospective longitudinal studies will determine how much the ASD diagnosis has been improved by these new criteria and whether the best threshold is eight rather than a different number of symptoms.

ADJUSTMENT DISORDERS

ADs are an important addition to the proposed DSM-5 category (or subcategory) of Anxiety Disorders, which encompass clinically meaningful syndromes preceded by a stressful or traumatic event (and which also include PTSD, ASD and dissociative disorders) [107]. ADs can be diagnosed at any time after an individual has been exposed to such events. Most precipitating events (e.g. rejections, failure, bankruptcy, etc.) are extremely distressing but do not exceed the threshold for a traumatic event, as in PTSD or ASD (see review by Strain [2]). If, however, an individual is exposed to a traumatic event but fails to meet other ASD or PTSD criteria, the proper diagnosis was AD in DSM-IV and will be the ASD/PTSD subtype of AD in DSM-5. Furthermore, if an individual exhibits the proposed DSM-5 ASD or PTSD symptoms without having been exposed to a traumatic event, he or she will also be diagnosed as the ASD/PTSD subtype of AD.

Because of its specificity, the ASD/PTSD subtype is an exception to all other AD subtypes in which the symptoms deliberately lack specificity. Strain [2] states that AD 'constitutes a "lynchpin" between normality, problems of living and pathological psychiatric states'. The lack of specificity allows the tagging of early or temporary mental states when the clinical picture is vague and indistinct but the morbidity is greater than expected in a normal reaction. The proposed DSM-5 Criterion B is unchanged from DSM-IV and stipulates that AD symptoms must exhibit either functioned impairment or disproportioned distress after exposure to the stressor.

It is possible that AD is the greatest example of gene × environment interaction in the DSM since an event that constitutes a temporary but surmountable challenge for resilient individuals may precipitate a severe adjustment reaction in more vulnerable individuals. Furthermore, DSM-III's six-month post-event window in which AD might be allowed (after which the diagnosis had to be dropped or changed to a more enduring psychiatric disorder) was changed in DSM-IV to a diagnosis of a chronic subtype if the stressor was still exerting its effects. It is proposed that this chronic subtype be retained in DSM-5.

A great advantage of AD is that its general nonspecificity has made it possible for clinicians to have a diagnosis that acknowledges the distressing and debilitating functional impairment of patients who require mental health treatment but do not meet criteria for any other psychiatric diagnosis. The problem is that because of such nonspecificity it has been very difficult to design epidemiological surveys, longitudinal studies or clinical treatment trials concerning people with this disorder. For the purposes of this review, addition of the uncharacteristically specific ASD/PTSD subtype may make it possible to conduct research regarding people who resemble ASD or PTSD patients but fail to meet full diagnostic criteria for either disorder. This is particularly useful since it is unlikely that a subsyndromal PTSD will be introduced into DSM-5.

PARTIAL/SUBSYNDROMAL PTSD

PTSD does not have a subsyndromal diagnosis comparable to dysthymia and cyclothymia in major depression and bipolar affective disorder, respectively. The argument for adding such a diagnosis is that considerable research indicates the likelihood of partial/subsyndromal PTSD and that it would have clinical utility by characterising people with clinically significant post-traumatic reactions who fail to exceed the PTSD diagnostic threshold (often for lack of one or two symptoms) and for whom a diagnosis of AD has previously been too nonspecific. The arguments against addition of a new subsyndromal category are: (i) that AD, especially with the proposed ASD/PTSD subtype, is the appropriate diagnosis for such individuals; and (ii) that it over-pathlogises normative reactions. Approximately 60 publications have reported on the prevalence and morbidity of 'partial/subsyndromal' PTSD among a wide assortment of traumatised individuals. Unfortunately, throughout these studies partial PTSD has been defined differently by different investigators [28].

In some studies, there is evidence that partial PTSD has a similar relationship to full PTSD as dysthymia has to major depressive disorder or cyclothymia has to bipolar disorder. People with partial PTSD exhibit significantly less symptom severity and functional impairment that those with the full syndrome, but significantly more than no-PTSD cohorts. There are also negative reports, however, in which few differences are detected between partial- and no-PTSD cohorts, although both differed significantly from full PTSD [28].

As stated previously, it is difficult to compare and interpret many of these findings because partial PTSD was defined differently in different studies. Therefore, future research should be based on a standard set of diagnostic criteria so that questions about the uniqueness and utility of partial PTSD can be addressed appropriately. At this time, however, it appears unlikely that partial subsyndromal PTSD will appear as a distinct diagnosis in DSM-5. It is more likely that the ASD/PTSD subtype of AD will be expected to fill this diagnostic niche.

DESNOS/COMPLEX PTSD

Since the work of Judith Herman [108], there have been complaints that the PTSD symptom clusters fail to encompass clinically significant problems often exhibited by individuals exposed to severe and protracted traumatic events (most notably victims of childhood sexual abuse and adult refugees and torture survivors). It's not that such individuals usually fail to meet PTSD diagnostic criteria, but, rather, that their most significant clinical symptoms are not included within the PTSD construct. These include: behavioural difficulties (such as impulsivity, aggression, sexual acting-out, alcohol/drug misuse and self-destructive actions), emotional difficulties (such as affective lability, rage, depression and panic), cognitive difficulties (such as dissociation and pathological changes in personal identity – dissociative identity disorder), interpersonal difficulties and somatisation [108–110].

In characterising the psychiatric sequelae of protracted child abuse, DESNOS (disorders of extreme stress not otherwise specified) has been considered a very useful construct as well as an appropriate diagnosis for the clinical pattern seen in adult (often) non-Western patients exposed to forced migration or torture [111, 112], although there has been little research in this area.

DESNOS was carefully considered for inclusion in DSM-IV and assessed during the DSM-IV Field Trials. Because only 8% of individuals with DESNOS did not also meet PTSD diagnostic criteria, it was considered too rare an occurrence to be classified as a separate diagnostic entity. Despite these findings, there is continued support for DESNOS in certain quarters and continued advocacy for its inclusion in DSM-5. During recent years, there has also been some research designed to clarify the prevalence and construct validity of DESNOS. Unfortunately, neither the quality nor quantity of such research has been persuasive [49].

Questions regarding the uniqueness and utility of DESNOS are far from settled. Given the strong belief among many seasoned clinicians that this is an important diagnosis that should be included in the DSM, we need rigorous research to determine whether exposure to trauma, especially during developmentally sensitive periods, may lead to a different pattern of symptoms than those included in PTSD. In a cross-cultural context, DESNOS may be especially useful because it emphasises both dissociation and somatisation, two symptoms not included in the DSM-IV PTSD diagnostic criteria that are frequently observed in traumatised non-Western cohorts [113]. It has also been reported that more complex cases of PTSD involve deficits in emotional regulation [114]. As a result, it has been proposed that in addition to the core PTSD symptoms, complex presentations are more difficult to treat because they involve acting-out, self-harm and self-destructive relationships and behaviours. Future research could usefully assess the extent to which emotion-regulation symptoms load on to a separate factor and do in fact characterise individuals with PTSD who also exhibit such self-destructive/emotional regulation problems. Identification of such a factor would be consistent with evidence that these patients benefit from specific treatments that precede traditional trauma-focused CBT with emotion-regulation training sessions [115].

Friedman *et al*. [28] suggest that another way to contextualise DESNOS might be to consider a spectrum of PTSD subtypes in which some people appear to have simple PTSD, some have additional internalising behaviours and symptoms, and some exhibit externalising behaviours along with their PTSD [71, 116]. It's possible that this approach might offer a more parsimonious construction of complex PTSD. Somatisation symptoms fall on the internalising dimension, along with depression and anxiety, while anger/aggression, substance abuse and behaviours indicative of cluster B axis II disorders fall on the externalising dimension. Both models can be tested empirically.

SUBTYPES OF PTSD

It has been proposed that there may be two subtypes of PTSD that involve (i) ongoing 'dissociative' versus (ii) 'hyperarousal' reactions [117, 118]. In this context, dissociation has been conceptualised as an avoidance strategy to reduce awareness of aversive emotions such as extreme anxiety [119]. For example, it has been shown that recent rape victims reporting high peritraumatic dissociation showed a decrease in heart rate and skin conductance while talking about the trauma, compared to an increase in physiological responding among those with low peritraumatic dissociation [119]. Neuroimaging studies have provided additional evidence that there may be distinctive prefrontal responses to trauma memories in individuals with dissociative and nondissociative PTSD responses [120]. For example, the 'hyperarousal' PTSD response to traumatic narratives was associated with reduced bilateral medial frontal activity and left anterior cingulate activity relative to controls [121]. In contrast, individuals displaying a 'dissociative' PTSD response had reduced amygdala but significantly increased right medial frontal, right medial prefrontal and right anterior cingulate activity relative to controls [122]. Lanius *et al.* have hypothesised that the heightened prefrontal activity in dissociative PTSD may reflect greater emotional regulation and inhibition of limbic emotional networks, including amygdala [122]. Other neuroimaging findings that distinguish dissociative from nondissociative PTSD have also been reported [28].

These findings are controversial. Several studies have not found differences in autonomic arousal between dissociative and nondissociative individuals with PTSD [123–125]. It appears that our current understanding of the role of dissociation in relation to arousal is very limited, and it is unclear whether there is sufficient evidence to include a unique dissociative subtype of PTSD in DSM-5.

CROSS-CULTURAL FACTORS

PTSD has been criticised as a culture-bound Euro-American construct that has little relevance to the rest of the world, especially to traditional societies [126]. For example, somatisation and dissociation, two common expressions of post-traumatic distress in traditional societies [113], are missing from DSM-IV PTSD diagnostic criteria (but not DESNOS). Whereas there may be culture-specific idioms of distress that provide a better characterisation of PTSDs found in one ethnocultural context or another [127], PTSD has been documented throughout the world [128–130]. Specifically, high prevalence rates have been reported in non-Western nations such as Algeria, Cambodia, Lebanon, Palestine, Nepal and the former Yugoslavia [131–133]. Furthermore, comparable PTSD prevalence has been found among Russian and American adolescents [134].

Unfortunately, direct comparisons in which similar traumatic events affected people from widely different cultures (Western versus non-Western) are rare. A notable exception is a study by North *et al.* [135], who compared psychiatric morbidity among Kenyan survivors of the bombing of the American embassy in Nairobi with American survivors of the bombing of the Federal Building in Oklahoma City. Kenyans and Americans exposed to these events exhibited remarkably similar impacts with respect to death, injury, destruction and other consequences. In addition, PTSD prevalence among Africans and Americans exposed to the events was also very similar.

DEVELOPMENTAL ISSUES

Maturational biological and psychological changes affect the appraisal of and reaction to traumatic events and cause differences in the expression of post-traumatic distress at either end of the life span [136, 137]. For children and adolescents who have experienced traumatic events, the developmental context must incorporate the dynamic and evolving relationship between experience, neurological processing, brain development and affect regulation [138]. The proposed criteria for children and adolescents have incorporated developmental manifestations of PTSD criteria for adults [139]. Scheeringa *et al.* [140] have previously reported on the inadequacy of DSM-IV PTSD criteria to adequately characterise post-traumatic symptoms with regard to infants and children less than four years old. They suggest that criteria anchored in observable behaviours should replace reports of subjective experiences or behaviours. Based on these observations, and others, a developmental pre-school PTSD subtype has been proposed for DSM-5 [139].

In contrast to an expanding literature for children and adolescents, PTSD among the elderly has received very little attention. Here too a developmental approach must address age-specific psychosocial, behavioural and neurobiological factors that mediate and moderate trauma-related symptom expression and clinical course [136]. PTSD among the elderly is often expressed within a context of negative health perceptions, primary care utilisation and suicidal ideation [141]. Traumatic events may result in different responses if they occurred many decades ago rather than recently. Differences in developmental and physiological factors in effect either at the time of the trauma or at the present time may influence the clinical expression of PTSD and post-traumatic distress. This has not been examined in research carried out thus far.

To summarise, a comprehensive, longitudinal developmental approach is needed to explicate how traumatic memories are differentially encoded, stored and retrieved by both immature and ageing individuals, how such differences affect the clinical expressions of PTSD, and what implications this has for treatment.

CONCLUSION

1. Empirical evidence regarding the PTSD DSM-IV diagnostic criteria suggest that: (i) Criterion A1 has proved ambiguous with respect to where/how to draw the line between traumatic and nontraumatic events; (ii) Criterion A2 has failed to demonstrate diagnostic utility; and (iii) confirmatory factor analysis strongly suggests that the latent structure of PTSD is best characterised by a four-factor model.
2. Proposed provisional criteria for DSM-5 (which may change after this review is published) are: (i) retain Criterion A1 but attempt to remove some of its ambiguity; (ii) eliminate Criterion A2; and (iii) propose a four-factor PTSD model, consisting of reexperiencing symptoms, avoidance behavior, negative alterations in cognitions and mood, and alterations in arousal and reactivity. In addition to DSM-IV PTSD symptoms consistent with a fear-conditioning model, the proposed new criteria are consistent with evidence that traumatic exposure may also be followed by a variety of non-fear-based anxiety symptoms such as dysphoric anhedonic symptoms, aggressive/externalising symptoms, guilt/shame symptoms, dissociative symptoms and negative appraisals about oneself and the future.
3. Proposed DSM-5 symptoms for ASD have eliminated the requirement that an individual must exhibit dissociative symptoms in order to meet diagnostic criteria. Although it is recognised that some acutely traumatised individuals may exhibit peritraumatic dissociation, it is proposed that ASD criteria may also be met by the presence of reexperiencing, avoidance and arousal symptoms without the presence of dissociative symptoms.
4. An ASD/PTSD subtype of AD has been proposed for DSM-5. This should provide a diagnostic niche for severely distressed individuals (i) who have been exposed to a traumatic event but do not meet full PTSD diagnostic criteria and (ii) who have been exposed to a very upsetting nontraumatic event but who exhibit the full range of PTSD symptoms.
5. It has been proposed for DSM-5 that PTSD, ASD, AD and dissociative disorders be clustered into a unique diagnostic category or subcategory (as part of Anxiety Disorders) for stress/trauma-induced disorders. Other candidate disorders currently under consideration are a dissociative subtype of PTSD, DESNOS/complex PTSD, prolonged/complicated grief and developmental trauma disorder. All were under consideration at the time this review was written.
6. There has been an effort in DSM-5 to make PTSD criteria developmentally and culturally sensitive.

After DSM-5 is finalised, we will all await empirical data and clinical experience to tell us whether the proposed new criteria are an improvement over DSM-IV. Whether they are or aren't, they will certainly be grist for the mill of DSM-6.

REFERENCES

1. American Psychiatric Association (2000) *Diagnostic and Statistical Manual of Mental Disorders*, 4th edn, Text Revision, American Psychiatric Association, Washington, DC.
2. Strain, J. and Friedman, M.J. (in press) Considering adjustment disorders as stress response syndromes for DSM-5. *Depression and Anxiety*, Published Online doi 10.1002/da.20782.
3. American Psychiatric Association (1980) *Diagnostic and Statistical Manual of Mental Disorders*, 3rd edn, American Psychiatric Association, Washington, DC.
4. Kolb, L.C., Ciccone, P.E., Burstein, A. *et al*. (1989) Heterogeneity of PTSD [letter]. *American Journal of Psychiatry*, **146** (6), 811–812.
5. Keane, T.M., Fairbank, J.A., Caddell, J.M. *et al*. (1985) A behavioral approach to assessing and treating post-traumatic stress disorder in Vietnam veterans, in *Trauma and its Wake*, The Study and Treatment of Post-traumatic Stress Disorder, Vol. I (ed. C.R. Figley), Brunner/Mazel, New York, pp. 257–294.
6. Foa, E.B. and Kozak, M.J. (1986) Emotional processing of fear: exposure to corrective information. *Psychological Bulletin*, **99** (1), 20–35.
7. Charney, D.S. (2004) Psychobiological mechanisms of resilience and vulnerability: implications for successful adaptation to extreme stress. *American Journal of Psychiatry*, **161** (2), 195–216.
8. Davis, M. and Whalen, P.J. (2001) The amygdala: vigilance and emotion. *Molecular Psychiatry*, **6** (1), 13–34.
9. Neumeister, A., Henry, S. and Krystal, J.H. (2007) Neurocircuitry and neuroplasticity in PTSD, in *Handbook of PTSD: Science and Practice* (eds M.J. Friedman, T.M. Keane and P.A. Resick), Guilford Press, New York, pp. 151–165.
10. Pitman, R.K., van der Kolk, B.A., Orr, S.P. *et al*. (1990) Naloxone-reversible analgesic response to combat-related stimuli in posttraumatic stress disorder: a pilot study. *Archives of General Psychiatry*, **47** (6), 541–544.
11. Lifton, R.J. (1967) *Death in Life: Survivors of Hiroshima*, vol. viii, Random House, New York, p. 594.
12. Janoff-Bulman, R. (1992) *Shattered Assumptions: Towards a New Psychology of Trauma*, vol. xii, Free Press, New York, p. 256.
13. Trimble, M.R. (1985) Post-traumatic stress disorder: history of a concept, in *Trauma and its Wake*, The Study and Treatment of Post-traumatic Stress Disorder, Vol. I (ed. C.R. Figley), Brunner/Mazel, New York, pp. 5–14.
14. Shay, J. (1994) *Achilles in Vietnam: Combat Trauma and the Undoing of Character*, vol. xxiii, Atheneum, New York, p. 246.

15. van der Kolk, B.A. (2007) The history of trauma in psychiatry, in *Handbook of PTSD: Science and Practice* (eds M.J. Friedman, T.M. Keane and P.A. Resick), Guilford Press, New York, pp. 19–36.
16. Monson, C.M., Friedman, M.J. and La Bash, H.A.J. (2007) A psychological history of PTSD, in *Handbook of PTSD: Science and Practice* (eds M.J. Friedman, T.M. Keane and P.A. Resick), Guilford Press, New York, pp. 37–52.
17. Friedman, M.J., Resick, P.A. and Keane, T.M. (2007) PTSD: twenty-five years of progress and challenges, in *Handbook of PTSD: Science and Practice* (eds M.J. Friedman, P.A. Resick and T.M. Keane), Guilford Press, New York, pp. 3–18.
18. American Psychiatric Association (1968) *Diagnostic and Statistical Manual of Mental Disorders*, 2nd edn, American Psychiatric Association, Washington, DC.
19. American Psychiatric Association (1952) *Diagnostic and Statistical Manual Mental Disorders*, 1st edn, American Psychiatric Association, Washington, DC.
20. Morgan, L., Scourfield, J., Williams, D. *et al*. (2003) The Aberfan disaster: 33-year follow-up of survivors. *British Journal of Psychiatry*, **182**, 532–536.
21. Neria, Y., Nandi, A.K. and Galea, S. (2008) Post-traumatic stress disorder following disasters: a systematic review. *Psychological Medicine*, **38** (4), 467–480.
22. Norris, F.H. and Slone, L.B. (2007) The epidemiology of trauma and PTSD, in *Handbook of PTSD: Science and Practice* (eds M.J. Friedman., T.M. Keane and P.A. Resick., Guilford Press, New York, pp. 78–98.
23. Whalley, M.G. and Brewin, C.R. (2007) Mental health following terrorist attacks [editorial]. *British Journal of Psychiatry*, **190** (2), 94–96.
24. Kessler, R.C., Sonnega, A., Bromat, E. (1995) Posttraumatic stress disorder in the National Comorbidity Survey. *Archives of General Psychiatry*, **52** (12), 1048–1060.
25. American Psychiatric Association (1994) *Diagnostic and Statistical Manual of Mental Disorders*, 4th edn, American Psychiatric Association, Washington, DC.
26. American Psychiatric Association (1987) *Diagnostic and Statistical Manual of Mental Disorders*, 3rd edn revised, American Psychiatric Association, Washington, DC.
27. Weathers, F.W. and Keane, T.M. (2007) The criterion A problem revisited: controversies and challenges in defining and measuring psychological trauma. *Journal of Traumatic Stress*, **20** (2), 107–121.
28. Friedman, M.J., Resick, P.A., Bryant, R.A. and Brewin, C.R. (in press) Considering PTSD for DSM-V, Depression and Anxiety. Published Online doi 10.1002/da.20767.
29. Haglund, M.E., Nestadt, P.S., Cooper, N.S. *et al*. (2007) Psychobiological mechanisms of resilience: relevance to prevention and treatment of stress-related psychopathology. *Development and Psychopathology*, **19**, 889–920.
30. McNally, R.J. (2009) Can we fix PTSD in DSM-V? *Depression and Anxiety*, **26** (7), 597–600.
31. Kilpatrick, D.G., Resnick, H.G., Freedy, J.R. *et al*. (1998) Posttraumatic stress disorder field trial: evaluation of the PTSD construct: criteria A through E, in *DSM-IV Sourcebook* (ed. T.A. Widiger), American Psychiatric Press, Washington, DC, pp. 803–844.

32. Kilpatrick, D.G., Resnick, H.S. and Acierno, R. (2009) Should PTSD Criterion A be retained? *Journal of Traumatic Stress*, **22**, 374–378.
33. Rosen, G.M. and Lilienfeld, S.O. (2008) Posttraumatic stress disorder: an empirical evaluation of core assumptions. *Clinical Psychology Review*, **28** (5), 837–868.
34. Breslau, N. and Kessler, R.C. (2001) The stressor criterion in DSM-IV posttraumatic stress disorder: an empirical investigation. *Biological Psychiatry*, **50** (9), 699–704.
35. Brewin, C.R., Lanius, R.A., Novac, A. *et al*. (2009) Reformulating PTSD for DSM-V: life after Criterion A. *Journal of Traumatic Stress*, **22**, 366–373.
36. Dohrenwend, B.P. (2006) Inventorying stressful life events as risk factors for psychopathology: toward resolution of the problem of intracategory variability. *Psychological Bulletin*, **132** (3), 477–495.
37. Davidson, J.R.T. and Foa, E.B. (1991) Diagnostic issues in posttraumatic stress disorder: considerations for the DSM-IV. *Journal of Abnormal Psychology*, **100** (3), 346–355.
38. Schnurr, P.P., Ford, J.D., Friedman, M.J. *et al*. (2000) Predictors and outcomes of posttraumatic stress disorder in World War II veterans exposed to mustard gas. *Journal of Consulting and Clinical Psychology*, **68** (2), 258–268.
39. Karam, E.G., Andrews, G., Bromet, E. *et al*. (2010) The role of Criterion A2 in the DSM-IV diagnosis of post-traumatic stress disorder. Biological Psychiatry. Advance online publication.doi:10.1016/j.biopsych.2010.04.032.
40. O'Donnell, M.L. *et al*. (2010) Should A2 be a diagnostic requirement for posttraumatic stress disorder in DSM-V? *Psychiatry Research*, **176** (2/3), 257–260.
41. Creamer, M.C., McFarlane, A.C. and Burgess, P.M. (2005) Psychopathology following trauma: the role of subjective experience. *Journal of Affective Disorders*, **86** (2/3), 175–182.
42. Rizvi, S.L., Kaysen, D.L., Gutner, C.A. *et al*. (2008) Beyond fear: the role of peritraumatic responses in posttraumatic stress and depressive symptoms among female crime victims. *Journal of Interpersonal Violence*, **23** (6), 853–868.
43. Bryant, R.A. (2001) Posttraumatic stress disorder and mild brain injury: controversies, causes and consequences. *Journal of Clinical and Experimental Neuropsychology*, **23** (6), 718–728.
44. Bryant, R.A., Marosszeky, J.E., Crooks, J. *et al*. (2000) Posttraumatic stress disorder after severe traumatic brain injury. *American Journal of Psychiatry*, **157** (4), 629–631.
45. Harvey, A.G. and Bryant, R.A. (2000) Memory for acute stress disorder symptoms: a two-year prospective study. *Journal of Nervous and Mental Disease*, **188** (9), 602–607.
46. Brewin, C.R., Andrews, B. and Rose, S. (2000) Fear, helplessness, and horror in posttraumatic stress disorder: investigating DSM-IV criterion A2 in victims of violent crime. *Journal of Traumatic Stress*, **13** (3), 499–509.
47. Resick, P.A. and Miller, M.W. (2009) Posttraumatic stress disorder: anxiety or traumatic stress disorder? *Journal of Traumatic Stress*, **22** (5), 384–390.
48. Friedman, M.J., Keane, T.M. and Resick, P.A. (2007) PTSD: twenty-five years of progress and challenges, in *Handbook of PTSD: Science and Practice* (eds M.J. Friedman, T.M. Keane and P.A. Resick), Guilford Press, New York, pp. 3–18.

49. Friedman, M.J. *et al*. (2009) PTSD and other posttraumatic syndromes, in *Current Perspectives on Anxiety Disorders: Implications for DSM-V and Beyond* (ed. D.W. McKay), Springer, New York, pp. 377–410.
50. Foy, D.W., Wood, J.L., King, D.W. *et al*. (1997) Los Angeles Symptom Checklist: psychometric evidence with an adolescent sample. *Assessment*, **4** (4), 377–384.
51. Krueger, R.F. and Markon, K.E. (2006) Reinterpreting comorbidity: a model-based approach to understanding and classifying psychopathology. *Annual Review of Clinical Psychology*, **2**, 111–133.
52. Watson, D. (2005) Rethinking the mood and anxiety disorders: a quantitative hierarchical model for DSM-V. *Journal of Abnormal Psychology*, **114** (4), 522–536.
53. Brewin, C.R., Gregory, J.D., Lipton, M. *et al*. (2010) Intrusive images and memories in psychological disorders: characteristics, neural basis, and treatment implications. *Psychological Review*, **117**, 210–232.
54. Ehlers, A., Hackmann, A. and Michael, T. (2004) Intrusive re-experiencing in post-traumatic stress disorder: phenomenology, theory, and therapy. *Memory*, **12** (4), 403–415.
55. Michael, T., Ehlers, A., Halligan, S.L. *et al*. (2005) Unwanted memories of assault: what intrusion characteristics are associated with PTSD? *Behaviour Research and Therapy*, **43** (5), 613–628.
56. Michael, T., Halligan, S., Clark, D. *et al*. (2007) Rumination in posttraumatic stress disorder. *Depression and Anxiety*, **24** (5), 307–317.
57. Speckens, A.E.M. *et al*. (2007) Intrusive images and memories of earlier adverse events in patients with obsessive compulsive disorder. *Journal of Behavior Therapy and Experimental Psychiatry*, **38** (4), 411–422.
58. Craske, B., Rauch, S.L., Ursano, R. *et al*. (2009) What is an anxiety disorder? *Depress Anxiety*, **47**, 285–293.
59. Simms, L.J., Watson, D. and Doebbeling, B.N. (2002) Confirmatory factor analyses of posttraumatic stress symptoms in deployed and nondeployed veterans of the Gulf war. *Journal of Abnormal Psychology*, **111** (4), 637–647.
60. Kashdan, T.B., Elhai, J.D. and Frueh, B.C. (2006) Anhedonia and emotional numbing in combat veterans with PTSD. *Behaviour Research and Therapy*, **44** (3), 457–467.
61. Ehlers, A., Clark, D.M., Dunmore, E. *et al*. (1998) Predicting response to exposure treatment in PTSD: the role of mental defeat and alienation. *Journal of Traumatic Stress*, **11** (3), 457–471.
62. Feiring, C. and Cleland, C. (2007) Childhood sexual abuse and abuse-specific attributions of blame over 6 years following discovery. *Child Abuse and Neglect*, **31** (11/12), 1169–1186.
63. Resick, P.A., Nishith, P., Weaver, T.L. *et al*. (2002) A comparison of cognitive-processing therapy with prolonged exposure and a waiting condition for the treatment of chronic posttraumatic stress disorder in female rape victims. *Journal of Consultting and Clinical Psychology*, **70** (4), 867–879.
64. Bryant, R.A. and Guthrie, R.M. (2007) Maladaptive self-appraisals before trauma exposure predict posttraumatic stress disorder. *Journal of Consulting and Clinical Psychology*, **75** (5), 812–815.

65. Dalgleish, T., Meiser-Stedman, R. and Smith, P.A. (2005) Cognitive aspects of posttraumatic stress reactions and their treatment in children and adolescents: an empirical review and some recommendations. *Behavioural and Cognitive Psychotherapy*, **33** (4), 459–486.
66. Ehring, T., Ehlers, A. and Glucksman, E. (2008) Do cognitive models help in predicting the severity of posttraumatic stress disorder, phobia, and depression after motor vehicle accidents: a prospective longitudinal study. *Journal of Consulting and Clinical Psychology*, **76** (2), 219–230.
67. Karl, A., Rabe, S., Zollner, T. *et al*. (2009) Negative self-appraisals in treatment-seeking survivors of motor vehicle accidents. *Journal of Anxiety Disorders*, **23** (6), 775–781.
68. Moser, J.S., Hajcak, G., Simons, R.F. *et al*. (2007) Posttraumatic stress disorder symptoms in trauma-exposed college students: the role of trauma-related cognitions, gender, and negative affect. *Journal of Anxiety Disorders*, **21** (8), 1039–1049.
69. Owens, G.P., Chard, K.M. and Cox, T.A. (2008) The relationship between maladaptive cognitions, anger expression, and posttraumatic stress disorder among veterans in residential treatment. *Journal of Aggression, Maltreatment and Trauma*, **17** (4), 439–452.
70. Resick, P.A., Galovski, T.E., Uhlmansick, M.O. *et al*. (2008) A randomized clinical trial to dismantle components of cognitive processing therapy for posttraumatic stress disorder in female victims of interpersonal violence. *Journal of Consulting and Clinical Psychology*, **76** (2), 243–258.
71. Miller, M.W. and Resick, P.A. (2007) Internalizing and externalizing subtypes in female sexual assault survivors: implications for the understanding of complex PTSD. *Behavior Theraphy*, **38** (1), 58–71.
72. Andrews, B., Brewin, C.R., Rose, S. *et al*. (2000) Predicting PTSD symptoms in victims of violent crime: the role of shame, anger, and childhood abuse. *Journal of Abnormal Psychology*, **109** (1), 69–73.
73. Orth, U., Cahill, S.P., Foa, E.B. *et al*. (2008) Anger and posttraumatic stress disorder symptoms in crime victims: a longitudinal analysis. *Journal of Consulting and Clinical Psychology*, **76** (2), 208–218.
74. Riggs, D.S., Dancu, C.V., Gershuny, B.S. *et al*. (1992) Anger and post-traumatic stress disorder in female crime victims. *Journal of Traumatic Stress*, **5** (4), 613–625.
75. Taft, C.T., Street, A.E., Marshall, A.D. *et al*. (2007) Posttraumatic stress disorder, anger, and partner abuse among Vietnam combat veterans. *Journal of Family Psychology*, **21** (2), 270–277.
76. Henning, K.R. and Frueh, B.C. (1997) Combat guilt and its relationship to PTSD symptoms. *Journal of Clinical Psychology*, **53** (8), 801–808.
77. Kubany, E.S., Abueg, F.R., Owens, J.A. *et al*. (1995) Initial examination of a multidimensional model of trauma-related guilt: applications to combat veterans and battered women. *Journal of Psychopathology and Behavioral Assessment*, **17** (4), 353–376.
78. Nishith, P., Nixon, R.D.V. and Resick, P.A. (2005) Resolution of trauma-related guilt following treatment of PTSD in female rape victims: a result of cognitive

processing therapy targeting comorbid depression? *Journal of Affective Disorders*, **86** (2/3), 259–265.

79. Leskela, J., Dieperink, M.E. and Thuras, P. (2002) Shame and posttraumatic stress disorder. *Journal of Traumatic Stress*, **15** (3), 223–226.
80. Street, A.E. and Arias, I. (2001) Psychological abuse and posttraumatic stress disorder in battered women: examining the roles of shame and guilt. *Violence and Victims*, **16** (1), 65–78.
81. Lanius, R.A., Williamson, P.C., Bluhm, R. *et al*. (2005) Functional connectivity of dissociative responses in posttraumatic stress disorder: a functional magnetic resonance imaging investigation. *Biological Psychiatry*, **57** (8), 873–884.
82. Sar, V., Koyuncu, A., Ozturk, E. *et al*. (2007) Dissociative disorders in the psychiatric emergency ward. *General Hospital Psychiatry*, **29** (1), 45–50.
83. Jakupcak, M., Conybeare, D., Phelps, L. *et al*. (2007) Anger, hostility, and aggression among Iraq and Afghanistan war veterans reporting PTSD and subthreshold PTSD. *Journal of Traumatic Stress*, **20** (6), 945–954.
84. Lasko, N.B., Gurvits, T.V., Kuhne, A.A. *et al*. (1994) Aggression and its correlates in Vietnam veterans with and without chronic posttraumatic stress disorder. *Comprehensive Psychiatry*, **35** (5), 373–381.
85. Taft, C.T., Kaloupek, D.G., Schumm, J.A. *et al*. (2007) Posttraumatic stress disorder symptoms, physiological reactivity, alcohol problems, and aggression among military veterans. *Journal of Abnormal Psychology*, **116** (3), 498–507.
86. Taft, C.T., Vogt, D.S., Marshall, A.D. *et al*. (2007) Aggression among combat veterans: relationships with combat exposure and symptoms of posttraumatic stress disorder, dysphoria, and anxiety. *Journal of Traumatic Stress*, **20** (2), 135–145.
87. Taft, C.T., Monson, C.M., Schumm, J.A. *et al*. (2009) Posttraumatic stress disorder symptoms, relationship adjustment, and relationship aggression in a sample of female flood victims. *Journal of Family Violence*, **24**, 389–396.
88. Pat-Horenczyk, R., Peled, O., Miron, T. *et al*. (2007) Risk-taking behaviors among Israeli adolescents exposed to recurrent terrorism: provoking danger under continuous threat? *American Journal of Psychiatry*, **164** (1), 66–72.
89. Fear, N.T., Iverson, R.C., Chatterjee, A. *et al*. (2008) Risky driving among regular armed forces personnel from the United Kingdom. *American Journal of Preventive Medicine*, **35** (3), 230–236.
90. Lapham, S.C., C'De Baca, J., McMillan, G.P. *et al*. (2006) Psychiatric disorders in a sample of repeat impaired-driving offenders. *Journal of Studies on Alcohol*, **67** (5), 707–713.
91. Lowinger, T. and Solomon, Z. (2004) PTSD, guilt, and shame among reckless drivers. *Journal of Loss and Trauma*, **9** (4), 327–344.
92. Green, B.L., Krupnick, J.L., Stockton, P. *et al*. (2005) Effects of adolescent trauma exposure on risky behavior in college women. *Psychiatry*, **68** (4), 363–378.
93. Hutton, H.E., Treisman, G.J., Hunt, W.R. *et al*. (2001) HIV risk behaviors and their relationship to posttraumatic stress disorder among women prisoners. *Psychiatric Services*, **52** (4), 508–513.

94. Andrews, B., Brewin, C.R., Philpott, R. *et al*. (2007) Delayed-onset posttraumatic stress disorder: a systematic review of the evidence. *American Journal of Psychiatry*, **164** (9), 1319–1326.
95. Bryant, R.A. and Harvey, A.G. (2002) Delayed-onset posttraumatic stress disorder: a prospective evaluation. *Australian and New Zealand Journal of Psychiatry*, **36** (2), 205–209.
96. Solomon, Z. and Mikulincer, M. (2006) Trajectories of PTSD: a 20-year longitudinal study. *American Journal of Psychiatry*, **163** (4), 659–666.
97. Wolfe, J., Erickson, D.J., Sharkansky, E.J. *et al*. (1999) Course and predictors of posttraumatic stress disorder among Gulf War veterans: a prospective analysis. *Journal of Consulting and Clinical Psychology*, **67** (4), 520–528.
98. Norris, F.H., Murphy, A.D., Baker, C.K. *et al*. (2003) Severity, timing, and duration of reactions to trauma in the population: an example from Mexico. *Biological Psychiatry*, **53** (9), 769–778.
99. Riggs, D.S., Rothbaum, B.O. and Foa, E.B. (1995) A prospective examination of symptoms of posttraumatic stress disorder in victims of nonsexual assault. *Journal of Interpersonal Violence*, **10** (2), 201–214.
100. Blanchard, E.B., Hickling, E.J., Taylor, A.E. *et al*. (1995) Psychiatric morbidity associated with motor vehicle accidents. *Journal of Nervous and Mental Disease*, **183** (8), 495–504.
101. Bryant, R., Friedman, M.J., Spiegel, D. *et al*. (in press) A review of acute stress disorder in DSM-5. *Depression and Anxiety*. Published Online doi 10.1002/da.20753.
102. Koopman, C., Classan, C.C., Cardena, E. *et al*. (1995) When disaster strikes, acute stress disorder may follow. *Journal of Traumatic Stress*, **8** (1), 29–46.
103. Spiegel, D., Koopman, G., Cardena, E. *et al*. (1996) Dissociative symptoms in the diagnosis of acute stress disorder, in *Handbook of Dissociation: Theoretical, Empirical, and Clinical Perspectives* (eds L.K. Michelson and W.J. Ray), Plenum, New York, pp. 367–380.
104. Bryant, R. (2011) Acute stress disorder as a predictor of posttraumatic stress disorder: a systematic review. *Journal of Clinical Psychiatry*, **72** (2), 233–239.
105. Bryant, R.A. (2003) Early predictors of posttraumatic stress disorder. *Biological Psychiatry*, **53** (9), 789–795.
106. Panasetis, P. and Bryant, R.A. (2003) Peritraumatic versus persistent dissociation in acute stress disorder. *Journal of Traumatic Stress*, **16** (6), 563–566.
107. Friedman, M.J., Resick, P.A., Bryant, R.A. *et al*. (Submitted) Classification of trauma and stressor-related disorders in DSM-5.
108. Herman, J.L. (1992) Complex PTSD: a syndrome in survivors of prolonged and repeated trauma. *Journal of Traumatic Stress*, **5** (3), 377–391.
109. Linehan, M.M., Tutek, D.A., Heard, I.H. *et al*. (1994) Interpersonal outcome of cognitive behavioral treatment for chronically suicidal borderline patients. *American Journal of Psychiatry*, **151** (12), 1771–1776.
110. van der Kolk, B.A., Roth, S., Pelcovitz, D. *et al*. (2005) Disorders of extreme stress: the empirical foundation of a complex adaptation to trauma. *Journal of Traumatic Stress*, **18** (5), 389–399.

111. De Jong, J.T.V.M., Komproe, I.H., Spinazzola, J. *et al*. (2005) DESNOS in three postconflict settings: assessing cross-cultural construct equivalence. *Journal of Traumatic Stress*, **18** (1), 13–21.

112. Söchting, I., Corrado, R., Cohen, I.M. *et al*. (2007) Traumatic pasts in Canadian Aboriginal people: further support for a complex trauma conceptualization? *British Columbia Medical Journal*, **49** (6), 320–326.

113. Kirmayer, L.J. (1996) Confusion of the senses: implications of ethnocultural variations in somatoform and dissociative disorders for PTSD, in *Ethnocultural Aspects of Posttraumatic Stress Disorder: Issues, Research, and Clinical Applications* (ed. A.J. Marsella), American Psychological Association, Washington, DC, pp. 131–163.

114. Cloitre, M., Miranda, R., Stovall-McClough, K.C. *et al*. (2005) Beyond PTSD: emotion regulation and interpersonal problems as predictors of functional impairment in survivors of childhood abuse. *Behavior Therapy*, **36**, 119–124.

115. Cloitre, M., Koenen, K.C., Cohen, L.R. *et al*. (2002) Skills training in affective and interpersonal regulation followed by exposure: a phase-based treatment for PTSD related to childhood abuse. *Journal of Consulting and Clinical Psychology*, **70** (5), 1067–1074.

116. Sellbom, M. and Bagby, R.M. (2009) Identifying PTSD personality subtypes in a workplace trauma sample. *Journal of Traumatic Stress*, **22** (5), 471–475.

117. Bremner, J.D. (1999) Acute and chronic responses to psychological trauma: where do we go from here? [editorial]. *American Journal of Psychiatry*, **156** (3), 349–351.

118. Lanius, R.A., Vermetten, E., Loewenstein, R.J., *et al*. (2010) Emotion modulation in PTSD: clinical and neurobiological evidence for a dissociative subtype. *American Journal of Psychiatry*, **167** (6), 640–647.

119. Griffin, M.G., Resick, P.A. and Mechanic, M.B. (1997) Objective assessment of peritraumatic dissociation: psychophysiological indicators. *American Journal of Psychiatry*, **154** (8), 1081–1088.

120. Lanius, R.A., Bluhm, R., Lanius, U. *et al*. (2006) A review of neuroimaging studies in PTSD: heterogeneity of response to symptom provocation. *Journal of Psychiatric Research*, **40** (8), 709–729.

121. Lanius, R.A., Williamson, P., Densmore, M. *et al*. (2001) Neural correlates of traumatic memories in posttraumatic stress disorder: a functional MRI investigation. *American Journal of Psychiatry*, **158** (11), 1920–1922.

122. Lanius, R.A., Williamson, P., Boksman, K. *et al*. (2002) Brain activation during script-driven imagery induced dissociative responses in PTSD: a functional magnetic resonance imaging investigation. *Biological Psychiatry*, **52** (4), 305–311.

123. Griffin, M.G., Nishith, P. and Resick, P.A. (2002) Peritraumatic dissociation in domestic violence victims. 18th Annual Meeting of the International Society for Traumatic Stress Studies, Baltimore, MD.

124. Kaufman, M.L., Kimble, M.O., Kaloupek, D.G. *et al*. (2002) Peritraumatic dissociation and physiological response to trauma-relevant stimuli in Vietnam combat

veterans with posttraumatic stress disorder. *Journal of Nervous and Mental Disease*, **190** (3), 167–174.

125. Nixon, R.D.V. and Bryant, R.A. (2005) Physiological arousal and dissociation in acute trauma victims during trauma narratives. *Journal of Traumatic Stress*, **18** (2), 197–113.
126. Summerfield, D.A. (2004) Cross-cultural perspectives on the medicalization of human suffering, in *Posttraumatic Stress Disorder: Issues and Controversies* (ed. G.M. Rosen), John Wiley & Sons, Ltd, Chichester, pp. 233–245.
127. Hinton, D. and Lewis-Fernåndez, R. (in press) A critical review of DSM-IV-TR's diagnosis of PTSD from a cross-cultural perspective. *Depression and Anxiety*, Published Online doi 10.1002/da.20753.
128. Green, B.L., Friedman, M.J., deJong, J.T.V.M. *et al*. (2003) *Trauma Interventions in War and Peace: Prevention, Practice, and Policy*, Kluwer Academic/Plenum Publishers, New York, p. xxiii, 388.
129. Marsella, A.J., Friedman, M.J., Gerrity, E.T. and Scurfield, R.M. (1996) *Ethnocultural Aspects of Posttraumatic Stress Disorder: Issues, Research, and Clinical Applications*, American Psychological Association, Washington, DC, p. xxii, 576.
130. Osterman, J.E. and De Jong, J.T.V.M. (2007) Cultural issues and trauma, in *Handbook of PTSD: Science and Practice* (eds M.J. Friedman, T.M. Keane and P.A. Resick), Guilford Press, New York, pp. 425–446.
131. De Jong, J.T.V.M., Komproe, I.H., Van Ommeren, M.H. *et al*. (2001) Lifetime events and posttraumatic stress disorder in 4 postconflict settings. *Journal of the American Medical Association*, **286** (5), 555–562.
132. Hinton, D.E., Chhean, D., Pich, V. *et al*. (2006) Assessment of posttraumatic stress disorder in Cambodian refugees using the Clinician-Administered PTSD Scale: psychometric properties and symptom severity. *Journal of Traumatic Stress*, **19** (3), 405–409.
133. Thapa, S.B. and Hauff, E. (2005) Psychological distress among displaced persons during an armed conflict in Nepal. *Social Psychiatry and Psychiatric Epidemiology*, **40** (8), 672–679.
134. Ruchkin, V.V., Schwab-Stone, M., Jones, S. *et al*. (2005) Is posttraumatic stress in youth a culture-bound phenomenon? A comparison of symptom trends in selected US and Russian communities. *American Journal of Psychiatry*, **162** (3), 538–544.
135. North, C.S., Pfefferbaum, B., Narayanan, P. *et al*. (2005) Comparison of post-disaster psychiatric disorders after terrorist bombings in Nairobi and Oklahoma City. *British Journal of Psychiatry*, **186** (6), 487–493.
136. Cook, J.M. and Niederehe, G. (2007) Trauma in older adults, in *Handbook of PTSD: Science and Practice* (eds M.J. Friedman, T.M. Keane and P.A. Resick), Guilford Press, New York, pp. 252–276.
137. Fairbank, J.A., Putnam, F.W. and Harris, W.W. (2007) The prevalence and impact of child traumatic stress, in *Handbook of PTSD: Science and Practice* (eds M.J. Friedman, T.M. Keane and P.A. Resick), Guilford Press, New York, pp. 229–251.

138. Saxe, G.N., MacDonald, H.Z., Ellis, B.H. *et al*. (2007) Psychosocial approaches for children with PTSD, in *Handbook of PTSD: Science and Practice*, Guilford Press, New York, pp. 359–375.
139. Scheeringa, M.S., Zeanah, C.H. and Cohen, J.A. (in press) PTSD in children and adolescents: towards an empirically based algorithm. *Depression and Anxiety*. Published Online doi 10.1002/da.20736.
140. Scheeringa, M.S., Zeanah, C.H., Drell, M.J. *et al*. (1995) Two approaches to the diagnosis of posttraumatic stress disorder in infancy and early childhood. *Journal of the American Academy of Child and Adolescent Psychiatry*, **34** (2), 191–200.
141. Rauch, S.A.M., Morales, K.H., Zubritsky, C. *et al*. (2006) Posttraumatic stress, depression, and health among older adults in primary care. *American Journal of Geriatric Psychiatry*, **14** (3), 316–324.

COMMENTARY

1.1 Walking the Line in Defining PTSD: Comprehensiveness Versus Core Features

Chris R. Brewin
Clinical Educational and Health Psychology, University College London, London, UK

The inclusion of post-traumatic stress disorder (PTSD) in the Diagnostic and Statistical Manual III (DSM-III) was a considerable achievement that has vastly enriched our knowledge of reactions to traumatic events and our ability to offer appropriate care to survivors. Nevertheless, limitations created by the way in which PTSD belatedly entered the diagnostic canon continue to create problems today. One problem was created by the assumption, subsequently proven incorrect, that PTSD was fully explained by exposure to an event outside the range of usual human experience. This resulted in the stressor criterion, Criterion A, assuming a central role in the diagnosis. The realisation that PTSD can follow more mundane traumatic events such as motor-vehicle accidents that nevertheless have the potential to create intense fear and helplessness, and the confirmation that individual vulnerability is as important in PTSD as in other psychiatric disorders, has led inevitably to subsequent problems in defining exactly what does and does not comprise a traumatic event.

In the late 1970s there was also far less appreciation than there is today concerning the role of stressful life events in the onset and maintenance of many psychiatric disorders. In seeking to introduce a condition that was defined in terms of the aetiological role of extreme stress, it may therefore not have been so evident to those crafting the DSM-III definition that traumatic stressors would produce a range of psychopathological reactions, and that it would be necessary

Post-traumatic Stress Disorder, First Edition. Edited by Dan Stein, Matthew Friedman, and Carlos Blanco.

to single out those features that made PTSD a unique syndrome. This aspect (i.e. discriminant validity) is key to defining psychiatric diagnoses and guarantees that the putative disorder is not simply a different but overlapping expression of another condition [1]. In contrast, the approach taken in DSM-III appears to have been one of assuming the uniqueness of the syndrome and seeking to provide a comprehensive description of its features. It is ironic in this regard that the ideas behind the PTSD diagnosis borrowed so much from the work of Mardi Horowitz (e.g. [2]), who, in drawing on earlier research on bereavement, has done more than most to emphasise the similarities between stress-response syndromes following a variety of challenging life events (see [3] for further discussion).

Although the strategy adopted in DSM-III was effective in helping mental health professionals to identify the condition in their practice, one legacy has been the complexity of the diagnosis relative to depression and other anxiety disorders. This complexity is not just created by the stressor criterion but by specifying three different groups of symptoms all possessed of different thresholds (PTSD currently requires one reexperiencing symptom, three avoidance/numbing symptoms and two hyperarousal symptoms). Perhaps as a result, PTSD is often still poorly recognised in primary care [4]. It is unlikely that the proposal to increase the number of symptom clusters from three to four, although this is consistent with the results of factor analyses, will alleviate this problem.

It can also be argued that this complexity has to some extent impeded the development of a scientific understanding of the condition. For example, the degree of overlap between the symptoms of PTSD and other disorders has been frequently remarked upon, and has left the field unable to determine whether the very substantial comorbidity associated with PTSD is a real effect or an artefact of similarity in the definition of the various diagnoses. Similarly, the fact that it is possible to receive the PTSD diagnosis on the basis of so many different combinations of symptoms makes it difficult to define the core nature of the disorder and to generalise the results of individual investigations. The lack of core symptoms of the kind found in other anxiety disorders is a major stumbling block to developing adequate biological models of PTSD.

The proposal to introduce new symptoms, for example those addressing the existence of a pervasive negative emotional state and persistent distorted blame of self or others, continues the strategy of comprehensively describing the features of the condition and will further increase heterogeneity. Although these additional symptoms do characterise many cases of PTSD they are also commonly encountered in other disorders such as depression, and hence will not assist in differentiating PTSD from the other disorders that share these features.

It is a source of disappointment that the DSM-5 Work Group has not had a more extensive knowledge base upon which to draw in considering its options. Analyses of the PTSD construct have largely consisted of factor analyses of the existing DSM-III-R and DSM-IV sets of 17 symptoms. There have been few if any systematic attempts to investigate the effect of varying the thresholds of the different symptom clusters, or to test whether the predictive value of the avoidance and numbing symptoms [5] is due to the higher threshold required. Nor have investigators conducted factor analyses on a broader range of possible symptoms, or used factor analysis to see which symptoms of PTSD, depression or pathological grief are distinctive and which overlap (but for recent exceptions see [6, 7]).

The proposed revisions for DSM-5 will provide a framework in which better research can be done in future. Clustering several stress- or trauma-induced disorders together is helpful in making explicit the substantial similarity between the different conditions that follow these events. As depressive reactions are also a major consequence of stress and trauma, these should probably form a new category of disorders, rather than a subcategory of Anxiety Disorders. The improved focus of the reexperiencing symptom cluster on memories rather than thoughts of the trauma will provide greater homogeneity and exclude individuals who solely report the depressive symptom of rumination. The separation of deliberate avoidance and numbing symptoms is an essential first step towards properly investigating these very different types of response. The addition of new symptoms, including the externalising features of aggressive and risk-taking behaviours, will hopefully provide additional ways of discriminating PTSD from other stress-response syndromes using factor-analytic and other methods.

The proposed revisions should also bring with them a number of clinical advantages. As Friedman notes, there is a tension between formulating Criterion A sufficiently broadly to include everyone who may benefit from trauma-focused treatment and making it narrow enough to define a homogeneous group of patients. The removal of Criterion A2 will allow people who for various very good reasons did not experience peritraumatic fear, helplessness or horror to be diagnosed with the disorder. Also, by introducing the ASD/PTSD subtype of AD, DSM-5 ensures that those not meeting the current Criterion A may nevertheless qualify for a diagnosis and for treatment. The introduction of additional PTSD symptoms to the diagnosis will alert clinicians to important aspects of the condition such as self-blame and risk-taking behaviour that good management needs to take into account. We are still learning much about stress- and trauma-related disorders, and it is to be hoped that the same open-minded and empirically-grounded spirit that has characterised the DSM-5 consideration of PTSD will also inform the development of DSM-6 in due course.

COMMENTARY

1.2 Trauma-Related Disorders in the Clinical and Legal Settings

Elie G. Karam
Department of Psychiatry and Clinical Psychology; Balamand University Medical School and St Georges Hospital University Medical Center; Institute for Development Research Advocacy and Applied Care (IDRAAC); Medical Institute for Neuropsychological Disorders (MIND), Beirut, Lebanon

INTRODUCTION

The diagnosis of PTSD has been an important topic of research by our group [8–10] and we are pleased that our recommendations might be finding echoes in the final formulation of DSM-5. This commentary addresses the 'clinical' (rather than research) aspects of PTSD. We will present here our reflections in two parts: the first draws on our practice of clinical psychiatry and psychology, and the second on our forensic experience.

ARE WE MISSING PTSD IN THE CLINICAL SETTING?

While the diagnosis of PTSD is quite straightforward for all members of our department (because of our ongoing field research), we do not make such a diagnosis as often as might be expected. This is also the case in many treatment settings around the world. We have pondered on the reasons for the relative rarity of this diagnosis.

The possible explanations that occurred to us are: patients with PTSD consult our centre less or consult less in general, or else we are not looking hard enough for PTSD. We intuitively dismiss the first two reasons. Our practice is vibrant and draws on all of Lebanon and the entire Middle East region and we are well

Post-traumatic Stress Disorder, First Edition. Edited by Dan Stein, Matthew Friedman, and Carlos Blanco.

known for our work on trauma and post-traumatic experiences, offer our services for free at times of big disasters, and have publicised it on radio, TV and so on for the past 30 years. Furthermore, even if patients with PTSD avoid coming to mental health specialists for fear of reliving their trauma, we would at least expect those with severe impairment in their daily lives to be brought by relatives and family, as occurs very frequently for other disorders in this part of the world.

It is possible, then, that we are not looking 'aggressively' enough for PTSD. We have had similar internal discussions on why adult ADHD was not as commonly diagnosed by our group (despite the fact that again we had published on that condition) [11, 12]; we decided we had not been used to looking for it, and the more we did, the more we found it, without falling into the trap of over-diagnosis. Reflecting on this for the purpose of this commentary, it seems to be true too for PTSD. Under-diagnosis at our centre appears to be more common during the first visit, especially when the examining clinician is a psychiatrist. Diagnosis is higher when patients are referred (independently or by the psychiatrists themselves) to our psychologists, or when a second opinion is requested, or during bedside rounds with interns and residents where a mandatory full history is taken.

Systematically, there are five situations which lead us to consider this diagnosis:

1. If the setting (geographically or temporally) favours the focus on the stressor criterion: war, earthquake, plane crash and so on.
2. If the presenting complaint by the patient or the informant is clearly and spontaneously announced to be linked to a trauma.
3. When the patient complains spontaneously of reexperiencing and avoidance symptoms.
4. If the presenting clinical picture is overwhelmingly that of severe anxiety with possible dissociative states and fear.
5. If the treatment provider is interested (for reasons other than the above) in the diagnosis of PTSD.

As stated above, we think this state of affairs is common in most treatment settings across the globe. With more clinical awareness, with more public knowledge, we could gather more data on the wide panoply of PTSD 'presentations' that are probably missed today.

Why is it that some patients have symptoms after trauma and others do not? Looking at risk factors, *specifically* in the case of PTSD, is not entirely satisfactory to clinicians. Risk factors are not automatically thought of as explaining the emergence of any disorder when the disorder has *a readily identifiable 'cause'*. If a person is hit by a car, and has a brain haemorrhage, we are not likely to consider risk factors; he or she has simply had a car accident. We think about risk factors only when an uncommon clinical picture is produced by the accident, such as generalised bleeding (was the patient already on anticoagulants before the accident?). The recent tendency to be more cautious about the word 'cause' in PTSD will have an impact on research (treatment and prevention) and move the debate in novel directions.

The possible mechanisms involved in the emergence of PTSD and its treatment carry a huge potential not only for improving understanding of why we react the way we do but also for future possibilities in recoding our memories. In the future we might be able not only to modify the emotional tone surrounding the trauma but also to change specifics of it [13, 14]; these are only glimpses of how far research in PTSD could propel us. Ultimately we could build resilience and modify memories: limits would be pushed further in the evolution of Homo sapiens. Undoubtedly, as with many scientific breakthroughs, this would raise a plethora of ethical issues.

Additionally, PTSD is a relative newcomer and consequently does not have the benefit of well-established (and trimmed) entities such as depression and mania; more so, it must earn its reputation before joining the club, especially since embedded in it is the bold contention of linking trauma to a disorder, something that psychiatric nosology has veered away from in the past 25 years, during the relative decline of psychoanalysis. This brings us to the second part of this commentary: the forensic experience.

DOES PTSD ADEQUATELY COVER TRAUMA-RELATED DISORDERS IN THE FORENSIC SETTING?

Our group has recently been called to assess dozens of prisoners of war from another country who claimed to have been tortured or abused. We had never before seen such a large number of patients with PTSD back to back. We worked as a group and naturally exchanged our impressions as we went along. We will not dwell here on the general misery that this group of subjects shared with us: listening to the atrocities they endured is akin to the experience reported by body handlers in situations of mass disasters [15]. The impairment these ex-prisoners claimed varied and was pervasive: professional, marital, social and so on. Most frequently the trauma had occurred months or years earlier; they did not look scared or horrified and did not volunteer complaints of nightmares or flashes.

Avoidance, anger, shame and irritability were the cardinal symptoms. Many of them heard a voice calling them or felt someone was following them. A large number attempted suicide. While they admitted having the other symptoms of PTSD, their complaints were tilted in favour of these cardinal symptoms. Should emotional dysregulation/regulation, as anger, still be thought of only as an associated feature?

Many of the victims were still ‘intra-traumatic’: they were confronted not by reminders, but by the actual alleged perpetrators (or their representatives); thus not only did they react to reminders but also to their ‘persecutors’. How does PTSD symptomatology differ in such cases?

We wondered what to make of the very frequent and more pervasive major depression that followed the trauma. Was this part of the PTSD? PTSD was not constructed so as to give particular weight to depressive symptoms. Yet in this large group of ex-prisoners, depression symptoms looked at least as important as the classical PTSD symptoms. Are we talking here of multiple comorbid pathologies? Is it a matter of severity or of perspective?

In short, the present DSM-IV criteria of PTSD did not adequately mirror the complaints of this subset of the population. We think PTSD should be part of a larger category, namely trauma-related disorders. As a side note: we wondered at times if these ex-prisoners were fabricating the stories for compensation; but they had not been questioned previously, to our knowledge, on the DSM symptoms of PTSD; an indirect proof being that they overwhelmingly reported irritability, shame and anger as major emotional states, which are not cardinal in the present DSM nosology. We expect this issue (moving from PTSD to trauma-related disorders) to be of importance not only in future developments of psychiatric nosologies but also in giving a new impetus to environmentally induced mental health pathologies. On the other hand, verifying the symptomatology from neurobiological perspectives will be of paramount importance in the continuing debate over the validity of trauma-related disorders in legal circles [16].

CONCLUSION

We think some of the problems with PTSD lie in its bold revival of linking a mental disorder to an event; this means that clinicians might expect that all symptoms secondary to trauma (albeit 'severe') can be encompassed under the umbrella of PTSD. They cannot. There are several subsets of symptoms that arise following trauma. It is true that many individuals present more with the classical symptoms of PTSD while many others, though fulfilling these criteria, still present a plethora of other symptoms (including major depression and psychotic symptoms); still others relate the onset of their symptomatology to a variety of trauma that cooccurred or followed each other, leading to a complex picture not readily identifiable under the present concept of PTSD. Others still are constantly exposed to the 'traumatic' experience. It would be simplistic to think that we could find a criteria-based category that will address all these issues; however, and by analogy, it would be as simplistic to find an entity that would encapsulate all symptoms secondary to direct 'physical' trauma; these range from bruises to wounds, fracture of the spleen, subdural haematoma, chronic pain, broken bones, blindness and so on. To think that trauma will affect only one area of the brain with a highly specific set of symptoms is not realistic. On the other hand, since physiology is essential in developing novel treatments, an understanding of how the brain responds to psychological trauma would undoubtedly contribute to better treatment; furthermore, the future might witness a revolution not only in the way we handle memories but also in how to code them or even change them, a path that is all too clear to those who observes the evolution of this field.

COMMENTARY

1.3 Redefining PTSD in DSM-5: Conundrums and Potentially Unintended Risks

Alexander C. McFarlane
Department of Psychiatry, University of Adelaide Node, Centre for Military and Veterans' Health, University of Adelaide, Adelaide, Australia

There are few opportunities that will provide us such a substantial opportunity for shaping the future of the study of traumatic stress as that created by the publication of DSM-5. The challenge involved is how to best distill the epidemiological and longitudinal research, published since the formulation the DSM-IV PTSD diagnostic criteria in 1994, without causing any major unintended consequences. In his discussion of the proposed criteria, Friedman states how at its core, PTSD is a condition manifest during an individual's interaction with interpersonal and physical environments; in essence, an information-processing disorder. A test of diagnostic criteria is the need for a high degree of inter-rater reliability and diagnostic specificity and sensitivity, different properties than describing the core characteristics of a disorder. These requirements represent a difficult goal.

Considerable thought has gone into how to reformulate the stressor criterion because it is the critical entry to the diagnosis. In particular, the dropping of Criterion A2 is welcomed because of the complexity of the affective response at the times of trauma exposure and particularly amongst groups such as police and combat troops whose training is likely to suppress the nature of their immediate awareness of affect [17]. Furthermore, the importance of the range of emotions related to traumatic events, such as guilt, shame, disgust and horror, has been underexplored. In this vein, Panksepp [18] has stressed the need for a clearer elucidation of the precise categorisation of the nature of emotion because it logically, from an evolutionary perspective, underpins cognition.

A caution needs to be made about one of the proposed modifications that emphasise the temporal rather than the aetiological relationship between the A1

Post-traumatic Stress Disorder, First Edition. Edited by Dan Stein, Matthew Friedman, and Carlos Blanco.

and B–F PTSD symptoms. A recent meta-analysis of delayed-onset PTSD [19] reviewed longitudinal studies and in the combined population found that 24.8% had delayed-onset PTSD. These data showed that the proportion of individuals with delayed-onset PTSD was larger when the duration of follow-up was longer, particularly amongst military populations. Hence, the wording of the temporal relationship between traumatic exposure and symptom development needs to be carefully sculptured to address the importance of delayed-onset PTSD, and minimising this delayed temporal relationship and symptom development would be a mistake.

A related issue that appears to have had little attention in the deliberations about the stressor criterion is the role of multiple trauma exposures as a cause of PTSD. Evidence demonstrates that individuals who have repeated exposure to traumatic stresses have an increased probability of suffering from PTSD through further exposure [20–22]. The evidence supports the role of an underlying sensitisation with subsequent trauma exposures [23, 24]. Hence the definition of the stressor criterion needs to consider the role of sensitisation in those groups that have multiple trauma exposures, such as emergency service workers and military personnel exposed to combat.

The proposal to include the AD/PTSD subtype in order to address the issue of subsyndromal PTSD is critically dependent on the definition of 'disproportional distress' following exposure to a traumatic event. Such a definition demands consensus about what is typical in the aftermath of traumatic events. The benchmark presented by Friedman is that 'most people exhibit distress during the acute aftermath of traumatic exposure', a position partly and erroneously based on longitudinal studies [25] of a treatment-seeking population. Such a patient population is not a valid group for drawing conclusions about normal patterns of distress after events as these are the individuals who are predictably going to have high levels of acute symptoms: the motivation to seek assistance. Further research has examined symptom progression from the acute post-trauma phase and shows clearly that the majority of injury survivors have low symptom levels in the acute setting and that this pattern persists over time [26]. Further evidence from aggregated data sets of disasters [27] shows that a stable mild reaction is the most common symptomatic pattern, being present in 34.5% of the combined samples, and that symptoms often escalate in those with higher levels of symptoms [26–28]. If an AD subtype is to be included, a more considered definition of the expected 'normal' response is required.

The gatekeeper to PTSD DSM-IV was the avoidance criterion, as these symptoms had the lowest rates of endorsement, an issue that created substantial differences in prevalence estimates from ICD-10 [29]. Therefore, reformulation of the avoidance and estrangement symptoms will be a benchmark against which the new criteria are likely to be judged, given that will be compared with the competing ICD-10 diagnostic criteria. An important departure from DSM-IV is the decision to separate the avoidance symptoms (C1 and C2) from those indicative of catastrophic or maladaptive appraisals. Friedman refers to the role of cognitive behaviour theory in informing this decision. However, the introduction of theoretic models takes the field back to the era of DSM-I and II, which were dominated by the psychoanalytical concept of neurosis, a relationship actively broken in DSM-III. This decision may also have unintended consequences that perhaps require more consideration from a theoretical and clinical perspective. First, True *et al.* [30] showed that individuals who develop PTSD in the military and emergency services temperamentally tend to place themselves in harm's way. Such individuals do not characteristically use avoidance as a coping mechanism. Hence, requiring such symptoms in the diagnostic criteria may lead to an underestimation of PTSD in these groups, a dilemma addressed in ICD-10 by introducing the concept of 'preferred' avoidance.

Second, identifying avoidance linked to a trauma can lead to problems in interrater reliability. The ability of individuals to accurately report avoidance directly linked to the trauma in question presumes explicit knowledge of the association. For example, in a 21-year longitudinal follow-up study of children exposed to a bushfire disaster [31], many participants did not understand the link between their weather phobia and the exposure to the storm that caused the bushfires, the origin of these symptoms. Hence, avoidance phenomena have the substantial potential to have high rates of false negatives because individuals often do not recognise the traumatic origins of their avoidance behaviour.

A further phenomenological issue is that avoidance phenomena are only one of the secondary responses to the distress arising from traumatic memories and hyperarousal [32]. Other phenomena that mitigate the arousal response include dissociation and numbing. Creating avoidance as a necessary symptom cluster has the potential to exclude individuals from the PTSD diagnosis (e.g. police) who temperamentally do not avoid highly distressing circumstances, even though they may have substantial levels of other symptoms. Designating the primacy of avoidance behaviour as a separate set of criteria is also partially driven by the conceptual importance placed on addressing avoidance in behaviour therapy, potentially opening it up to the criticism that it is not atheoretical.

A related issue is the welcomed introduction of post-traumatic reckless behaviour and post-traumatic aggressive behaviour into the hyperarousal criterion. The question arises as to whether, alternatively, these should be included as part of the avoidance criterion. From a psychodynamic perspective, aggression is an emotional state that tends to suppress fear. Similarly, reckless behaviour is a counterphobic response, demonstrating a disregard for consequences and seeking increased arousal, replacing avoidance with risk-taking. As these behaviours may potentially represent the opposite polarity of avoidance, it would be clinically more logical to include them in the new specific avoidance criterion.

Perhaps, before avoidance behaviour is separated into a specific subcategory, this decision should be assessed in epidemiological samples. Introducing the proposed avoidance criterion may have the unintended consequence of increasing false-negative rates for PTSD, particularly in emergency service and military populations. Friedman's chapter is the welcomed entrance into a brave new age with all its unanticipated risks and possibilities.

REFERENCES

1. Robins, E. and Guze, S.B. (1970) Establishment of diagnostic validity in psychiatric illness – its application to schizophrenia. *American Journal of Psychiatry*, **126**, 983–987.
2. Horowitz, M.J. (1976) *Stress Response Syndromes*, Jason Aronson, New York.
3. Brewin, C.R., Dalgleish, T. and Joseph, S. (1996) A dual representation theory of posttraumatic stress disorder. *Psychological Reviews*, **103**, 670–686.
4. Ehlers, A., Gene-Cos, N. and Perrin, M. (2009) Low recognition of post-traumatic stress disorder in primary care. *London Journal of Primary Care*, **2**, 36–42.
5. North, C.S., Suris, A.M., Davis, M. and Smith, R.P. (2009) Toward validation of the diagnosis of posttraumatic stress disorder. *American Journal of Psychiatry*, **166**, 34–41.
6. Golden, A.M.J. and Dalgleish, T. (2010) Is prolonged grief distinct from bereavement-related posttraumatic stress? *Psychiatry Research*, **178**, 336–341.
7. Kassam-Adams, N., Marsac, M.L. and Cirilli, C. (2010) Posttraumatic stress disorder symptom structure in injured children: functional impairment and depression symptoms in a confirmatory factor analysis. *Journal of the American Academy of Child and Adolescent Psychiatry*, **49**, 616–625.
8. Karam, E.G. (1997) Comorbidity of posttraumatic stress disorder and depression, in *Posttraumatic Stress Disorder. Acute and Long-Term Responses to Trauma and Disaster* (eds R.J. Ursano and C.S. Fullerton), American Psychiatric Association Press, Washington, DC, pp. 77–90.
9. Karam, E.G., Andrews, G., Bromet, E. *et al*. (2010) The role of Criterion A2 in the DSM-IV diagnosis of post-traumatic stress disorder. *Biological Psychiatry*, **68**, 465–473.
10. Karam, E.G., Mneimneh, Z., Karam, A.N. *et al*. (2006) Prevalence and treatment of mental disorders in Lebanon: a national epidemiological survey. *The Lancet*, **367**, 1000–1006.
11. Farah, L., Fayyad, J., Eapen, V. *et al*. (2009) Attention deficit hyperactivity disorder (ADHD) in the Arab world: a review of epidemiologic studies. *Journal of Attention Disorders*, **13**, 211–222.
12. Fayyad, J.A., De Graaf, R., Kessler, R.C. *et al*. (2007) Cross national prevalence and correlates of adult attention deficit hyperactivity disorder. *The British Journal of Psychiatry*, **190**, 402–409.
13. Holmes, E.A., Arntz, A. and Smucker, M.R. (2007) Imagery rescripting in cognitive behaviour therapy: images, treatment techniques and outcomes. *Journal of Behavior Therapy and Experimental Psychiatry*, **38**, 297–305.

14. Ehlers, A. and Clark, D.M. (2000) A cognitive model of posttraumatic stress disorder. *Behaviour Research and Therapy*, **38**, 319–345.
15. Ursano, R.J., Fullerton, C.S., Kao, T.C. *et al*. (1995) Longitudinal assessment of posttraumatic stress disorder and depression after exposure to traumatic death. *Journal of Nervous and Mental Disease*, **183**, 36–42.
16. Large, M.M. and Nielssen, O. (2008) Factors associated with agreement between experts in evidence about psychiatric injury. *Journal of the American Academy of Psychiatry and Law*, **36**, 515–521.
17. Adler, A.B., Wright, K.M., Bliese, P.D. *et al*. (2008) A2 diagnostic criterion for combat-related posttraumatic stress disorder. *Journal of Traumatic Stress*, **21** (3), 301–308.
18. Panksepp, J. (1998) *Affective Neuroscience: The Foundations of Human and Animal Emotions*, Oxford University Press, New York.
19. Smid, G., Mooren, T.T., van der Mast, R.C. *et al*. (2009) Delayed posttraumatic stress disorder: systematic review, meta-analysis, and meta-regression analysis of prospective studies. *The Journal of Clinical Psychiatry*, **70** (11), 1572–1582.
20. Post, R.M. and Weiss, S.R. (1998) Sensitisation ad kindling phenomena in mood, anxiety and obsessive compulsive disorders: the role of serotonergic mechanisms in illness progression. *Biological Psychiatry*, **44**, 193–206.
21. Bremner, J.D., Southwick, S.M., Johnson, D.R. *et al*. (1993) Childhood physical abuse and combat-related posttraumatic stress disorder in Vietnam veterans. *The American Journal of Psychiatry*, **150**, 235–239.
22. Yehuda, R., Kahana, B., Schmeidler, J. *et al*. (1995) Impact of cumulative lifetime trauma and recent stress on current posttraumatic stress disorder symptoms in holocaust survivors. *The American Journal of Psychiatry*, **152**, 1815–1818.
23. Copeland, W.E., Keeler, G., Angold, A. and Costello, E.J. (2007) Traumatic events and posttraumatic stress in childhood. *Archives of General Psychiatry*, **64**, 577–584.
24. Breslau, N., Chilcoat, H.D., Kessler, R.C. and Davies, G.C. (1999) Previous exposure to trauma and PTSD effects of subsequent trauma: results from the Detroit area survey of trauma. *The American Journal of Psychiatry*, **156** (6), 902–907.
25. Riggs, D.S., Rothbaum, B.O. and Foa, E.B. (1995) A prospective examination of symptoms of posttraumatic stress disorder in victims of nonsexual assault. *Journal of Interpersonal Violence*, **10** (2), 201–214.
26. O'Donnell, M.L., Elliott, P., Lau, W. and Creamer, M. (2007) PTSD symptom trajectories: from early to chronic response. *Behaviour Research and Therapy*, **45** (3), 601–609.
27. Orcutt, H.K., Erickson, D.J. and Wolfe, J. (2004) The course of PTSD symptoms among gulf war veterans: a growth mixture modeling approach. *Journal of Traumatic Stress*, **17**, 195–202.
28. Norris, F.H., Tracy, M. and Galea, S. (2009) Looking for Resilience: understanding the longitudinal trajectories of responses to stress. *Social Science and Medicine*, **68**, 2190–2198.
29. Peters, L., Issakidis, C., Slade, T. and Andrews, G. (2006) Gender differences in the prevalence of DSM-IV and ICD-10 PTSD. *Psychology Medicine*, **36** (1), 81–89.

30. True, W.R., Rice, J., Eisen, S.A. *et al*. (1994) Twin study of genetic and environmental contributions to liability for posttraumatic stress disorder symptoms. *Archives of General Psychiatry*, **51**, 838–839.
31. McFarlane, A.C. and Van Hoof, M. (2009) Adult outcomes of childhood exposure to a disaster: a cohort study of the Ash Wednesday Bushfires of 1983. *British Journal of Psychiatry*, **152**, 142–148.
32. McFarlane, A.C. (1992) Avoidance and intrusion in posttraumatic stress disorder. *Journal of Nervous and Mental Disease*, **180** (7), 439–445.

CHAPTER 2

Epidemiology of PTSD

Carlos Blanco
Department of Psychiatry, Columbia University, New York, NY, USA

INTRODUCTION

Although trauma-related disorders have gained increased recognition since their inclusion in the Diagnostic and Statistical Manual III (DSM-III) in 1980, interest in reactions to stressful events goes back to much earlier times. Samuel Pepys described his experience of the Great Fire of London in 1666, with details of events, social behaviours, feelings, insights and ideas that would probably currently be understood as symptoms of post-traumatic stress disorder (PTSD). By the end of World War I, the concept of 'shell shock' was used to describe the reaction to exposure to a traumatic event, hypothesising that the impact of physical forces on the central nervous system generated a temporary disconnection that led to the development of distressing symptoms [1]. Despite a growing body of information, it was not until the nineteenth and twentieth centuries that enough data on the consequences of exposure to a traumatic event were available to construct a coherent syndrome.

A large number of terms have been used to describe the disorder, including 'spinal concussion' [2, 3], 'soldier's heart' [4, 5], 'cardiac weakness' [6], 'traumatic shock' [7], 'traumatic neurosis' [8], 'nervous shock' [9], 'effort syndrome' [10], 'shell shock' [11], 'war psychoneurosis' [11, 12] and 'combat exhaustion' [13].

PTSD was first included in the diagnostic nomenclature in 1980 in the DSM-III [14] as an Anxiety Disorder, aetiologically linking traumatic events to a specific disorder. Diagnostic criteria introduced included a gateway criterion (Criterion A), which suggested that only certain traumas qualified to produce PTSD. Traumatic experience was defined in this context as an overwhelming experience outside the usual range. DSM-III diagnosis also required the presence of one symptom that satisfied Criterion B (reexperiencing the trauma), such as nightmares or intrusive thoughts, one symptom that satisfied Criterion C (numbing or decreased responsiveness to the outside world) and two symptoms of

Post-traumatic Stress Disorder, First Edition. Edited by Dan Stein, Matthew Friedman, and Carlos Blanco.

those included under Criterion D (hyperarousal), such as anger, sleep disturbance or hypervigilance.

PTSD criteria were modified in the Revised Edition of DSM-III (DSM-III-R), which required three symptoms instead of one to meet Criterion C (avoidance and reexperiencing) and two instead of one symptom to meet Criterion D (hyperarousal). Furthermore, the duration of Criteria B–D had to be 'at least one month', as Criterion E. DSM-IV [15] not only broadened the stressor criterion but highlighted the clinical principle that people can perceive and respond differently to outwardly similar events. It modified the definition of Criterion A, requiring Criterion A1 and Criterion A2 to be met, such that: 'The person experienced, witnessed or was confronted with an event that involved actual or threatened death or serious injury or threat to the physical integrity of self or other (Criterion A1), and which evoked intense fear, helplessness or horror (Criterion A2)' [15]. DSM-IV is more inclusive than any previous edition regarding the traumas that qualify to meet Criterion A. The wider variety of events and the added subjective component in DSM-IV may have increased by about 20% the total number of qualifying events observed in previous DSM editions [16]. Finally, Criterion F, which involves clinically significant distress or impairment in social, occupational or other important areas of functioning, is also required to meet PTSD diagnosis.

The International Classification of Diseases (ICD) [17], used by the World Health Organization (WHO), is the international standard diagnostic classification of mental and behavioural disorders. Although DSM-IV and CIE-10 diagnostic criteria for PTSD are similar, there are some differences. Unlike DSM-IV, ICD-10 does not require the individual's response to the event to involve intense fear, helplessness or horror (DSM Criterion A2). Whereas CIE-10 requires PTSD symptoms to start within six months of experiencing the traumatic event, DSM-IV provides a specifier to describe the 'delayed onset' of the disorder. Additional criteria for the diagnosis of PTSD in DSM-IV not described in CIE-10 include the one-month duration of the symptoms and the clinical significance criterion.

In this chapter, we present a review of epidemiological studies of PTSD conducted in North America, Latin America, Europe, Lebanon and Australia. We focus on studies examining rates of exposure to traumatic events and prevalence of PTSD in the general population. We also summarise evidence on sociodemographic risk factors and describe available information on acute stress disorder (ASD).

TRAUMA EXPOSURE AND PTSD IN THE GENERAL POPULATION

Although many epidemiological reports of PTSD exist, most are based on studies of Vietnam veterans or specific populations exposed to circumscribed situations like conflicts [18], disasters [19, 20] or terrorist attacks [21]. It has been suggested that PTSD correlates may differ substantially by type of trauma (e.g. sexual abuse versus accident) and sample (e.g. military versus community) [22]. Due to space constraints, we limit our review to studies examining rates of trauma exposure and PTSD in the general population. Table 2.1 provides a brief summary of the studies reviewed in this chapter.

United States and Canada

The majority of epidemiological studies on PTSD have been conducted in the United States and Canada. Early studies examining the prevalence of PTSD in community samples in the USA reported very low PTSD rates. Data from the second wave of the St Louis, MO (n = 2493) and the North Carolina (n = 2985) sites of the Epidemiologic Catchment Area (ECA) estimated a lifetime prevalence of PTSD of 1.0% in St Louis and 1.3% in North Carolina [23, 24]. Additionally, the six-month prevalence of PTSD in the North Carolina site was 0.44%. The ECA used the Diagnostic Interview Schedule (DIS) version III, which was based on DSM-III criteria. Although the reasons for these low rates are not fully understood, they may be related to the restricted range of potential traumatic events probed (Vietnam combat and having been mugged).

Breslau *et al*. [25] assessed the prevalence of traumatic events and PTSD in a random sample of young adults aged 21–30 years (n = 1007) in Detroit, MI, using the DIS-III-R, which assesses DSM-III-R criteria [26]. Of the total sample, 39.2% (n = 394) reported at least one lifetime exposure to traumatic events that fit the PTSD 'stressor definition'. Among those who had experienced a traumatic event, 67.3% had been exposed to one event, 23.3% to two events and 9.4% to three events. The most commonly reported traumatic experiences included sudden injury or serious accident (9.34%), physical assault (8.3%), seeing someone seriously hurt or killed (7.1%) and hearing news of the sudden death of a loved one (5.7%). Of the 394 respondents with exposure to a traumatic event (39.2% of the whole sample), 23.6% met full criteria for lifetime PTSD, yielding a lifetime prevalence of 9.2% among the full sample. PTSD rates did not vary significantly across types of event experienced (11.6–24.0%), with the exception of sexual abuse, which caused PTSD in 80% of sexually abused women.

Resnick *et al*. [26] conducted a telephone survey of a US national probability household sample of 4088 adult women. Specific crime or other traumatic event history and PTSD were examined using the National Women's Study (NWS) PTSD module, which was modified from the DIS used in the National Vietnam Veterans Readjustment Study. Diagnoses were based on DSM-III-R criteria. The authors reported a lifetime exposure to any type of traumatic event of 69%. Lifetime and six-month prevalence rate of PTSD were reported as 12.3% and 4.6% respectively. Additionally, the conditional prevalence of PTSD (i.e. the prevalence among those exposed to a traumatic event) was reported as 17.9% in a lifetime and 6.7% in the past six months.

Table 2.1 Summary of general population studies and estimates of lifetime and 12-month PTSD.

Country	Author	Study and sample	Interview	PTSD diagnosis	Lifetime PTSD			12-month PTSD		
					Total	Male	Female	Total	Male	Female
USA	Helzer *et al.* [23]	ECA St Louis Age not provided n = 2493	DIS	DSM-III	1.0%	–	–	–	–	–
USA	Davidson *et al.* [24]	ECA North Carolina Age 18–45 n = 2985	DIS	DSM-III	1.3%	–	–	0.44%[a]	–	–
USA	Breslau *et al.* [25]	Michigan Age 21–30 n = 1007	DIS	DSM-III-R	9.2%	6%	11.3%	–	–	–
USA	Resnick *et al.* [26]	NWS Adult women Age 18–34 n = 4008	PTSD interview sched-ule/PTSD module NWS[b]	DSM-III-R (Criterion F not included)	–	–	12.3%	–	–	4.6%[a]
USA	Kessler *et al.* [27]	NCS Age 15–54 n = 5877	Modified version of PTSD modules of CIDI and DIS	DSM-III-R	7.8%	5%	10.4%	–	–	–
USA	Breslau *et al.* [28]	PMSA Detroit Age 18–45 n = 2181	WHO-CIDI[b]	DSM-IV	9.2%	6.2%	13%	–	–	–

USA	Breslau *et al.* [29]	Mid-Atlantic city Age 18–45 n = 2311	WHO-CIDI	DSM-IV	7.1%	–	–	–	–	–
USA	Kessler *et al.* [30]	NCS-R Age ≥15 n = 9282	WHO-CIDI	DSM-IV	–	–	–	3.5%	–	–
Canada	Stein *et al.* [31]	Winnipeg, MB Age ≥18 n = 1002	Modified PTSD symptom scale[b]	DSM-IV	–	–	–	–	Full PTSD: 1.2%[c]; Partial PTSD: 0.3%[c]; Full/ partial: 1.5%[c]	Full PTSD: 2.7%[c]; Partial PTSD: 3.4%[c] Full/ partial: 6%[c]
Canada	van Ameringen *et al.* [32]	Age ≥18 n = 2991	Modified version of CIDI PTSD module[b]	DSM-IV	Full PTSD: 9.2%; Partial PTSD: 2.2%	Full PTSD: 5.3%; Partial PTSD: 1.5%	Full PTSD: 12.8%; Partial PTSD: 2.9%	Full PTSD: 2.4%[c]; Partial PTSD: 2.2%[c]	Full PTSD: 1.3%[c]; Partial PTSD: 1.8%[c]	Full PTSD: 3.3%[c]; Partial PTSD: 5.0%[c]
Mexico	Norris *et al.* [33]	Four Mexican cities Age ≥18 n = 2509	WHO-CIDI	DSM-IV	11.2%	7.2%	14.5%	–	–	–
Chile	Zlotnick *et al.* [34]	CPPS Age ≥15 n = 2390	WHO-CIDI	DSM-III-R	4.4%	2.5%	6.2%	–	–	–
Six Western European countries	Alonso *et al.* [35]	ESEMeD project Age ≥18 n = 21425	WMH-CIDI	DSM-IV	1.9%	0.9%	2.9%	0.9%	0.4%	1.3%

(*continued overleaf*)

Table 2.1 (*continued*)

Country	Author	Study and sample	Interview	PTSD diagnosis	Lifetime PTSD			12-month PTSD		
					Total	Male	Female	Total	Male	Female
Germany	Perkonigg *et al.* [36]	EDSP Age 14–24 n = 3021	CIDI	DSM-IV	1.3%	0.4%	2.2%	0.75%	0.1%	0.00%
Germany	Darves-Bornoz *et al.* [37]	ESEMeD project Age ≥18 n = 3555	WMH-CIDI	DSM-IV	–	–	–	0.68%	–	–
Sweden	Frans *et al.* [38]	Age 18–70 n = 3000	DSM-IV PTSD symptom scale[d]	DSM-IV	5.6%	3.6%	7.4%	–	–	–
Belgium	Darves-Bornoz *et al.* [37]	ESEMeD project Age ≥18 n = 2419	WMH-CIDI	DSM-IV	–	–	–	0.76%	–	–
Switzerland	Hepp *et al.* [39]	Zurich 1993: Age 34–35 1999: Age 41–42 n = 4547	SPIKE + PTSD module from DSM	1993: DSM-III-R 1999: DSM-IV	–	–	–	Full PTSD: 0% Partial PTSD: 1993: 1.90%; 1999:1.3%	Full PTSD: 0% Partial PTSD: 1993: 2.9%; 1999: 0.26%	Full PTSD: 0% Partial PTSD: 1993:0.9%; 1999: 2.21%
The Netherlands	Darves-Bornoz *et al.* [37]	ESEMeD project Age ≥18 n = 2372	WMH-CIDI	DSM-IV	–	–	–	2.56%	–	–
The Netherlands	de Vries and Olff [40]	Age 18–80 n = 1087	CIDI[b]	DSM-IV	7.4%	4.3%	8.8%	–	–	–

France	Lepine *et al.* [41]	ESEMeD project Age ≥18 n = 2894	WMH-CIDI	DSM-IV	3.9%	–	–	2.2%	–	–
Italy	de Girolamo *et al.* [42]	ESEMeD project Age ≥18 n = 4712	WMH-CIDI	DSM-IV	2.3%	1.1%	3.3%	0.8%	0.7%	0.9%
Spain	Haro *et al.* [43]	ESEMeD project Age ≥18 n = 5473	WMH-CIDI	DSM-IV	1.95%	1.06%	2.79%	0.5%	0.25%	0.94%
Lebanon	Karam *et al.* [44, 45]	Age ≥18 n = 2857	WHO-CIDI	DSM-IV	3.4%	–	–	2.0%	–	–
Australia	Creamer *et al.* [46]	NSMHWB Age ≥18 n = 10641	CIDI modified version	DSM-IV	–	–	–	1.33%	1.2%	1.4%

[a]Six-month PTSD prevalence.
[b]Telephone interview.
[c]One-month PTSD prevalence.
[d]Mailed questionnaire.
WHO-CIDI, Composite International Diagnostic Interview; DIS, Diagnostic Interview Schedule; ECA, Epidemiologic Catchment Area Program; WHM, World Mental Health; NCS, National Comorbidity Survey; NWS, National Women's Study; SPIKE, Structured Psychopathological Interview and Rating of the Social Consequences for Epidemiology; ESEMeD, European Study of the Epidemiology of Mental Disorders; NSMHWB, National Survey of Mental Health and Wellbeing.

Because previous studies examining the prevalence of PTSD in the general population focused only on 'worst traumas', the 1996 Detroit Area Survey of Trauma [28] examined the conditional risk of PTSD based on the representative sample of traumas. The sample in this study comprised 2181 respondents aged between 18 and 45, randomly selected and interviewed by telephone using the DIS-IV and the WHO Composite International Diagnostic Interview (CIDI) version 2.1 [48]. The lifetime history of exposure to any type of trauma in this sample was 89.6%. The conditional prevalence of PTSD was 9.2%. The conditional prevalence, based on the randomly selected traumas, was about one third lower than that based on the 'worst trauma'. Using the 'worst trauma', the lifetime prevalence of PTSD was 13.6% [49]. Within types of traumatic events, assaultative violence had the highest risk of developing PTSD (20.9%). Furthermore, 31% of PTSD cases were from the sudden unexpected death of a loved one. In the majority of the cases, PTSD persisted for at least six months and duration was longer in women than in men.

Important information on PTSD in the United States comes from the National Comorbidity Survey (NCS) [27], which used the modified version of the DSM-III-R PTSD module from the DIS and the CIDI. The NCS, conducted between 1990 and 1992, included 5877 respondents aged 15–54. It reported the PTSD prevalence in the United States, the types of trauma associated, demographic correlates and the clinical course. Results showed that 60.7% of men and 51.2% of women experienced at least one traumatic event during their lifetimes. The most common types of traumatic event were witnessing someone being badly injured or killed (35.6% of men and 14.5% women), being in a fire, flood or natural disaster (18.9% of men and 15.2% for women) and being involved in a life-threatening accident (25% of men and 13.8% of women). Whereas the lifetime prevalence of PTSD in the general population was 5% for males and 10.4% for females (7.8% of the total sample), the prevalence among those exposed to trauma was 8.2% for men and 20.4% for women.

Because the NCS only reported rates of lifetime PTSD, the subsequent National Comorbidity Survey Replication (NCS-R) [30] examined the 12-month prevalence in the US general population. The NCS-R was a nationally representative face-to-face household survey conducted between 2001 and 2003, applying the completed structured diagnostic interview, the WHO-CIDI [50]. The sample comprised 9282 English-speaking respondents aged 18 years and older. The 12-month PTSD prevalence reported was 3.5%.

Another study using a population-based sample in the USA [29] explored the characteristics and lifetime prevalence of PTSD in 2311 subjects recruited from 1985 to 1986 at entry into first grade of the public school system of a large mid-Atlantic city. Between 2000 and 2002, the original sample was traced and interviewed when their mean age was 21 (n = 1698). PTSD diagnoses were based on DSM-IV criteria. Of the sample, 82.5% had experienced at least one traumatic event. The most common events were sudden unexpected death of a close friend or relative by homicide or murder (26.1%), assaultative violence (47.2%) and being held up or threatened with a weapon (35.9%). On the other hand, the event most associated with PTSD development was rape, with over 40% of those exposed meeting PTSD criteria. The lifetime PTSD prevalence rate in the whole sample was 7.1%, while among those reporting exposure to trauma the rate was 8.8% (7.4% for men, 10.2% for women).

To date, only two Canadian surveys have examined the current prevalence of PTSD in the general population. A cross-sectional study [31] conducted in Winnipeg, MB (located in Midwest Canada) administered the Modified PTSD Symptom Scale, a reliable DSM-IV PTSD checklist, via telephone to a random sample of 1002 people. This was the first study in which a comparison of 'full' and 'partial' PTSD was attempted in an epidemiological sample. Subjects were classified as having full PTSD if they met all DSM-IV criteria for the disorder and 'partial' PTSD if they met DSM-IV criteria but lacked one or two of the necessary three Criterion C symptoms and/or one of the required two Criterion D symptoms. Subjects needed to meet at least one symptom in each category to qualify for a 'partial' PTSD. The lifetime prevalence of exposure to traumatic events was 81.3% for men and 74.2% for women. The most commonly traumatic experiences were the violent death of a friend or family member and being physically attacked. The estimated prevalence of full one-month PTSD was 1.2% for men and 2.7% for women, while the prevalence of partial one-month PTSD was 0.3% for men and 3.4% for women. Interference with work or school was significantly more pronounced in persons with full current PTSD than in those experiencing only partial symptoms, although the latter group was significantly more occupationally impaired than those exposed to trauma without PTSD.

A second study in Canada [32] used a nationally representative sample of 2991 individuals aged 18 and older. Individuals were assessed with a modified version of the CIDI PTSD module via telephone. Diagnosis of PTSD was based on the worst event. In the general population, 75.9% reported lifetime exposure to trauma (78.5% for men and 73.4% for women). The most common forms of trauma resulting in PTSD included the unexpected death of a loved one, sexual assault and seeing someone badly injured or killed. The lifetime and one-month prevalence rates of PTSD in this study were 9.2% and 2.4%, respectively.

In general, studies conducted in the United States and Canada have found high rates of trauma exposure and prevalence of PTSD. However, the changing definitions of PTSD across different DSM editions and differences in the range of traumatic events probed in the studies make it difficult to compare the findings of studies conducted over recent years. Studies based on DSM-III criteria yielded the lowest rates of exposure. Results from the ECA project using the DSM-III trauma definition [23] reported a prevalence of trauma exposure of 39.2%, whereas estimates from the NCS [30] (using DSM-III-R) were of 60.7% for men and

51.2% for women. The highest rate of trauma exposure was obtained from the 1996 Detroit Area Survey of Trauma study, which used DSM-IV criteria to evaluate trauma [28]. Breslau *et al*. [28] reported that 89.6% of the entire sample experienced at least one trauma in their lifetime. PTSD prevalence rates in the general population ranged from 1.0% in the ECA study [23] to 12.3% in a sample of adult women [26]. The conditional lifetime prevalence of PTSD also varied between studies, ranging from 8.8% (based on DSM-IV) among young adults in a mid-Atlantic city [29] to 23.6% (based on DSM-III-R) among young adults in Detroit [25]. This difference in the conditional prevalence for PTSD may be explained by the differences in the inclusiveness of the stressor criterion between versions of the DSM used. As described previously, the DSM-III-R stressor criterion was more restrictive than that of DSM-IV as it required that traumatic events were 'distressing to almost everyone' and 'generally outside the range of usual human experience', such as being attacked or raped, or being in a fire or flood. It is natural to find higher rates of PTSD if only these most 'severe' traumatic experiences are considered.

Latin America

To our knowledge, only two studies examining PTSD rates in the general population in Latin American countries have been published.

Norris *et al*. [33] estimated PTSD lifetime prevalence from a probability sample of 2509 adults in four cities in Mexico between 1999 and 2001. PTSD was assessed according to DSM-IV criteria using the WHO-CIDI Spanish Version. PTSD was assessed only for a single worst event. The lifetime prevalence of trauma exposure was 76%, whereas the lifetime prevalence of PTSD was 11.2% in the whole sample (7% for men and 15% for women). The conditional probability of PTSD in this Mexican sample was 15%.

A recent study in Chile [34] used data from the Chile Psychiatric Prevalence Study (CPPS) to estimate the lifetime prevalence of PTSD based on a household-stratified sample of individuals from the general population. Lifetime PTSD was assessed using the DIS-III-R in 2390 individuals aged 15 years and older. Over one third (39.7%) of the population reported trauma exposure (46.7% for men and 33.2% for women). The estimated lifetime prevalence of PTSD in the entire sample was 4.4% (2.5% for men and 6.2% for women). Rape was the most common event associated with PTSD.

Methodological differences such as the use of different diagnostic criteria may account for the differences in the lifetime estimates of PTSD between these Latin American countries. Moreover, the better socioeconomic conditions of the Chilean population compared with Mexicans (e.g. less inequality between the wealthy and the poor, and lower rates of violence, crime and poverty) may have also played a role [34].

Europe

A significant proportion of studies in European countries have also reported rates of exposure to traumatic events and PTSD in the general population. A study conducted in Germany [36] examined the prevalence rates of PTSD using data from the Early Developmental Stages of Psychopathology (EDSP) Study. This study included 3021 young individuals from the community aged 14–24 years interviewed with the Munich-CIDI [51], based on DSM-IV criteria. The prevalence of traumatic exposure in the sample was 21.4% (26% for men and 17.7% for women). The most frequent traumatic events were physical attacks (7.5%), serious accidents (5.4%), witnessing traumatic events happening to others (3.6%) and sexual abuse in childhood (2.0%). Prevalence of PTSD in this community sample was 1% for males and 2.2% for women, whereas among those reporting a qualifying traumatic event prevalence rates were 14.5% for women and 2.2% for men. In this study, if a respondent reported more than one qualifying event, the worst event method previously described was used. Development of PTSD was strongly associated with sexual abuse or rape as well as with the number of traumatic events experienced and with being younger than age 12 when the event took place.

The cross-national European Study of the Epidemiology of Mental Disorders (ESEMeD) also examined rates of PTSD in six Western European countries (Belgium, France, Germany, Italy, the Netherlands and Spain) [52]. The sample comprised 21 425 respondents aged 18 and older assessed in their homes between January and August 2003 with the WMH-CIDI, which was developed and adapted by the Coordinating Committee of the WHO-World Mental Health 2000 Initiative [52]. Overall lifetime PTSD prevalence was 1.9% (0.9% of men, 2.9% of women) and 12-month PTSD prevalence was 0.9% (0.4% of men, 1.3% of women) [35]. Twelve-month prevalence rates of PTSD were higher in the Netherlands (2.56%) and France (2.32%) and lower in the rest of the countries (0.76% in Belgium and 0.68% in Germany). Independent reports are available for the ESEMeD project samples from Spain and Italy. Haro *et al.* [43] reported the lifetime and 12-month prevalence of PTSD in the Spanish population (n = 5473) using DSM-IV; estimates were 1.9% (1.06% for men and 2.79% for women) and 0.5% (0.25% for men and 0.94% for women), respectively. In Italy (n = 4712) lifetime and 12-month PTSD estimates derived from the ESEMeD project were reported as 2.3% (1.1% for men and 3.3% for women) and 0.8% (0.7% for men and 0.9% for women), respectively [42].

Another study conducted in Switzerland examined the rates of exposure to traumatic events and PTSD in a representative community-based cohort from the canton of Zurich. In this study, the initial sample of the Zurich cohort included 4547 young adults screened in 1978 using the Symptoms Checklist 90 Revised (SCL-90-R). Following the screening, two thirds of the sample with a score above percentile 85 was randomly selected, resulting in a final sample of 2599 subjects.

Subthreshold (partial) PTSD was established according to Stein *et al*. [31] if the symptoms for Criterion B (reexperiencing cluster, ≥1 symptom) plus either Criterion C (avoidance cluster, ≥3 symptoms) *or* D (hyperarousal cluster, ≥2 symptoms) were fulfilled, but not C *and* D. In 1993, the weighted lifetime prevalence of exposure to a traumatic event was 28% and none of the respondents met full PTSD criteria. The prevalence of subthreshold 12-month DSM-III-R PTSD was 1.9% in the total sample (2.9% for men and 0.9% for women). The same pattern was observed in 1999. No single case of PTSD was found in the sample. The subthreshold rate of 12-month DSM-IV PTSD was 1.3% in the total sample (0.26% for men and 2.21% for women). The authors [39] argued that the socioeconomic and political situation in Switzerland could have contributed to these findings.

Frans *et al*. [38] conducted a study to examine the prevalence of traumatic experiences and the lifetime prevalence of PTSD in the general adult population in Sweden. A sample of 1500 male and 1500 female subjects, aged 18–70, was randomly selected from the general population using a population-based registry. Individuals were mailed a questionnaire which included the PTSD checklist (PCL) [53], used in diagnosing PTSD. The diagnostic procedure followed the DSM-IV. Only a total of 1824 subjects (60.8%) were qualified for analyses. Traumatic experiences were highly common, with 80.8% of the sample having experienced at least one traumatic event in their lives. The authors reported that the highest PTSD risk was associated with sexual and physical assault, robbery and multiple trauma experiences. Also, while the prevalence of lifetime PTSD was 5.6% of the full sample (3.6% for men and 7.4% for women), the conditional probability of PTSD given at least one trauma was 6.9% [38].

Additionally, since the ESEMeD only reported the 12-month rate of PTSD, Vries *et al*. [54] examined the lifetime PTSD prevalence in a nationally representative sample of the Netherlands. The sample of 1087 adults aged 18–80 years old were selected using a random digit dialing procedure and interviewed via telephone between 2004 and 2005 using CIDI version 2.1 [55], which is based on the DSM-IV criteria. Traumatic exposure was estimated to be 80.7% and did not differ by gender. The lifetime prevalence of PTSD in the general population was 7.4% (4.3% for men and 8.8% for women). Of the respondents, 3.3% reported symptoms within the last 12 months and 1.3% reported symptoms in the last month. If the 3.3% estimate is considered an approximation of the 12-month prevalence of PTSD in this study, it would be in agreement with the 2.6% 12-month PTSD prevalence found in the ESEMeD project for the same country [35]. The PTSD prevalence among those exposed to trauma was 14.1% (8.5% of men and 19.7 of women).

In summary, estimates of lifetime prevalence of PTSD in Europe range from 1.3% in Spain to 7.4% in the Netherlands, whereas the 12-month prevalence of PTSD ranges from 0% in Zurich (Switzerland) and 0.5% in Spain to 2.56% in the Netherlands. The higher rates of PTSD in the Netherlands may be explained by higher exposure rates to physical and sexual violence (previously reported to have the strongest associations with development of PTSD) in this country compared with other Western European countries.

Lebanon

A cross-sectional study in a community sample in Lebanon [44] used WHO-CIDI version 3.0 [50], which generates ICD-10 and DSM-IV diagnosis. The study was a nationally representative psychiatric epidemiological survey of 2875 adults aged 18 and older. The survey was conducted between September 2002 and 2003. The 12-month prevalence of PTSD was 2.0% in the overall sample, while the lifetime prevalence was 3.4% [45]. The study suggested that psychiatric disorders were common in Lebanon and that prevalence rates were similar to those of Western European countries, described above.

Australia

To our knowledge, only one population survey has been conducted in Australia [46]. This study examined the current prevalence of PTSD in 10 641 participants. The diagnostic interview was the National Survey of Mental Health and Wellbeing (NSMHWB) [56], a modified version of CIDI.

The prevalence of traumatic exposure was 64.6% for men and 49.5% for women. The most common types of traumatic event were witnessing someone being badly injured or killed (37.8% for men and 16.1% for women), being in a life-threatening accident (28.3% for men and 13.6% for women) and being involved in a natural disaster (19.9% for men and 12.7% for women). The traumatic events most likely to be associated with the development of PTSD were physical assault and rape. The 12-month prevalence of PTSD was 1.3% in the Australian general population (1.2% for men and 1.4% for women).

Summary

General population samples have been used in a wide range of studies examining the epidemiology of PTSD across the world. Lifetime and 12-month prevalence from the USA and Canada are consistently higher than those in Lebanon, Australia, Chile and Western European countries, with the exception of the Netherlands. However, prevalence rates of PTSD among those exposed (i.e. conditional prevalence) are quite similar across countries, suggesting that differences in PTSD prevalence across countries may be at least partially explained by differences in exposure rates to traumatic events.

SOCIODEMOGRAPHIC RISK FACTORS

Although most community residents have experienced one or more traumatic events in their lifetime, only a relatively small portion of victims develop PTSD. Findings from recent studies have shed light on some sociodemographic factors that confer a higher risk for trauma exposure and PTSD in the general population.

Gender

A significant number of studies [25, 37, 38, 57], although with some exceptions [27, 33, 40], have found that women are less likely than men in the general population to have experienced a traumatic event. However, females have been consistently shown to have higher rates of PTSD than men [25, 27, 31–33, 36–38, 58], with women probably having at least twice the risk of developing PTSD than men [26, 27]. Part of the explanation may lie in the high rates of sexual trauma among women [59], which are associated with high rates of PTSD [25, 26]. It is also possible that women may have been exposed recurrently to the same traumatic events. Results from the Australian NSMHWB showed that although female gender was a significant predictor of PTSD, when analyses were controlled for type and number of trauma, and for the passage of time, gender ceased to be a significant contributor to the risk of PTSD [57]. Factors accounting for gender differences in the risk for PTSD remain speculative. It is likely that biological, genetic, social and cultural aspects may also play an important role.

Age

Although PTSD can develop early in childhood, some studies have suggested that older age may be strongly associated with PTSD. In a community sample of individuals 14–24 years old from Germany, those in the 18–24 age group were 50% more likely to report lifetime trauma exposure and twice as likely to report lifetime prevalence of PTSD than those in the 14–17 age group. Interestingly, the authors also reported that development of PTSD was associated with age below 12 when the event took place [36]. The NCS [27] found a higher risk for lifetime PTSD among those in the 35–44 age group than among those in the 15–24 (the youngest) age group. Studies from Sweden [38] and the Netherlands [40] found that an increased prevalence of trauma exposure was associated with younger age. However, only in the latter study, as well as in that conducted in the Australian population [57], younger age was a risk factor for developing PTSD after trauma exposure. Future studies on the differential risk among age groups are needed to draw more definitive conclusions.

Race and ethnicity

There is still a lack of consistency across studies in the differences in risk of developing PTSD among ethnic minority groups. An early study conducted by Breslau *et al.* [25] reported that there were no differences in the risk for exposure to traumatic events between racial groups. Additionally, a latter study, using data from the NCS-R (n = 5424) [60], examined race-ethnic differences in risk for psychiatric disorders. Lifetime prevalence of PTSD was 5.9% for Hispanics, 7.1% for non-Hispanic blacks and 6.8% for non-Hispanic whites. When PTSD rates of Hispanics and Non-Hispanic blacks were compared separately with the PTSD rate obtained among Non-Hispanic Whites no differences were found to be significant.

To our knowledge, only one study, conducted in Sweden, has found a significant association between PTSD and ethnicity [38]. This study found that foreign-born individuals had about three-fold increased risk of reporting exposure to at least one trauma and that the conditional prevalence of PTSD was also significantly increased among those born outside Sweden. Providing partial support to these results, Breslau *et al.* [28], using data from the 1996 Detroit Area Survey of Trauma, revealed that rates of one trauma type – assaultative violence – were higher among non-whites compared to whites.

In summary, no consistent evidence from general population studies exists at present regarding the relationship between race and ethnicity and the risk for PTSD.

Marital status

Whereas Breslau *et al.* [25] found that marital status was not associated with exposure to traumatic events, results from the NCS [27] and from a Canadian study [32] suggest that among women, lifetime prevalence of PTSD is over three times higher among those separated, divorced or widowed than those currently married. In men, the prevalence of PTSD is significantly higher among married than never-married individuals [27]. Also, de Vries and Olff, using a community sample from the Netherlands, found that exposure was twofold higher for singles and previously married people than for those living together. Moreover, the authors found a threefold risk for developing PTSD after trauma exposure among those formerly married compared with those living together [40].

Overall, there is some evidence from general population studies from different countries suggesting that those not currently married are at higher risk for PTSD. Longitudinal studies have yet to clarify whether not being married is a risk factor or a consequence of PTSD.

Socioeconomic status

Numerous studies have reported a relationship between socioeconomic status (SES) and PTSD. A study from Australia found that living in poorer areas was associated with an increased risk for trauma exposure. In the same line, two studies [28, 36] suggested assaultative violence to be higher in individuals with low SES. At the same time, higher risk for PTSD development after trauma exposure was observed in the Australian study [57] and higher rates of lifetime PTSD among those with lower SES have been reported in Germany [36, 46].

Education

A general population study conducted in the USA [25] and another conducted in six European countries [37] found that respondents with low levels of education were more likely to have been exposed to traumatic events, but when considering only those exposed to a traumatic event, educational level was not a risk factor for the development of PTSD. Similarly, data from an Australian survey found that lower levels of education were associated with increased odds of developing PTSD after exposure to traumatic events [46].

Conflicting evidence comes from the results of studies conducted in Sweden [38] and Mexico [33]. These studies reported that increased prevalence of trauma exposure was associated with higher educational levels. Nonetheless, education level was not found to be a risk factor for PTSD development among those with a history of exposure to traumatic events in either of the studies.

In summary, contradictory evidence from different countries exists regarding the association between education level and exposure to trauma. However, no general population study has found education level to be a risk factor for PTSD development after trauma exposure.

PSYCHIATRIC COMORBIDITY

Several studies have documented strong associations between PTSD and comorbid psychiatric disorders [61]. In a community sample of adolescents and young adults aged 14–24, Pekonigg *et al*. [36] found that 87.5% of those with lifetime PTSD had at least one additional psychiatric diagnosis and 77.5% had two or more additional diagnoses. Psychiatric disorders most strongly associated with PTSD include dysthymia, major depressive disorder (MDD), somatisation symptoms, panic disorder, bipolar disorder, specific phobias and dissociative disorders. Having had a psychiatric disorder before a trauma increases the risk for developing PTSD, while having PTSD seems to increase the risk for developing an additional psychiatric disorder as well. In the study by Pekonigg *et al*. [36], individuals with previous somatoform, dysthymic and social anxiety disorders were four to five times more likely to develop PTSD later. The most common disorder cooccurring with PTSD is MDD, with about 35–50% of cases of PTSD in the general population being comorbid with MDD [25, 27, 28, 62]. Alcohol abuse and dependence are also common; rates are approximately 31.2% among individuals with PTSD in the NCS [27].

It has been argued that the comorbidity of PTSD would be expected since criteria from the C and D symptoms overlap with those of MDD or generalised anxiety disorder (GAD) and Criterion D6 of PTSD also overlaps with social anxiety disorder, specific phobia and panic disorder [63] criteria. Further prospective studies are needed to clarify the associations of PTSD with other psychiatric disorders.

In a more recent study, using data from a longitudinal epidemiological study of young adults in southeast Michigan, Breslau *et al*. [64] found an increased risk for presenting a drug-use disorder and nicotine dependence among those with PTSD. Analyses of the prospective and retrospective data suggest that PTSD might be the cause of nicotine dependence and other drug-use disorders, or, alternatively, that PTSD and the subsequent onset of these disorders are caused by shared risk factors other than the exposure to trauma [64]. In samples of substance users the presence of comorbid PTSD has been associated with poorer substance-use disorder outcomes.

COURSE OF PTSD

The onset of PTSD symptoms usually begins within the first months after experiencing the triggering traumatic event, although there may be a delay of months before symptoms become noticeable. DSM-IV-TR describes delayed onset as a specifier for PTSD, where 'at least 6 months have passed between the traumatic event and the onset of the symptoms' [15]. In a systematic review, Andrews *et al*. [65] found that delayed-onset cases that represented exacerbations or reactivations of prior symptoms accounted for 38.2% and 15.3%, respectively, whereas delayed-onset PTSD among individuals with no prior symptoms was rare.

DSM-IV includes two specifiers for the duration of PTSD. It suggests that PTSD cases that lasts less than three months should be considered as 'acute', whereas cases of PTSD lasting longer should be considered 'chronic'. Although PTSD is widely recognised as a generally chronic disorder, knowledge of the course of PTSD is limited by the use of samples who have experienced a specific type of traumatic event and by inconsistent timeframes used to assess the evolution and course of the disorder. However, the stipulations of a chronic course do not necessarily mean that the person affected meets diagnostic criteria for PTSD continuously. In fact, variations in severity around the diagnostic threshold (shifts from supra- to subthreshold expressions and vice versa) appear to be quite frequent. Furthermore, in some cases, the course of PTSD is characterised by a decrease of symptoms, with specific symptoms fluctuating over time and sometimes even increasing in intensity after several years of declined severity [66]. Symptom reactivation may occur in response to reminders of the original trauma, life stressors or new traumatic events.

A study suggested that complete recovery occurs within three months in approximately 50% of cases and that a significant proportion of individuals have persisting symptoms for longer than 12 months after the trauma. Through survival analysis based on retrospective data, findings from the Detroit Area survey Trauma of 1996 estimated that the median time to remit from PTSD was 24.9 months. The median time to remission was 48.1 months in women versus 12.0 months in men [28]. Approximately 26% of PTSD cases remitted by 6 months and 40% by 12 months.

Data from the US general population also showed that PTSD persisted over 60 months in at least one third of subjects [27]. Survivors of assault, man-made disasters and combat frequently meet criteria for PTSD even several years after the original trauma [67, 68]. Some studies show that anxiety and somatoform disorders, depressive symptoms after the onset of PTSD [69, 70], occurrence of new traumatic events and avoidant symptoms during the onset of the disorder [71] are associated with a chronic course of PTSD.

ACUTE STRESS DISORDER

Like PTSD, ASD is a condition that can develop after trauma exposure. Unfortunately, epidemiological information regarding ASD in community samples is lacking. In this section we will briefly describe this trauma-related disorder and its relationship with PTSD.

ASD was first introduced in 1994 and was classified among the Anxiety Disorders in the DSM-IV [15] in response to the need for a diagnostic entity that defines acute reactions to traumatic stressors as something more than an adjustment disorder. It was introduced to describe the development of anxiety symptoms, reexperiencing of the event, avoidance of stimuli and increased arousal with an emphasis on the dissociative reactions to the trauma. While PTSD acknowledges possible inclusion of amnesia of the trauma or feelings of detachment, these symptoms are not necessary for a diagnosis of PTSD. On the other hand, the diagnosis of ASD requires that the individual experiences at least three of the following five dissociative symptoms: (i) a subjective sense of numbing or detachment; (ii) reduced awareness of their surroundings; (iii) derealisation; (iv) depersonalisation; and (v) dissociative amnesia (e.g. inability to recall an important part of the traumatic experience).

Additionally, whereas ASD diagnosis requires that symptoms persist for a minimum of two days and up to a month after the trauma, PTSD diagnosis can be given only after one month of the symptoms being present. Thus, whereas ASD describes the reaction that occurs immediately in the early aftermath of a trauma, the persistence of symptoms after one month receives the diagnosis of PTSD.

Incidence of ASD has been reported among individuals exposed to a specific trauma. For example, it has been estimated that among assault victims, 19% are diagnosed with ASD [72]; among motor-vehicle accident (MVA) survivors, 13% are diagnosed [73]; and among mildly head-injured MVA survivors, 14% have ASD [74].

A major reason for the emphasis on dissociative symptoms in ASD is their prognostic value. Numerous studies have shown that severe early reactions to trauma predict the development and chronicity of PTSD [75–78]. About a dozen prospective studies have assessed the relationship between ASD in the initial month after trauma and development of subsequent PTSD (for a review, see [75]). For example, in a longitudinal study (n = 187), Koopman [77] examined the relationship between dissociative symptoms and PTSD in the immediate aftermath of the Oakland/Berkeley firestorm. Results suggested that the presence of dissociative symptoms in the initial reactions after a traumatic event increased the risk for the development of PTSD after seven months. In the same line, several studies among individuals suffering MVAs have found that ASD predicts the subsequent development of PTSD in 42%–78% of participants [73, 74, 79, 80].

In victims of terrorist attacks, 44% of the sample diagnosed with ASD developed PTSD symptoms after four months [78]. In victims of assault, between 83% and 89% of the individuals with ASD ultimately developed PTSD [72, 81]. However, a lower proportion of victims of health-related traumatic events developed PTSD (17%–33%) seven months and one year later [82–84]. Results from different studies showed that 75% of victims of MVAs, 46% of assault victims and 12% of cancer patients diagnosed with ASD ultimately met PTSD criteria [79, 81, 84, 85]. Other studies have suggested that using less stringent scores of ASD could increase the identification of individuals at risk of developing PTSD from 28% to 44% [86], further increasing the sensibility of ASD as a PTSD predictor.

ASD has triggered considerable debate in the field [87, 88]. Although the majority of individuals with ASD develop PTSD, the utility of the ASD diagnosis is less evident when one considers that the percentage of individuals who have ASD among all people who eventually develop PTSD is actually a minority. For example, a study on adult individuals who sustained mild traumatic brain injury after MVA found that only 40% of those with PTSD after six months of the trauma exposure met ASD diagnosis at the first month [74]. This has led to suggestions that ASD does not achieve the important objective of providing adequate clinical coverage for individuals with acute post-traumatic symptomatology and the utility of requiring peritraumatic dissociative symptoms as a core feature has been questioned [88, 89].

Although the relevance of the predictive relation between ASD and PTSD symptoms is yet to be further determined, detailed information on the pathways from ASD to PTSD and the protective and resilience factors may still be relevant for implementation of preventive interventions, especially among individuals from higher-risk sociodemographic groups and those reporting sexual and physical violence.

CONCLUSION

Epidemiological studies on PTSD in the general population have grown remarkably around the world over the past 30 years. Although some of the differences in rates of trauma exposure and prevalence of PTSD across studies may be due to methodological differences, differences in the economic, political and social context are also likely to play an important role. At present, a wide variability of exposure to traumatic events appears to exist throughout different continents. Whereas in some countries such as Switzerland, lifetime rates of exposure to traumatic events in the population are reported to be very low (28%), in countries such as the United States, rates as high as 89% have been reported. Nonetheless, studies seem to indicate that the minority of individuals exposed to traumatic events develop PTSD as a consequence. While most research has consistently found female gender to be a risk factor for PTSD development, studies on other demographic factors such as age, socioeconomic condition and marital status are less consistent. Finally, evidence for ethnic and racial differences in the risk for PTSD in the general population is limited at present.

As most of the information comes from cross-sectional studies, longitudinal epidemiological research may help increase our knowledge of PTSD. Areas of particular importance will include the relationship between risk factors and the development of PTSD and the existence of gender differences in trauma exposure and the development of PTSD. Finally, knowledge of subthreshold PTSD and ASD might contribute greatly to our understanding of the wider range of reaction to traumatic events.

REFERENCES

1. Turnbull, G.J. (1998) A review of post-traumatic stress disorder. Part I: historical development and classification. *Injury*, **29** (2), 87–91.
2. Erichsen, J.E. (1866) *On Railway and Other Injuries of the Nervous System*, Walton and Maberly, London.
3. Putnam, J. (1883) Recent investigations into the pathology of so-called concussion of the spine. *Boston Medical and Surgical Journal*, **CIX**, 217–220.
4. Myers, A. (1870) *On the Aetiology and Prevalence of Disease of the Heart Among Soldiers*, J. Churchill, London.
5. World Health Organization (1955–1957) International Classification of Diseases, 7th Revision, WHO, Geneva.
6. Hood, P. (1875) On cardiac weakness as a remote consequence of injures by railway collisions and other accidents. *Lancet*, **i**, 299–301.
7. Neale, R. (1882) *The Medical Digest, or Busy Practicioner's Vademecum*, Ledger, Smith and Co, London.
8. Clevenger, S. (1889) *Spinal Concussion*, F.A Davis, Philadelphia, PA.

9. Page, H. (1885) *Injuries of the Spinal Cord without Apparent Mechanical Lesion and Nervous Shock in ther Surgical and Medicolegal Aspects*, JandA Churchill, London.
10. Wood, P. (1941) Da Costa's Syndrome (or effort syndrome). *British Medical Journal*, **i**, 767–851.
11. Mott, F. (1918) War psychoneurosis (1) Neuraesthenia: the disorders and disabilities of fear. *Lancet*, **i**, 127–129.
12. Mackenzie, J. (1916) Discussion on the Soldier's Heart. *Proceedings of the Royal Society of Medicine, Therapeutical and Pharmacological Section*, **9**, 60.
13. Kardiner, A. and Spiegel, H. (1947) *War Stress and Neurotic Illness*, Paul B. Hoeber, New York.
14. American Psychiatric Association (1987) *Diagnostic and Statistical Manual of Mental Disorders*, 3rd edn, American Psychiatric Association, Washington, DC.
15. American Psychiatric Association (2000) *Diagnostic and Statistical Manual of Mental Disorders*, 4th edn, Text revision, American Psychiatric Association, Washington, DC.
16. Breslau, N. and Kessler, R.C. (2001) The stressor criterion in DSM-IV posttraumatic stress disorder: an empirical investigation. *Biological Psychiatry*, **50** (9), 699–704.
17. World Health Organization (1992) The ICD-10 Classification of Mental and Behavioural Disorders, World Health Organization, Geneva, Switzerland.
18. de Jong, J.T., Komproe, I.H., Van Ommeren, M. *et al*. (2001) Lifetime events and posttraumatic stress disorder in 4 postconflict settings. *Journal of Amercian Medical Association*, **286** (5), 555–562.
19. Carr, V.J., Lewin, T.J., Webster, R.A. *et al*. (1995) Psychosocial sequelae of the 1989 Newcastle earthquake: I. Community disaster experiences and psychological morbidity 6 months post-disaster. *Psychological Medicine*, **25** (3), 539–555.
20. Goenjian, A.K., Molina, L., Steinberg, A.M. *et al*. (2001) Posttraumatic stress and depressive reactions among Nicaraguan adolescents after hurricane Mitch. *American Journal of Psychiatry*, **158** (5), 788–794.
21. Galea, S., Ahern, J., Resnick, H. *et al*. (2002) Psychological sequelae of the September 11 terrorist attacks in New York City. *The New England Journal of Medicine*, **346** (13), 982–987.
22. Wittchen, H.U., Gloster, A., Beesdo, K. *et al*. (2009) Posttraumatic stress disorder: diagnostic and epidemiological perspectives. *CNS Spectrums*, **14** (1, Suppl. 1), 5–12.
23. Helzer, J.E., Robins, L.N. and McEvoy, L. (1987) Post-traumatic stress disorder in the general population: findings of the epidemiologic catchment area survey. *The New England Journal of Medicine*, **317** (26), 1630–1634.
24. Davidson, J.R.T., Hughes, D., Blazer, D.G. and George, L.K. (1991) Posttraumatic stress disorder in the community: an epidemiological study. *Psychological Medicine*, **21** (3), 713–721.
25. Breslau, N., Davis, G.C., Andreski, P. and Peterson, E. (1991) Traumatic events and posttraumatic stress disorder in an urban population of young adults. *Archives of General Psychiatry*, **48** (3), 216–222.

26. Resnick, H.S., Kilpatrick, D.G., Dansky, B.S. *et al.* (1993) Prevalence of civilian trauma and posttraumatic stress disorder in a representative national sample of women. *Journal of Consulting and Clinical Psychology*, **61** (6), 984–991.
27. Kessler, R.C., Sonnega, A., Bromet, E. *et al.* (1995) Posttraumatic stress disorder in the National Comorbidity Survey. *Archives of General Psychiatry*, **52** (12), 1048–1060.
28. Breslau, N., Kessler, R.C., Chilcoat, H.D. *et al.* (1998) Trauma and posttraumatic stress disorder in the community: the 1996 Detroit Area Survey of Trauma. *Archives of General Psychiatry*, **55** (7), 626–632.
29. Breslau, N., Wilcox, H.C., Storr, C.L. *et al.* (2004) Trauma exposure and posttraumatic stress disorder: a study of youths in urban America. *Journal of Urban Health-Bulletin of the New York Academy of Medicine*, **81** (4), 530–544.
30. Kessler, R.C., Berglund, P., Demler, O. *et al.* (2005) Lifetime prevalence and age-of-onset distributions of DSM-IV disorders in the National Comorbidity Survey Replication. *Archives of General Psychiatry*, **62** (6), 593–602.
31. Stein, M.B., Walker, J.R., Hazen, A.L. and Forde, D.R. (1997) Full and partial posttraumatic stress disorder: findings from a community survey. *Archives of General Psychiatry*, **154** (8), 1114–1119.
32. van Ameringen, M., Mancini, C., Patterson, B. and Boyle, M.H. (2008) Post-traumatic stress disorder in Canada. *CNS Neuroscience and Therapeutics*, **14** (3), 171–181.
33. Norris, F.H., Murphy, A.D., Baker, C.K. *et al.* (2003) Epidemiology of trauma and posttraumatic stress disorder in Mexico. *Journal of Abnormal Psychology*, **112** (4), 646–656.
34. Zlotnick, C., Johnson, J., Kohn, R. *et al.* (2006) Epidemiology of trauma, post-traumatic stress disorder (PTSD) and co-morbid disorders in Chile. *Psychological Medicine*, **36** (11), 1523–1533.
35. Alonso, J., Angermeyer, M.C. and Lepine, J.P. (2004) The European Study of the Epidemiology of Mental Disorders (ESEMeD) project: an epidemiological basis for informing mental health policies in Europe. *Acta Psychiatrica Scandinavica*, **109** (Suppl. 420), 5–7.
36. Perkonigg, A., Kessler, R.C., Storz, S. and Wittchen, H.U. (2000) Traumatic events and post-traumatic stress disorder in the community: prevalence, risk factors and comorbidity. *Acta Psychiatrica Scandinavica*, **101** (1), 46–59.
37. Darves-Bornoz, J.M., Alonso, J., de Girolamo, G. *et al.* (2008) Main traumatic events in Europe: PTSD in the European study of the epidemiology of mental disorders survey. *Journal of Traumatic Stress*, **21** (5), 455–462.
38. Frans, O., Rimmo, P.A., Aberg, L. and Fredrikson, M. (2005) Trauma exposure and post-traumatic stress disorder in the general population. *Acta Psychiatrica Scandinavica*, **111** (4), 291–299.
39. Hepp, U., Gamma, A., Milos, G. *et al.* (2006) Prevalence of exposure to potentially traumatic events and PTSD: the Zurich Cohort Study. *European Archives of Psychiatry and Clinical Neuroscience*, **256**, 151–158.

40. de Vries, G.J. and Olff, M. (2009) The lifetime prevalence of traumatic events and posttraumatic stress disorder in the Netherlands. *Journal of Traumatic Stress*, **22** (4), 259–267.
41. Lepine, J.P., Gasquet, I., Kovess, V., Arbabzadeh-Bouchez, S., Negre-Pages, L., Nachbaur, G., and Gaudin, A.F. (2005) Prevalence and comorbidity of psychiatric disorders in the French general population. *Encephale* **31** (2): 182–194.
42. de Girolamo, G., Polidori, G., Morosini, P. *et al*. (2006) Prevalence of common mental disorders in Italy: results from the European Study of the Epidemiology of Mental Disorders (ESEMeD). *Social Psychiatry and Psychiatric Epidemiology*, **41** (11), 853–861.
43. Haro, J.M., Palacin, C., Vilagut, G. *et al*. (2006) Prevalence of mental disorders and associated factors: results from the ESEMeD-Spain study. *Medicina Clinica (Barc)*, **126** (12), 445–451.
44. Karam, E.G., Mneimneh, Z.N., Karam, A.N. *et al*. (2006) Prevalence and treatment of mental disorders in Lebanon: a national epidemiological survey. *Lancet*, **367**, 1000–1006.
45. Karam, E.G., Mneimneh, Z.N., Dimassi, H. *et al*. (2008) Lifetime prevalence of mental disorders in Lebanon: first onset, treatment, and exposure to war. *PLoS Medicine*, **5** (4), e61.
46. Creamer, M., Burgess, P. and McFarlane, A.C. (2001) Post-traumatic stress disorder: findings from the Australian National Survey of Mental Health and Well-being. *Psychological Medicine*, **31** (7), 1237–1247.
47. Robins, L.N., Helzer, J.E., Cottler, L.B. and Golding, E. (1989) *NIMH Diagnostic Interview Schedule Version III, (revised)*, Washington University, St. Lous, MO.
48. World Health Organization (1997) Composite International Diagnostic Interview (CIDI Version 2.1), World Health Organization, Geneva, Switzerland.
49. Breslau, N. (2002) Epidemiologic studies of trauma, posttraumatic stress disorder, and other psychiatric disorders. *Canadian Journal of Psychiatry-Revue Canadienne De Psychiatrie*, **47** (10), 923–929.
50. Kessler, R.C. and Ustun, T.B. (2004) The World Mental Health Survey initiative version of WHO-CIDI. *International Journal of Methods in Psychiatric Research*, **13**, 95–121.
51. Wittchen, H. and Pster, H. (eds) (1997) *DIA-X-Interview: Manual für Screening-Verfahren und Interview; Interviewheft Längsschnittuntersuchung (DIA-X-Lifetime); Ergänzungsheft (DIA-X- Lifetime); Interviewheft Querschnittuntersuchung (DIA-X-12 Monate); Ergänzungsheft (DIA-X-12 Monate); PC-Programm zur Durchführung des Interviews (Längs- und Querschnittuntersuchung); Auswertungsprogramm*, Sweets and Zeitlinger, Frankfurt.
52. Alonso, J., Ferrer, M., Romera, B. *et al*. (2002) The European Study of the Epidemiology of Mental Disorders (ESEMeD/MHEDEA 2000) project: rationale and methods. *International Journal of Methods in Psychiatric Research*, **11** (2), 55–67.
53. Ruggiero, K.J., Del Ben, K., Scotti, J.R. and Rabalais, A.E. (2003) Psychometric properties of the PTSD Checklist-Civilian Version. *Journal of Traumatic Stress*, **16** (5), 495–502.

54. Vries, G.O.M. (2009) The lifetime prevalence of traumatic events and posttraumatic stress disorder in tne Netherlands. *Journal of Traumatic Stress*, **22** (4), 259–287.
55. Robins, L.N., Wing, J., Wittchen, H.U. *et al.* (1988) The Composite International Diagnostic Interview. an epidemiologic instrument suitable for use in conjuntion with different diagnostic systems and in different cultures. *Archives of General Psychiatry*, **45**, 1069–1077.
56. Andrews, G. and Peters, L. (1998) Psycometric properities of the CIDI. *Social Psychiatry and Psychiatric Epidemiology*, **33**, 80–88.
57. Rosenman, S. (2002) Trauma and posttraumatic stress disorder in Australia: findings in the population sample of the Australian National Survey of Mental Health and Wellbeing. *Australian and New Zealand Journal of Psychiatry*, **36** (4), 515–520.
58. Davidson, J.R.T., Hughes, D., Blazer, D. and George, L.K. (1991) Posttraumatic stress disorder in the community: an epidemiological study. *Psychological Medicine*, **21**, 1–19.
59. MacMillan, H.L., Fleming, J.E., Trocme, N. *et al.* (1997) Prevalence of child physical and sexual abuse in the community: results from the Ontario Health Supplement. *Journal of the American Medical Association*, **278**, 131–135.
60. Breslau, J., Aguilar-Gaxiola, S., Kendler, K.S. *et al.* (2006) Specifying race-ethnic differences in risk for psychiatric disorder in a USA national sample. *Psychological Medicine*, **36**, 57–68.
61. Kessler, R.C., Chiu, W.T., Demler, O. *et al.* (2005) Prevalence, severity, and comorbidity of 12-month DSM-IV disorders in the National Comorbidity Survey Replication. *Archives of General Psychiatry*, **62**, 617–627.
62. Breslau, N., Davis, G.C., Peterson, E.L. and Schultz, L. (1997) Psychiatric sequelae of posttraumatic stress disorder in women. *Archives of General Psychiatry*, **54** (1), 81–87.
63. Davidson, J.R.T. and Foa, E.B. (1991) Diagnostic issues in posttraumatic stress disorder: considerations for the DSM-IV. *Journal of Abnormal Psychology*, **100** (3), 346–355.
64. Breslau, N., Davis, G.C. and Schultz, L.R. (2003) Posttraumatic stress disorder and the incidence of nicotine, alcohol, and other drug disorders in persons who have experienced trauma. *Archives of General Psychiatry*, **60** (3), 289–294.
65. Andrews, B., Brewin, C.R., Philpott, R. and Stewart, L. (2007) Delayed-onset posttraumatic stress disorder: a systematic review of the evidence. *American Journal of Psychiatry*, **164** (9), 1319–1326.
66. McFarlane, A.C. (2000) Posttraumatic stress disorder: a model of the longitudinal course and the role of risk factors. *Journal of Clinical Psychiatry*, **61** (Suppl. 5), 15–20; discussion 21–13.
67. Dirkzwager, A.J., Bramsen, I. and van der Ploeg, H.M. (2001) The longitudinal course of posttraumatic stress disorder symptoms among aging military veterans. *Journal of Nervous and Mental Disease*, **189** (12), 846–853.
68. Green, B.L., Lindy, J.D., Grace, M.C. and Leonard, A.C. (1992) Chronic posttraumatic stress disorder and diagnostic comorbidity in a disaster sample. *Journal of Nervous and Mental Disease*, **180** (12), 760–766.

69. Goenjian, A.K., Steinberg, A.M., Najarian, L.M. *et al*. (2000) Prospective study of posttraumatic stress, anxiety, and depressive reactions after earthquake and political violence. *American Journal of Psychiatry*, **157** (6), 911–916.
70. Shalev, A.Y., Freedman, S., Peri, T. *et al*. (1998) Prospective study of posttraumatic stress disorder and depression following trauma. *American Journal of Psychiatry*, **155** (5), 630–637.
71. Perkonigg, A., Pfister, H., Stein, M.B. *et al*. (2005) Longitudinal course of posttraumatic stress disorder and posttraumatic stress disorder symptoms in a community sample of adolescents and young adults. *American Journal of Psychiatry*, **162** (7), 1320–1327.
72. Brewin, C.R., Andrews, B., Rose, S. and Kirk, M. (1999) Acute stress disorder and posttraumatic stress disorder in victims of violent crime. *American Journal of Psychiatry*, **156** (3), 360–366.
73. Harvey, A.G. and Bryant, R.A. (1999) Predictors of acute stress following motor vehicle accidents. *Journal of Traumatic Stress*, **12** (3), 519–525.
74. Harvey, A.G. and Bryant, R.A. (1998) The relationship between acute stress disorder and posttraumatic stress disorder: a prospective evaluation of motor vehicle accident survivors. *Journal of Consulting and Clinical Psychology*, **66** (3), 507–512.
75. Bryant, R.A. (2003) Early predictors of posttraumatic stress disorder. *Biological Psychiatry*, **53** (9), 789–795.
76. Foa, E. and Rothbaum, B.A. (1998) *Teating the Trauma of Rape Cognitive-Behavioral Therapy for PTSD*, The Guildford Press, New York, London.
77. Koopman, C., Classen, C. and Spiegel, D. (1994) Predictors of posttraumatic stress symptoms among survivors of the Oakland/Berkeley, Calif., firestorm. *American Journal of Psychiatry*, **151** (6), 888–894.
78. Kutz, I. and Dekel, R. (2006) Follow-up on victims of a terrorist attack in Israel: ASD, PTSD, and the perceived threat of Iraqui missile attacks. *Personality and Individual Differences*, **40**, 1579–1583.
79. Hamanaka, S., Asukai, N., Kamijo, Y. *et al*. (2006) Acure stress disorder an posttramatic stressdisorder among patients severely injured in motor vehicle accidents in Japan. *General Hospital Psychiatry*, **28**, 234–241.
80. Holeva, V., Tarrier, N., Wells, A. (2001) Prevalence and predictors of acute stress disorder and PTSD following road traffic accidents: thought control strategies and social support. *Behavioral Therapy*, **32**, 65–83.
81. Elkit, A. and Brink, O. (2004) Acute stress disorder as a predictor of post-traumatic stress disorder in physical assault victims. *Journal of Interpersonal Violence*, **19**, 709–726.
82. Creamer, M., O'Donnell, M.L. and Pattison, P. (2004) The relationship between acute stress disorder and posttraumatic stress disorder in severely injured trauma survivors. *Behaviour Research and Therapy*, **42** (3), 315–328.
83. Ginzburg, K., Solomon, Z., Koifman, B. *et al*. (2003) Trajectories of postraumatic stress disorder following myocardial infarction: A prospective study. *Journal of Clinical Psychiatry*, **64**, 1370–1376.

84. Kangas, M., Henry, J.L. and Bryant, R.A. (2005) The course of psychological disorders in the 1st year after cancer diagnosis. *Journal of Consulting and Clinical Psychology*, **73**, 763–768.
85. Bryant, R.A., Moulds, M.L. and Guthrie, R.M. (2000) Acute stress disorder scale: a self report measure of acute stress disorder. *Psychological Assessment*, **12**, 61–68.
86. Fuglsang, A.K., Moergeli, H. and Schnyder, U. (2004) Does acute stress disorder predict posttraumatic stress disorder in traffic accident victims? Analysis of self report inventory. *Nordic Journal of Psychiatry*, **161**, 223–229.
87. Bryant, R.A. and Harvey, A.G. (2000) New DSM-IV diagnosis of acute stress disorder. *American Journal of Psychiatry*, **157** (11), 1889–1891.
88. Marshall, R.D., Spitzer, R. and Liebowitz, M.R. (1999) Review and critique of the new DSM-IV diagnosis of acute stress disorder. *American Journal of Psychiatry*, **156** (11), 1677–1685.
89. Bryant, R.A. (2007) Does dissociation further our understanding of PTSD? *Journal of Anxiety Disorders*, **21** (2), 183–191.

COMMENTARY

2.1 Challenges and Future Horizons in Epidemiological Research into PTSD

Abdulrahman M. El-Sayed and Sandro Galea
Department of Epidemiology, Mailman School of Public Health, Columbia University, New York, NY, USA

INTRODUCTION

In Commentry of Chapter 1, Blanco provides an excellent review of studies of the epidemiology of post-traumatic stress disorder (PTSD), summarising findings from epidemiological studies into PTSD by continent, as well as synthesising findings about predictors and trajectories of PTSD following traumatic event exposure. In this commentary, building on Blanco's work, we discuss the methodological challenges to our understanding of the epidemiology of PTSD, and suggest horizons for future research in this area.

We will discuss the following challenges in research into PTSD epidemiology, addressing how and why they impose limitations on our understanding of PTSD: (i) the lack of sufficiently cogent, sensitive and specific definitions of traumatic stressors; (ii) the relative paucity of longitudinal studies into PTSD in the general population; and (iii) our limited understanding of the breadth of psychopathology following exposure to traumatic stressors.

Moreover, we will examine the following horizons for future research into PTSD epidemiology, outlining each area's potential to address the above limitations: (i) expanded longitudinal study of PTSD and other psychopathologies among groups particularly vulnerable to 'chronic', rather than acute, traumatic event exposures; (ii) baseline surveys in contexts that are particularly prone to acute traumatic exposures, in order to support longitudinal studies into the causes and clinical trajectories of PTSD and other psychopathologies following exposure

Post-traumatic Stress Disorder, First Edition. Edited by Dan Stein, Matthew Friedman, and Carlos Blanco.

to acute stressors; and (iii) the use of complex systems approaches to modelling PTSD and other psychopathologies following traumatic event exposure.

CHALLENGES

The insufficiency of current criteria for traumatic stressors, and the need for a cogent, adequately sensitive and adequately specific definition of exposure to traumatic events that encompasses the universe of potentially traumatic acute and chronic stressors is a substantial challenge to current PTSD research. Blanco discusses the history of definitions for Criterion A, the gateway criterion, throughout iterations of the Diagnostic and Statistical Manual (DSM). The most current DSM-IV [1] modifies Criterion A into two parts, Criterion A1 and Criterion A2, requiring that 'the person experienced, witnessed or was confronted with an event that involved actual or threatened death or serious injury or threat to the physical integrity of self or other' (Criterion A1), and that this 'evoked intense fear, helplessness or horror' (Criterion A2). Blanco also notes that the inclusivity and exclusivity of stressor criteria may substantially influence conditional prevalence in studies into the epidemiology of PTSD – findings in studies defining traumatic event exposures based on either DSM-III-R [2] or DSM-IV criteria have differed by almost 15% in the conditional prevalence of PTSD noted [3, 4]. Indeed, some authors have suggested the removal of Criterion A from the definition of PTSD, in large part because of the limitations in its measurement [5].

Of interest here is the conceptual inclusivity and exclusivity of the approach to defining a traumatic stressor. Most well-studied traumatic stressors are acute, as they are defined and well-contained within time and space, facilitating epidemiological definitions for 'exposure'. More chronic traumatic event exposures may be systematically excluded from formal traumatic event criteria, as they often lack a formal 'beginning' and 'end' and may not be confined within a particular space. Moreover, because Criterion A requires intensity by definition, these more chronic exposures may not reach adequate levels of intensity to meet Criterion A at any given point in time, but may exert cumulative effects over time that still elicit psychopathological sequelae. As Blanco highlights, such chronic traumatic event exposures may be epidemiologically important [6]. Moreover, indirect exposures to traumatic stressors, which have only recently been included in Criterion A definitions, may also affect PTSD risk. For example, several studies following the 11 September 2001 terrorist attacks suggest that watching televised coverage of the attacks, speaking on the phone with someone who was affected, hearing the attacks or feeling their physical impact, and being within blocks of the sight of the attacks were predictors of PTSD symptomatology, despite being indirect exposures [7, 8]. These findings challenge our current understanding of the aetiology of PTSD, suggesting that traumatic stressors associated with PTSD may not require threat of harm to self.

Another challenge highlighted by Blanco's work is the relative need for longitudinal studies of PTSD in the general population. It is particularly difficult to study PTSD longitudinally because traumatic events – particularly acute events – are almost never expected, making baseline data almost impossible to collect. Therefore, attributing causality, particularly with regard to historical events and preexposure factors such as underlying psychopathology, is challenging. Moreover, as Blanco suggests, the paucity of longitudinal studies among the general population limits our understanding of (i) differences in the aetiology of PTSD by traumatic exposure and (ii) PTSD trajectories, as present data are limited to findings among samples with inconsistent timeframes or who have experienced only one particular event.

A third challenge is the limited study of the breadth of psychopathology that may accompany PTSD after traumatic exposures. While some studies have found that nicotine and drug dependencies may be associated with PTSD, it is unclear whether PTSD predicts these psychopathologies or whether they arise from mutually shared risk factors with PTSD [9]. Extant research into the mental health effects of traumatic exposures has been limited by studies that have focused solely on PTSD as an outcome of interest. Few studies of the epidemiology of PTSD following traumatic exposure have adjusted for other psychopathologies when assessing the onset of PTSD after exposure.

FUTURE HORIZONS

We suggest three directions that may help address the present challenges in our understanding of PTSD epidemiology and the psychopathological sequelae of traumatic exposures. First, there is a need for expanded longitudinal research into PTSD and other psychopathology among groups particularly vulnerable to 'chronic' traumatic event exposures (e.g. the homeless, women in domestic relationships, service personnel, police officers, firefighters, etc.). Such research would clarify the psychopathological effects of less intense, cumulative chronic stressors, allowing for more appropriately framed inclusive or exclusive definitions of Criterion A traumatic event exposures. Moreover, further longitudinal study of this type may improve our heretofore limited understanding of the influence of historical events and preexposure factors, such as underlying psychopathology, on risk for PTSD following traumatic exposure. Finally, such studies would improve our understanding of the trajectories of PTSD and other psychopathologies following traumatic exposure.

Second, baseline studies in contexts that are particularly prone to acute traumatic stress exposures (e.g. hurricanes, earthquakes, volcanoes, battles, etc.) are needed to support longitudinal studies into the causes and clinical trajectories of PTSD and other psychopathologies following exposure to acute traumatic stress. These baseline studies would address a principal limitation discussed above: the limitation to longitudinal study imposed by the fundamentally unexpected nature of acute trauma. Following acute mass traumas, these baseline studies could be used to support longitudinal analyses of their psychopathological sequelae. Such longitudinal studies would improve our understanding of the influence of historical events and preexposure factors on risk for PTSD and other psychopathologies, and clarify the nature and extent of PTSD trajectories.

Third, epidemiological research into PTSD might benefit from an expanded toolkit, including the use of complex systems analytic tools, such as agent-based models and network analysis. Agent-based models allow investigators to simulate complex social phenomena using agents that behave according to programmed rules governing their baseline characteristics, distributions in space and interactions with one another and their simulated environment, and which can be parameterised according to available data. These tools are gaining ground in psychiatric epidemiology, and they have been used in previous epidemiological studies concerned with psychopathology [10, 11]. Agent-based models might allow for expanded research into the influence of different types of traumas, preexposure characteristics and historical events on risk for PTSD and other psychopathologies following simulated traumatic exposures. Additionally, agent-based models might also prove useful in understanding PTSD trajectories by allowing for their simulation and affording investigators an opportunity to manipulate key factors that inform PTSD trajectories with time.

Network analysis allows investigators to analyse the topologies and dynamics of real and simulated networks in order to understand how social interactions might influence an outcome of interest. This approach has been used in the psychiatric epidemiological literature to study adolescent risk behaviours [12], binge-drinking [13] and overall wellbeing [14] among densely interconnected populations. Network analysis may prove important in our understanding of the role of indirect exposure to traumatic events in the population-level aetiology of PTSD.

CONCLUSION

As well articulated by Blanco, several challenges to our understanding of PTSD epidemiology remain, including the lack of sufficiently cogent, sensitive and specific definitions of traumatic stressors, the relative paucity of longitudinal studies into PTSD in the general population, and a limited understanding of the breadth of psychopathology following exposure to traumatic stressors. Expanded longitudinal study of PTSD and other psychopathologies among groups particularly vulnerable to 'chronic', rather than acute, traumatic event exposures, baseline studies in contexts that are particularly prone to acute traumatic stress exposures and the use of complex systems approaches to modelling PTSD are future avenues for research into the epidemiology of PTSD that may help address these challenges.

COMMENTARY

2.2 Preventing Mental Ill-Health Following Trauma

Helen Herrman
Centre for Youth Mental Health, University of Melbourne, Victoria, Australia

How does the available epidemiological information help us to understand the possibilities for prevention of mental ill-health following trauma? Epidemiology is among other things the science of prevention [15]. Individual and community reactions to trauma are now recognised more clearly than in the past as major challenges to global health and mental health, especially trauma related to child maltreatment, road traffic accidents and disasters and civil emergencies, including war.

The systematic review of epidemiological evidence on PTSDs in general populations reveals important gaps in understanding the effects of stress on adult mental health. There are also gaps in understanding the effects of stress on the mental health of children and the patterns of stress-related disorders among children in populations. However, the extent of trauma from everyday life, including child maltreatment and neglect, is now becoming clear worldwide [16], and disasters in many forms touch the lives of millions of children each year [17]. One well-supported finding in the literature on trauma and its consequences is the dose-response effect. As exposure to extreme adversity rises or accumulates, including the effects on children via the effects on parents and parenting quality, there is an increase in symptoms of trauma, behaviour problems, mental anguish and many other kinds of problems observed in children as well as adults. There are also specific toxic experiences with lasting and distinct effects such as the experience of rape [17]. Acute distress after major disasters is common and expectable. Studies in Thailand after the 2004 tsunami showed that the rates of symptoms of PTSD, anxiety and depression in adults decreased by approximately one half after nine months. Children, on the other hand, showed little change in symptoms, perhaps because they continued to experience emotional isolation or grief following the loss of parents, although this was not measured in the studies [18–20].

Post-traumatic Stress Disorder, First Edition. Edited by Dan Stein, Matthew Friedman, and Carlos Blanco.

Authorities note that there is widespread uncertainty and confusion about the nature and effects of stress in childhood or at any life stage [16]. For example, mastery of minor adversity by children is important for developing resilience to later challenges. The public and professions are less aware, however, that levels of stress associated with excessive, persistent or uncontrollable adversity, without the protection of stable adult support, are associated with disruptive effects on brain function (and multiple organ systems) that can lead to lifelong disease and behavioural problems. Early experiences can affect adult health in two ways [16], either by cumulative effects over time or by the biological embedding of adversities or advantages during sensitive developmental periods. Overall, insufficient attention is paid to health-promotion and disease-prevention strategies for vulnerable children and their parents, or older and marginalised groups, based on either reducing significant stressors or ameliorating the effects of these stressors [16, 21].

The vulnerability or resilience of any child or adult is determined by a complex interplay of individual attributes and the social context [22, 23]. Strong evidence exists that supportive, sensitive early caregivers in infancy and childhood can increase resilience and reduce the effects of 'toxic' environments and that there may be sensitive periods when interventions work best [24]. Resilience is an interactive concept, referring to a relative resistance to environmental risk experiences or the overcoming of stress or adversity, and it is thus differentiated from positive mental health [25]. Michael Rutter has described the cumulative and interactive effects of life stresses in children and young people and the turning points that positive events may represent [25].

Researchers are increasingly aware of the need for developmentally informed prevention, and investigation into the mechanisms underlying resilient functioning, using multiple levels of analysis ranging from DNA sequences to cultural analysis. The findings can then support the design of interventions promoting positive change during adversity or trauma, especially at periods of developmental change and transitions, and help evaluate them through randomised controlled trials [23] and other means.

Awareness that PTSD affects pregnant women (between 3 and 14% in one study) brings other opportunities to prevent a range of adverse effects [26]. Pregnant women with PTSD are likely to have had exposure to childhood abuse and traumatic reproductive events including rape, and to have sociodemographic disadvantages and comorbid anxiety and depression. This group is also at high risk of adverse perinatal health behaviours. For these women, trauma-informed interventions may be more effective than separately applied substance abuse, primary depression and domestic violence interventions [26].

Examples of population-based interventions across the lifespan that are likely to support resilience include social policies and support for parents of infants, early childhood intervention programmes, school-based interventions, workplace and unemployment programmes and activity programmes for older adults; all with attention to environment, gender, culture, life cycle and the special vulnerabilities of population groups [22]. Particularly relevant is the scaling up and evaluation of effective participatory community-based programmes to support early child development [27].

There is relatively little experience or information to support efforts to address the needs of adults, children and youth in the context of disasters. Nonetheless, a consensus is developing about the responses desirable after disasters [28]. Culturally appropriate social strategies developed with the recipient group are recommended to protect vulnerable people, reunite families and communities wherever possible, create meaningful roles and livelihoods and reestablish institutions and services (religious, cultural, mental health) that promote communal cohesion and a sense of order [28]. Future research needs to examine more closely the extent to which these broad social interventions influence individual and communal recovery from traumatic stress reactions and prevent more sustained morbidity. Research is also needed to identify more accurately the personal, social and cultural factors that encourage natural recovery from immediate stress reactions and those that predict chronicity and disability [20].

Other needs for research in any context include the following: understanding indigenous concepts and terms for describing stress; and including assessments of a wider range of stress reactions such as complicated grief, separation anxiety, somatoform disorders, feelings of anger, hatred and revenge, impulse control disorders and substance abuse [20]. Epidemiological studies need to be complemented by psychological, biological and intervention studies of the consequences of trauma in the general population and in population subgroups in countries of all types. Psychiatrists and health professionals have an important role to play in the process of building and applying knowledge relevant to population-based and clinic-based prevention, contributing to the transfer of knowledge from research to policy and practice, as well as the reverse.

COMMENTARY

2.3 PTSD Epidemiology with Particular Reference to Gender

Marianne Kastrup
Videnscenter for Transkulturel Psykiatri, Psykiatrisk Center København, Strandboulevarden, Denmark

INTRODUCTION

There are valid reasons to focus on gender-specific problems in relation to PTSD as women and men face different life situations, cope differently with traumata and receive different treatments thereof. Besides being exposed to traumas in the same ways as men, women are subjected to a variety of forms of sexual abuse. Refugee women run particular risks, and this commentary will focus on PTSD among them.

PREVALENCE

Males and females may experience different kinds of traumas [29]. As Blanco notes, numerous studies (e.g. [30]) report that men are more likely than women to experience at least one traumatic event. As an example of sex differences, some work [31] reports that men have a higher prevalence of exposure to injuries and natural disasters, which may explain their overall higher prevalence of traumatic experiences.

Consistently, however, women report PTSD more frequently than men (e.g. [30]). In fact, women exposed to a given trauma are four times more likely to develop PTSD [29], and neither the character of the event nor how the event was perceived seem to explain these differences. Blanco demonstrates how the majority of epidemiological studies report gender differences in PTSD prevalence. Of particular interest are differences following a qualifying traumatic event. Here,

Post-traumatic Stress Disorder, First Edition. Edited by Dan Stein, Matthew Friedman, and Carlos Blanco.

the US National Comorbidity Survey [32] reported that the prevalence of PTSD among those exposed was 8% for men and 20% for women, and Wittchen and Pfister [33] found PTSD rates of 2% for men and 14% for women.

Gender differences in relation to treatment are not systematically studied and we do not have thorough data on whether gender is predictive of treatment outcome [29]. The literature suggests that women are more responsive to treatment, but women with PTSD also tend to exhibit a more chronic course and the World Mental Health Report states disability-adjusted life years (DALYs) among women with PTSD to be 6% compared to 3% in men [34].

Blanco summarises our present knowledge by underlining that many factors contribute to observed gender differences in the risk for PTSD, including biological, genetic, social and cultural, but that findings are still speculative.

GENDER, REFUGEE STATUS AND PTSD

Regardless of culture, women fulfil the role of nurturers, which following traumatic events may result in their overloading their coping capacity by their preoccupation with the needs of others [35]. This is notably the case in traumatised refugee women. Yet few studies have focused on refugees and findings are inconsistent. Some report a relatively higher level of psychological distress in females and relate this to the accumulation of stressors refugee women face in exile.

Findings of gender differences in PTSD among non-Western adults exposed to violence differ. Some studies, for example one into Bosnian refugees in Sweden [36] and another into Cambodian refugees in the USA, revealed no sex differences [37]. Others reported that women run a greater risk of war-related PTSD, for example Reppesgaard's [38] study of Tamil refugees. Among Kosovar refugees in the USA, 60% showed PTSD, with higher female PTSD scores [39].

Refugee women with young children have an increased vulnerability to stress and a heightened risk of mental disorders including PTSD [40]. In Cambodian refugee women in Australia the number of trauma events prior to childbirth was related to psychological morbidity subsequently.

The different social roles and expectations of the two sexes are reflected in findings among Bosnian refugee couples in the USA [41].Women's marital satisfaction was predicted by their husbands' PTSD, whereas the opposite was not the case for the husbands, arguably indicating that women are more orientated towards others.

ACCESS TO CARE

The report from the WHO European Ministerial Conference [42] lists several vulnerable groups facing treatment gap but makes no mention of gender, which may be due to a lack of gender focus. Yet women are in many cultures [43] more likely to experience stigma when accessing health care, and mental health programmes specifically targeting traumatised women are rare [44].

Despite awareness of gender discrimination, women continue to suffer differential treatment. Civil society and governments need to pay attention to changing community and societal norms, and with increasing globalisation, new directions for action are needed [45].

CONCLUSION

Research into the role of gender with respect to PTSD has tended to focus almost exclusively on individual vulnerability. It is characteristic that there is a scarcity of studies viewing the issue from a more societal perspective and attributing the high level of PTSD to the multiple difficulties refugee women face in exile. If we want to fulfil the needs of refugee women with PTSD we must recognise the complex interrelationship of traumatic experiences, social relationships, gender roles and expectations and how this influences these women in their attempts to overcome trauma.

REFERENCES

1. American Psychiatric Association (2000) *Diagnostic and Statistical Manual of Mental Disorders*, 4th edn, Text Revision, American Psychiatric Association, Washington, DC.
2. American Psychiatric Association (1987) *Diagnostic and Statistical Manual of Mental Disorders*, 3rd edn, American Psychiatric Association, Washington, DC.
3. Breslau, N., Davis, G.C., Andreski, P. and Peterson, E. (1991) Traumatic events and posttraumatic stress disorder in an urban population of young adults. *Archives of General Psychiatry*, **48** (3), 216–222.
4. Breslau, N., Wilcox, H.C., Storr, C.L. *et al*. (2004) Trauma exposure and posttraumatic stress disorder: a study of youths in urban America. *Journal of Urban Health*, **81** (4), 530–544.
5. Brewin, C.R., Lanius, R.A., Novac, A. *et al*. (2009) Reformulating PTSD for DSM-V: life after Criterion A. *Journal of Traumatic Stress*, [epub].
6. Wittchen, H.U., Gloster, A., Beesdo, K. *et al*. (2009) Posttraumatic stress disorder: diagnostic and epidemiological perspectives. *CNS Spectrums*, **14** (1, Suppl 1), 5–12.
7. Schlenger, W.E., Caddell, J.M., Ebert, L. *et al*. (2002) Psychological reactions to terrorist attacks: findings from the National Study of Americans Reactions to September 11. *Journal of the American Medical Association*, **288** (5), 581–588.
8. Silver, R.C., Holman, E.A., McIntosh, D.N. *et al*. (2002) Nationwide longitudinal study of psychological responses to September 11. *Journal of the American Medical Association*, **288** (10), 1235–1244.

9. Breslau, N., Davis, G.C. and Schultz, L.R. (2003) Posttraumatic stress disorder and the incidence of nicotine, alcohol, and other drug disorders in persons who have experienced trauma. *Archives of General Psychiatry*, **60** (3), 289–294.
10. Galea, S., Hall, C. and Kaplan, G. (2009) Social epidemiology and complex system dynamic modelling as applied to health behavior and drug use research. *International Journal of Drug Policy*, **20**, 209–216.
11. Levy, D.T., Nikolayev, L. and Mumford, E. (2005) Recent trends in smoking and the role of public policies: results from the SimSmoke tobacco control policy simulation model. *Addiction*, **100** (10), 1526–1536.
12. Andrews, J.A., Tildesley, E., Hops, H. and Li, F. (2002) The influence of peers on young adult substance use. *Health Psychology*, **21** (4), 349–357.
13. Rosenquist, J.N., Murabito, J., Fowler, J.H. and Christakis, N.A. (2010) The spread of alcohol consumption behavior in a large social network. *Annals of Internal Medicine*, **152** (7), 426–433.
14. Christakis, N.A. and Fowler, J.H. (2008) The collective dynamics of smoking in a large social network. *New England Journal of Medicine*, **358** (21), 2249–2258.
15. Morris, J.N. (1975) *Uses of Epidemiology*, 3rd edn, Churchill Livingstone, New York.
16. Shonkoff, J.P., Boyce, W.T. and Mcewen, B.S. (2009) Neuroscience, molecular biology, and the childhood roots of health disparities: building a new framework for health promotion and disease prevention. *Journal of the American Medical Association*, **301**, 2252–2259.
17. Masten, A.S., and Osofsky, J.D. (2010) Disasters and their impact on child development: Introduction to the Special Section. *Child Development*, **81** (4), 1029–1039.
18. van Griensven, F., Chakkraband, M.L.S., Thienkrua, W. *et al*. (2006) Mental health problems among adults in tsunami-affected areas in southern Thailand. *Journal of the American Medical Association*, **296**, 537–548.
19. Thienkrua, W., Lopes Cardozo, B., Chakkraband, M.L.S. *et al*. (2006) Symptoms of posttraumatic stress disorder and depression among children in tsunami-affected areas of southern Thailand. *Journal of the American Medical Association*, **296**, 549–559.
20. Silove, D. and Bryant, R. (2006) Rapid assessment of mental health needs after disasters. *Journal of the American Medical Association*, **296**, 576–577.
21. Olsson, C.A., Bond, L. and Burns, J.M. (2003) Adolescent resilience: a concept analysis. *Journal of Adolescence*, **26**, 1–11.
22. Herrman, H., Stewart, D.E., Diaz-Granados, N. *et al*. (2010) What is resilience? *Canadian Journal of Psychiatry*, **56** (5).
23. Cicchetti, D. (2010) Resilience under conditions of extreme stress: a multilevel perspective. *World Psychiatry*, **9**, 145–154.
24. Gunnar, M.R. and Fisher, P.A. (2006) Bringing basic research on early experience and stress neurobiology to bear on preventive interventions for neglected and maltreated children. *Development and Psychopathology*, **18**, 651–677.
25. Rutter, M. (2006) Implications of resilience concepts for scientific understanding. *Annals of the New York Academy of Science*, **1094**, 1–12.

26. Seng, J., Low, L.K., Sperlich, M. *et al*. (2009) Prevalence, trauma history, and risk for posttraumatic stress disorder among nulliparous women in maternity care. *Obstetrics and Gynaecology*, **114**, 839–847.
27. Engle, P.L., Black, M.M. and Behrman, J.R. (2007) Strategies to avoid the loss of developmental potential in more than 200 million children in the developing world. *Lancet*, **369**, 229–242.
28. Silove, D. and Zwi, A.B. (2005) Translating compassion into psychosocial aid after the tsunami. *Lancet*, **365**, 269–271.
29. ISTSS (International Society Traumatic Stress Studies) (2000) Guidelines for Treatment of PTSD. *Journal of Traumatic Stress*, **13**, 539–588.
30. Darves-Bornoz, J.M., Alonso, J., de Girolamo, G. *et al*. (2008) Main traumatic events in Europe: PTSD in the European study of the epidemiology of mental disorders survey. *Journal of Traumatic Stress*, **21**, 455–462.
31. Creamer, M., Burgess, P. and McFarlane, A.C. (2001) Post-traumatic stress disorder: findings from the Australian National Survey of Mental Health and Well-being. *Psychological Medicine*, **31**, 1237–1247.
32. Kessler, R.C., Sonnega, A., Bromet, E. *et al*. (1995) Posttraumatic stress disorder in the National Comorbidity Survey. *Archives of General Psychiatry*, **52**, 1048–1060.
33. Wittchen, H. and Pfister, H. (eds) (1997) *DIA-X-Interview: Manual für Screening-Verfahren und Interview; Interviewheft Längsschnittuntersuchung (DIA-X-Lifetime); Ergänzungsheft (DIA-X- Lifetime); Interviewheft Querschnittuntersuchung (DIA-X-12 Monate); Ergänzungsheft (DIA-X-12 Monate); PC-Programm zur Durchführung des Interviews (Längs- und Querschnittuntersuchung); Auswertungsprogramm*, Sweets & Zeitlinger, Frankfurt.
34. Rupp, A. and Sorel, E. (2001) Economic models, in *The Mental Health Consequences of Torture* (eds E. Gerrity *et al*.), Kluwer Academic Publishers, New York.
35. Kastrup, M. and Arcel, L. (2004) Gender specific treatment of refugees with PTSD, in *Broken Spirits The Treatment of Traumatized Asylum Seekers Refugees War and Torture Victims* (eds J. Wilson and B. Drozdek), Brunner and Routledge, New York.
36. Thulesius, H. and Håkansson, A. (1999) Screening for posttraumatic stress disorder symptoms among Bosnian refugees. *Journal of Traumatic Stress*, **12**, 167–174.
37. Cheung, P. (1994) Posttraumatic stress disorder among Cambodian refugees in New Zealand. *International Journal of Social Psychiatry*, **40**, 17–26.
38. Reppesgaard, H. (1997) Studies on psychosocial problems among displaced people in Sri Lanka. *European Journal of Psychiatry*, **11**, 223–234.
39. Ai, A.L., Peterson, C. and Ubelhor, D. (2002) War-related trauma and symptoms of posttraumatic stress disorder among adult Kosovar refugees. *Journal of Traumatic Stress*, **15**, 157–160.
40. Matthey, S., Silove, D.M., Barnett, B. *et al*. (1999) Correlates of depression and PTSD in Cambodian women with young children: a pilot study. *Stress Medicine*, **15**, 103–107.
41. Spasojevic, J., Heffer, R.W. and Snyder, D.K. (2000) Effects of posttraumatic stress and acculturation on marital functioning in Bosnian refugee couples. *Journal of Traumatic Stress*, **13**, 205–217.

42. WHO (2005) Mental health: facing the challenges, building solutions. Report WHO European Ministerial Conference WHO.
43. Kastrup, M. and Niaz, U. (2009) The impact of culture on women's mental health, in *Contemporary Topics in Womens Mental Health* (eds P. Chandra *et al.*), John Wiley & Sons, Ltd, Chichester.
44. Patel, V. (2005) Gender in Mental Health Research, WHO, Geneva.
45. Ekblad, S., Kastrup, M., Eisenman, D. and Arcel, L. (2007) Interpersonal violence towards women: an overview and clinical direstions, in *Immigrant Medicine Philadelphia* (eds P. Walker and E. Barnett), Elsevier, Saunders.

CHAPTER 3

Neurobiology of PTSD

Arieh Y. Shalev,[1] Asaf Gilboa[2] and Ann M. Rasmusson[3]

[1] *Department of Psychiatry, Hadassah University Hospital, Jerusalem, Israel*
[2] *The Rotman Research Institute, Baycrest Centre, Toronto, ON, Canada*
[3] *Women's Health Sciences Division, National Center for PTSD, VA Boston Healthcare System; Boston University School of Medicine, Boston, MA, USA*

INTRODUCTION

From 'black box' tradition to sophisticated neuroscience

Well before the delineation of post-traumatic stress disorder (PTSD) by the Diagnostic and Statistical Manual III (DSM-III) (1980), debilitating combat stress reactions received the name 'physioneuroses' [1] because they consisted of bodily 'alarm' responses to reminders of stressful events. Studying physiological responses to reminders in Vietnam combat veterans, Kolb and Multipassi [2] equated PTSD with a 'conditioned emotional response' similar to those observed in animal experiments of fear conditioning. Kolb [3] further suggested that PTSD involves *permanent neuronal changes leading to impaired learning, habituation and stimulus discrimination*. Psychophysiological studies (reviewed by Orr [4]) established the universality of elevated physiological responses to trauma reminders and startling tones. Other studies uncovered and buttressed the association between PTSD and elevated heart-rate responses to the traumatic event itself (e.g. [5, 6]) – a surrogate of the full panoply of unconditioned responses.

From these modest technological beginnings (at a time when the brain was considered a 'black box' which only peripheral input and output measures could fathom) the exploration of PTSD has exploited every technical innovation in neuroscience. To cite but a few, current studies of PTSD use structural and functional brain imaging, advanced neuroendocrine challenges, gene-expression profiling and epigenetic gene-transcription recording. Inspired by the construct

Post-traumatic Stress Disorder, First Edition. Edited by Dan Stein, Matthew Friedman, and Carlos Blanco.

of traumatic stress, animal experiments of emotional learning and its regulation continue to provide fruitful analogies to human PTSD.

Notwithstanding their novelty, recent neurobiological studies remain focused on the same basic features of PTSD: the acquisition and maintenance of maladaptive responses resembling fear conditioning, and the emergence of hyperarousal, threat-biased perception and memory disturbances after trauma exposure. Effective psychological therapies have demonstrated the importance of 'top-down' brain processes in the acquisition, maintenance and treatment of the disorder, rightfully placing PTSD at the junction of external reality and a responsive brain: a bad outcome of a perverted host–environment interaction.

It is virtually impossible to do justice to the hundreds of published neurobiological studies of PTSD. One problem involves the different 'levels of analysis' of pertinent studies, which expand from molecular/cellular mechanisms, via brain structures and neural networks, to complex behaviour embedded in an individual and social context. Other difficulties stem from the frequent focus of studies on one regulatory system (e.g. hormonal), from divergent findings within any one system, and from the array of study designs and heterogeneity of study samples.

More than an account of cumulative work, this chapter is an effort to organise knowledge along conceptual lines. These lines, not surprisingly, resemble those outlined decades ago. We thus refer to the following research domains in PTSD: fear conditioning and extinction, neuroendocrine responses, genetic vulnerability, epigenetic regulation, structural functional brain abnormalities and a neural network perspective. To avoid 'laundry lists' of all published studies we have attempted to organise knowledge along relevant aetiopathogenic hypotheses. Thus, rather than 'explaining' PTSD, we hope to provide the reader with a framework for evaluating current and forthcoming neurobiological *knowledge about PTSD*.

Complexity and heterogeneity

To be diagnosed with PTSD, an individual must have experienced a traumatic event that posed a perceived threat to life or physical integrity, followed by the development of sustained reexperiencing, hyperarousal and avoidance symptoms of sufficient frequency and intensity [7]. The precise composition and severity of these symptoms vary among individuals with PTSD, but the disorder's symptom structure has been shown to be stable across samples, traumatic conditions and time-lags from the triggering trauma.

In contrast, several neurobiological perturbations have been associated with PTSD, but none has proven to be characteristic of the disorder for all individuals, or across different populations. Such variability may reflect variations in the underlying neurobiological perturbations (e.g. [8, 9]), thereby making PTSD the end result of several redundant and confluent disturbances.

For this reason, it is important to take a step back and reconsider how can deep neurobiological perturbations map on to higher-level changes in brain function expressed as symptoms characteristic of PTSD. Such mapping is reciprocal: deeper neurobiological components influence higher brain function and attendant thoughts, feelings and behaviours – while higher brain function and attendant thoughts, feelings and behaviours, in turn, influence changes in the deeper neurological layers.

This chapter considers both deep system neurochemical factors and emergent patterns of higher brain function. It emphasises the *complexities* and the *ultimate equilibrium* (adaptive or maladaptive) that neurobiological systems reach when the individual either recovers from early symptoms or continues to suffer from persisting, tenacious PTSD. The neural systems that govern the development of PTSD are inherently redundant and simultaneously synergetic *and* controlling, hence we emphasise interactions among them, rather than any one predominant component.

FEAR CONDITIONING AND EXTINCTION

Extensive animal and human research allows us to construct a reasonable model of dynamic central nervous system (CNS) processing of threat that informs studies of PTSD in humans. The core components of this model, namely *fear conditioning* and *extinction*, involve normal learning processes. A close examination of the mechanisms underlying these processes suggests that both real threat and contextual cues are key sensory elements incorporated into the neurocircuitry, subserving adaptive as well as maladaptive responses to traumatic experiences. An update on the mechanisms of fear conditioning and extinction is thus provided below.

Unconditioned defence responses and the acquisition of conditioned emotional responses

During exposure to extreme threat, previously neutral stimuli overlapping in time with unconditioned threat stimuli (US) pass through the thalamus to impinge on glutamatergic projection neurons of the basolateral nucleus of the amygdala (BLA). The BLA projection neurons, in turn, activate γ-amino butyric acid (GABA)-containing inhibitory interneurons located either in the intercalated cell mass between the BLA and the central nucleus (CE) of the amygdala or in the capsule of the CE. These interneurons impinge on GABA- and peptide-containing projection neurons of the CE to enable defensive responding [10]. A subset of CE projection neurons are also directly activated by unconditioned stress stimuli thought to be routed through downstream sources such as the pontine parabrachial nucleus (PB) [10, 11]. The net effects of the combined BLA-to-CE and direct-CE stimulation are to: (i) *induce an association between the US and previously neutral stimuli (now termed conditioned stimuli or CS)* at the single neuronal level within the BLA via long-term potentiation (LTP) [12]; and (ii) *activate the species-specific defence response (SSDR – see below)*.

Consequently, subsequent exposure to the CS alone can activate BLA projection neurons and the SSDR. Importantly, the balance between direct excitatory and indirect inhibitory inputs to the CE is thought to influence the nature of the SSDR [10], with sympathetic system activation prevailing during the initial unconditioned stress when both BLA-to-CE and direct-CE inputs are activated, and a mix of parasympathetic and sympathetic responses occurring during conditioned stress when inputs to the CE from the BLA prevail.

Importantly, both activation of the SSDR and the formation of conditioned associations between the US and CS can be restrained by glutamatergic inputs from the prefrontal cortex (PFC) to GABAergic interneurons of the BLA that, in turn, restrain BLA glutamatergic projection neurons [13]. Thus, a balance between the intensity of the US and the capacity of the PFC to integrate updated information with regard to potential threat and then counter the effects of the US within the amygdala may influence both risk for PTSD development and PTSD recovery. Neurotransmitter and neurohormone mechanisms affecting these critical interactions are discussed below.

The species-specific defence response (SSDR)

As noted above, the highly conserved mammalian SSDR, coordinated by the amygdala, includes sympathetic and parasympathetic system activation, as well as cardiovascular and respiratory reactions, activation of the hypothalamic–pituitary–adrenal (HPA) axis, defensive fight, flight and freezing behaviours, and changes in information processing [14]. The magnitude of the SSDR is modulated, in large part, by activation of brainstem monoaminergic neuronal cell bodies located in the ventral tegmental area (VTA), dorsal and median raphe nuclei, and locus coeruleus (LC) (reviewed by LeDoux [15]). Raphe serotonergic (5-HT) neurons and noradrenergic neurons from the LC project diffusely throughout the brain, while VTA dopaminergic neurons project to key limbic brain regions such as the PFC, amygdala and the shell of the nucleus accumbens (NA) and release dopamine (DA) in direct proportion to the intensity of incoming stress stimuli [16, 17]. These monoamine responses: (i) *influence the magnitude of unconditioned stress responses* by modulating PFC and amygdala excitability, as well as the function of downstream effectors; and (ii) *facilitate consolidation of US–CS associations*. The balance of neurotransmitters and neuromodulators activated during unconditioned responding also influences the extent to which contextual stimuli, more loosely associated in time with the US, may acquire affective salience and contribute to later overgeneralisation of threat stimuli (see below).

Monoaminergic modulation of prefrontal and amygdala responding

At the PFC

During stress, changing levels of monoamines in the PFC influence its function via concentration-dependent activation of monoamine receptors with different ligand affinities. Specifically, moderate levels of norepinephrine (NE) activate high-affinity noradrenergic α_2 receptors that enhance working memory, while higher NE levels engage low-affinity α_1 receptors that impair PFC function (Figures 3.1 and 3.2). High levels of DA and serotonin acting at DA_1 and $5\text{-}HT_{2A}$ receptors, respectively, have similar deleterious effects on PFC function (reviewed in [18]). As discussed above, glutamatergic pyramidal output neurons from the PFC tonically activate inhibitory interneurons within the BLA, which in turn suppress BLA outputs to the CE. Therefore, *during intense stress, interference with PFC pyramidal output to the amygdala by rising monoamine levels will promote expression of the amygdala-mediated SSDR*.

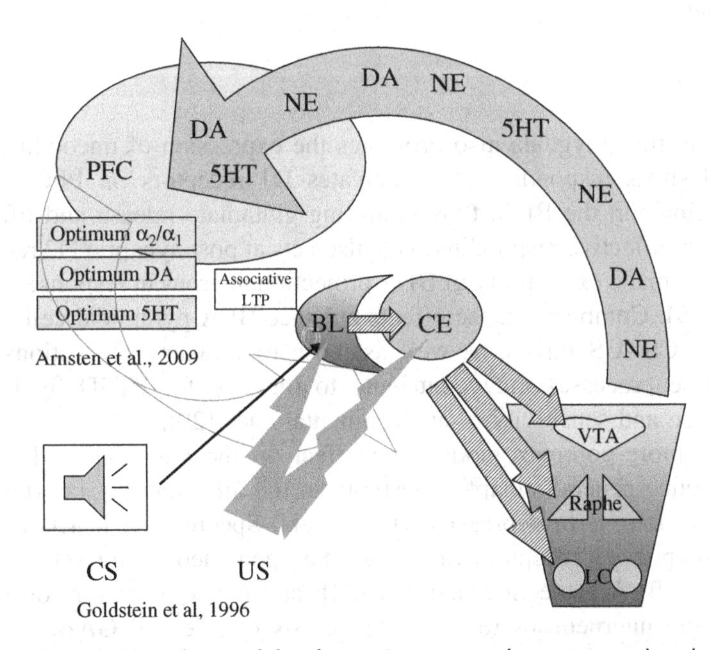

Figure 3.1 Processing of stressful information at moderate stress levels: moderate levels of monoamines and activation of high-affinity noradrenergic α_2 receptors enhance prefrontal cortex-mediated working memory and inhibition of amygdala reactivity.

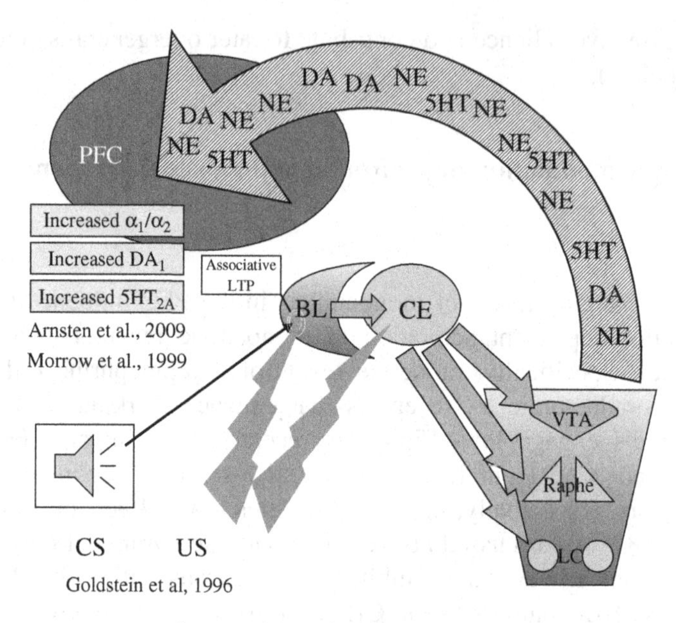

Figure 3.2 Processing of stressful information at high levels of stress: high monoamine levels and activation of low-affinity noradrenergic α_1 receptors impair prefrontal cortex-mediated working memory and lift prefrontal cortical inhibition of the amygdala.

In the amygdala

DA release in the amygdala also promotes the expression of unconditioned and conditioned stress responding. DA activates D1 receptors on PFC projection neuron terminals in the BLA, thus inhibiting glutamate release and lifting PFC suppression of affective responding. DA also acts at post-synaptic D2 receptors to increase the somatic excitability of BLA projection neurons in response to sensory inputs [13, 19]. Combined, these effects enhance BLA pyramidal cell responses to combined CS–US inputs, as well as those to weaker, adventitious sensory stimuli. These processes may contribute to the risk for PTSD by increasing hypervigilance and sensitivity to environmental cues [20].

NE has a more complex modulating effect on the amygdala. NE has been shown to reduce general synaptic plasticity in the amygdala by interfering with both LTP and long-term depression (LTD) [21]. Specifically, it acts at: (i) pre- and post-synaptic α_2 receptors to reduce the spontaneous and sensory-evoked excitability of BLA projection neurons [22]; and (ii) α_1 receptors on terminals of GABAergic interneurons to facilitate GABA release and $GABA_A$ receptor-mediated inhibition of BLA projection neurons [23]. In contrast, the spontaneous activity of a small subpopulation of BLA projection neurons is dramatically increased by activation of noradrenergic β-receptors. Together, these effects may increase a signal-to-noise ratio as follows [22]: *the primarily inhibitory effects of NE in the BLA can suppress activity within amygdalar circuits in which fear conditioning has not taken place, while its more restricted excitatory effects can enhance US–CS pairing.*

Finally, the monoaminergic effects are further modulated by neuroactive steroids and neuropeptides released by the adrenal gland during stress – a complement subject to significant interindividual variability. This could further magnify, mitigate or otherwise shape the nature of the SSDR, as well as the capacity for reintegrating and maintaining PFC modulatory capacities during fear extinction and recall.

Conditioned stress, extinction and extinction recall

Chronic stress and fear conditioning are accompanied by diminished GABA-mediated neurotransmission within the amygdala [24], as expressed by a decrease in α_1-stimulated GABA release from the terminals of interneurons within the BLA [23], as well as by downregulation of gephyrin (a protein that anchors synaptic $GABA_A$ receptors), synaptic $GABA_A$ receptors themselves, and expression of genes for GABA-synthesising enzymes [25, 26]. This decrease in GABAergic transmission could facilitate the conditioned activation of BLA projection neurons by CS in the absence of the US and promote sensitivity to newly encountered US.

Extinction involves a progressive reduction in the magnitude of the SSDR upon repeated exposure to CS without US. Notably, extinction does not involve a loss in the CS–US association or memory per se, but rather the introduction of *active inhibition of different components of the conditioned fear circuit*. Within the amygdala, GABA transmission is restored during extinction [26, 27] and could progressively restrain CE activation of monoamine input to the PFC, thus allowing PFC suppression of BLA projection neurons to be restored. As demonstrated by Milad and Quirk [28], PFC inhibitory input to the BLA is restored during extinction and is thereafter essential for *recall* of extinction. Reintegration of PFC inhibitory input to BLA has been shown to be subject to consolidation, requiring NMDA (*N*-methyl-D-aspartate) receptor-mediated bursting of ventromedial prefrontal cortex (vmPFC) neurons and protein synthesis [29, 30]; it is dependent on PFC DA D_4 receptor activation [31] and is enhanced by noradrenergic β-receptor activation [32]. Finally, PFC convergent information, such as contextual information from the hippocampus, is required to determine the circumstances under which the extinction of fear should be recalled [33]. Thus, it is possible to envision numerous pathophysiological factors with relevance to mechanisms that could interfere with extinction and contribute to PTSD.

For example, numerous studies have shown that chronic stress affects amygdala, PFC and hippocampal function in a manner that would increase PTSD risk. Chronic cold stress has been shown to sensitise CE and BLA neurons to excitation by foot shock [34], shift noradrenergic effects on spontaneous activity of BLA neurons from inhibitory to excitatory, facilitate BLA neuronal responses to hippocampal and sensory cortical inputs [22] and impair noradrenergic α^1 receptor-mediated facilitation of GABAergic transmission in the BLA [23]. This suggests that chronic stress may increase the risk for PTSD by *reducing the signal-to-noise ratio of sensory inputs tightly associated with the US while increasing responding to adventitious contextual stimuli, which would contribute to threat generalisation*.

As reviewed by Arnsten [35], chronic stress also compromises PFC function, with even brief chronic stress resulting in dendritic atrophy in PFC layers subserving working memory and attentional set-shifting, while dendrites of pyramidal cells in infralimbic areas that project directly to the amygdala are preserved. In addition, chronic stress interferes with the plasticity of hippocampal–PFC circuits likely needed to update the appropriateness of context-specific defensive responding [36]. The combined effects of high glucocorticoid and catecholamine responses experienced during acute and chronic stress have been shown to mediate these changes in neuronal structure [35]. This may help explain the significant contribution of stressors that follow the traumatic event to the likelihood of developing chronic PTSD [37].

Summary and clinical implications

Functionally mild stress increases arousal and enhances PFC function, thereby sustaining the PFC's tonic inhibition of the amygdala and creating a state in which finely discriminated sensory characteristics of the threat and threat environment remain available for decision-making. Consequently, spatiotemporal relationships among the sensory inputs can be integrated and compared with prior experience, allowing executive control over defensive behaviour as well as revision of experiential probabilities within plastic hippocampal circuits.

Stress exceeding a given threshold may, in contrast, lead to deactivation of PFC modulation of the amygdala [18] and thereby promote the expression of the full SSDR. Under severe stress, previously neutral cues that temporally overlap with incoming unconditioned threat cues become consolidated within amygdalar circuits, while less immediately relevant contextual details, as well as experiential and probability information relevant to the threat, remain unavailable for modulation of behavioural reactions.

Because the cytoarchitectonic structure of the BLA (which is part of the paleocortex – see below) limits its processing power, the BLA may only respond to broad differences in the frequency and amplitude of incoming stimuli. This may account for the precipitous and 'all-or-none' qualities of defensive reactions experienced during traumatic stress and in PTSD. The restriction of false-negative error in the prediction of threat by the amygdala may be protective because it creates a bias towards recruitment of alarm responses: neither context, nor probability, nor discrimination of fine detail are relevant to survival in the face of a sudden, unexpected and potentially lethal event.

In the aftermath of traumatic stress experiences, context and probability, as well as a capacity to discriminate details that bear on the reality of threat, are critical for successful readjustment. When inputs from the PFC and hippocampus are compromised during attempts at extinction (e.g. by continuous stress, absence of soothing contacts, mild traumatic brain injury or agents that heighten monoaminergic tone or diminish GABAergic tone such as nicotine, alcohol or hypnotic drugs [38]) extinction may fail. Interventions that facilitate activation and early engagement of the PFC and hippocampus during reexposure to conditioned cues may facilitate extinction and functional recovery from traumatic experiences.

NEUROENDOCRINE MODULATION OF CONDITIONED STRESS RESPONSES

The HPA axis and sympathetic nervous system are important stress-reactive systems. They contribute to brain information processing, energy regulation, immune defences and behaviour in response to threat. Research in PTSD has identified a number of neuroendocrine factors that appear to influence the risk for PTSD development and recovery. Many of these factors concern organ systems (e.g. brain, the peripheral nervous system, the adrenal gland, the reproductive organs) and interact at a number of levels, promoting or deterring each other and influencing the generation of other stress-responsive factors. This section will discuss the complex interactions among these broad-impact neuromodulatory factors, as they are relevant to the dynamic processing of threat by the brain and to PTSD.

Neuropeptide Y (NPY)

There is ample research demonstrating the beneficial effects of neuropeptide Y (NPY) on psychological and behavioural responses to stress. NPY activation of amygdalar NPY-Y_1 receptors (Y_1Rs) has been shown to exert anxiolytic and anticonflict effects in numerous animal models [39–44]. NPY stimulates neurogenesis in the hippocampus and subventricular zone of the brain, and in this way may support recovery from stress [45, 46]. In humans, NPY gene variants associated with increased NPY expression have been associated with reduced trait anxiety and reduced activation of the amygdala in response to emotionally provocative stimuli [47]. Higher plasma NPY levels achieved by male military personnel during intensely stressful training procedures were associated with less dissociation and emotional distress, as well as superior performance reliant on adequate prefrontal cortical function [48, 49]. Higher baseline plasma NPY levels and greater NPY release in response to the intravenous administration of the noradrenergic α_2 receptor antagonist yohimbine have been associated with reduced PTSD symptoms in combat-exposed veterans [50, 51]. Higher baseline plasma NPY levels have also been associated retrospectively with greater improvement in PTSD symptoms over time [52].

NPY also restores homeostasis and contributes to general recovery from stress over time. At rest, NPY exerts an NPY-Y_2 receptor (Y_2R)-mediated bradycardic effect in the nucleus tractus solitarius [53, 54]. When released during stress, NPY inhibits vagal action at the heart via presynaptic Y_2Rs to facilitate heart-rate increases [55, 56] and acts at Y_1Rs in the vasculature to amplify the effects of NE on blood pressure. However, dipeptidyl peptidase 4 then removes two amino acids from the NPY to produce NPY_{3-36}, a presynaptic Y_2R agonist that returns the firing rate of sympathetic neurons to baseline [57]. The NPY system likewise helps to maintain energy balance and promote recovery from stress-induced energy depletion by facilitating feeding and weight gain through effects in the brainstem [58] and promotion of lipogenesis in the periphery [59]. Finally, NPY has been shown to decrease sleep latency, increase stage 2 sleep and reduce nighttime HPA axis reactivity in healthy men [60, 61].

Alterations in NPY system function in response to extreme stress may contribute to the development of PTSD in some individuals

In male veterans and active-duty military personnel, baseline plasma NPY levels correlated negatively with combat exposure and previous exposure to life threat [51, 62], as well as NE reactivity [51, 63]. As previously discussed, elevated NE reactivity may diminish the efficacy of PFC function while facilitating amygdalar reactivity, processes that would contribute to fear conditioning and interfere with extinction [18, 64]. Perturbations in NE and NPY function may also mediate increases in blood-pressure reactivity seen in PTSD. Male combat veterans with PTSD who had reduced resting and stress-activated plasma NPY levels had enhanced and sustained increases in heart rate, blood pressure and NE release in response to sympathetic stimulation [51]. Systolic blood pressure increases were positively correlated with yohimbine-stimulated increases in plasma NPY, but not with NE in the veterans with PTSD, and conversely with increases in NE but not NPY in healthy comparison subjects – a situation that may contribute to ischaemic risk in PTSD since the half-life of NPY is substantially longer than that for NE.

Allopregnanolone/pregnanolone

Cerebrospinal fluid levels of the neuroactive steroids allopregnanolone and its equipotent enantiomer, pregnanolone (collectively termed ALLO), have been found to be low in PTSD and depression and to correlate negatively with PTSD reexperiencing and depression symptoms [8]. These steroids are the most potent and selective positive endogenous modulators of the action of GABA at brain $GABA_A$ receptors [65, 66]. Their effects at extrasynaptic $GABA_A$ receptors maintain a tonic inhibitory conductance that moderates gain in neuronal output during periods of increased excitation [67–69], as during stress. And indeed, a number of studies have shown that acute, physically threatening stress, such as swim stress in rats, increases brain ALLO levels [70, 71]. Multiple studies in animals have demonstrated their potent anxiolytic, sedative and anaesthetic effects [72] and their capacity to provide negative-feedback inhibition of the HPA axis [73]. In addition, allopregnanolone exerts neuroprotective actions, supporting neurogenesis, enhancing myelination [74] and reducing apoptosis and inflammation [75]. Experimental reduction of brain ALLO in rodents has been shown to increase anxious, aggressive and depressive behaviours [76], and to enhance contextual fear conditioning [77]. Low CNS levels of ALLO in persons with PTSD would also be expected, like low baseline NPY levels, to enhance sympathetic and HPA axis reactivity during stress. Studies are therefore currently underway to determine whether deficient activity of 3α-HSD (hydroxysteroid dehydrogenase) or dysfunction at other points in the synthetic pathway for ALLO production occur in humans. Such deficits may not only contribute to the risk for PTSD but could also explain the limited therapeutic effects of serotonin-selective reuptake inhibitors, which have been proposed to work in conditions like PTSD by enhancing allopregnanolone production [78].

Dehydroepiandrosterone (DHEA)

Dehydroepiandrosterone (DHEA), the immediate precursor for androgen synthesis, is secreted from the adrenal gland episodically and synchronously with cortisol in response to fluctuating adrenocorticotrophic hormone (ACTH) levels [79]. DHEA and its sulfated metabolite DHEAS, collectively termed DHEA(S), are detectable in the brain. However, peripherally derived DHEA is thought to be the source of brain DHEA(S) in humans [80]. As previously reviewed [81], DHEA(S) antagonises $GABA_A$ receptors and facilitates NMDA receptor function. It also protects against excitatory amino acid- and oxidative stress-induced neuronal damage, restores cortisol-induced decrements in LTP, regulates programmed cell death and promotes neurogenesis in the hippocampus. DHEA also enhances the activity of 11β-HSD 2 [82], which converts cortisol to the inactive glucocorticoid, cortisone.

Studies suggest that DHEA(S) is beneficial to humans; an increasing DHEA(S) level under stress appears to confer psychological and neurocognitive resilience and may protect against negative health outcomes. For example, in premenopausal women with PTSD, increased DHEA responses to ACTH were associated with lower PTSD symptoms. Gill *et al.* [9], however, found lower morning cortisol and higher DHEA : cortisol ratios in women with PTSD compared to trauma-exposed and unexposed healthy controls, but the lower DHEA levels were present in patients with comorbid PTSD/major depressive disorder (MDD).

There are similar findings in males. In a study of refugees from Kosovo, increasing DHEAS levels over time were associated with the development of PTSD without MDD, while lower DHEAS levels were associated with PTSD/MDD [83]. Increased morning plasma DHEAS levels were seen in male combat veterans with PTSD compared to those without PTSD [84], and in male combat veterans with lifetime PTSD compared to those without [85]. In the group with lifetime PTSD, higher plasma DHEAS levels were associated with greater improvements in PTSD symptoms over time. In healthy male military personnel, higher DHEAS : cortisol ratios at the peak of intense survival training predicted fewer dissociative symptoms and better military performance [86]. Higher DHEAS levels before and immediately after intense training stress in navy divers predicted better navigation skills that depended upon optimum hippocampus and frontal lobe function [87].

DHEA administration studies also suggest that DHEA contributes to mental and physical health. Subchronic DHEA administration enhances peak ACTH and cortisol responses to psychological stress and exercise without lengthening the time to return to baseline [88, 89]. Chronic low-dose DHEA reduces baseline cortisol levels and increases allopregnanolone levels in humans [90, 91]; it also reduces negative mood and depression, including among patients refractory to standard antidepressants [92, 93].

Cortisol

Given the critical role of cortisol in responses to extreme stress, researchers have extensively studied cortisol regulation in PTSD. A pattern of low cortisol output and/or increased sensitivity to glucocorticoid negative feedback has been seen in some populations with PTSD; other studies, however, have shown increased cortisol levels or output in populations with PTSD or have not shown a difference in cortisol indices between subjects with and without PTSD (reviewed in Yehuda, 2002 [94]; Rasmusson *et al*., 2003 [81]; Young and Breslau, 2004 [95]; Meewisse *et al*., 2007 [96]; Handwerger, 2009 [97]). Of note, a *large prospective* study of an unselected cohort of participants presenting after trauma to an emergency room [98] found no differences in cortisol levels between the groups that did and did not develop chronic PTSD, whether measured in urine, saliva, or blood immediately after the trauma or 10 days, 1 month, or 5 months later.

As previously argued [81], the sources of the variability in the outcome of these studies include different experimental designs, population characteristics such as ethnicity and/or individual genetic endowment, gender, menstrual cycle and the use of pharmacological agents, whether prescribed or unprescribed (such as nicotine and alcohol), that impact HPA axis function and/or cortisol levels.

Thus, cortisol appears to play a mediating role in the pathophysiology of PTSD within a broader neuroendocrine context that may vary from patient to patient. For example, cortisol responses to stress are potentiated by low allopregnanolone levels [71], which may result in increased cortisol reactivity to stressors. On the other hand, cortisol normally upregulates expression of the 3α-HSD gene, which mediates allopregnanolone synthesis [99]. It is thus conceivable that individuals with trait deficiencies in cortisol synthesis and release during stress may not appropriately upregulate allopregnanolone levels. Yehuda and Bierer [100] showed an association between lower cortisol levels in the healthy offspring of Holocaust survivors and PTSD diagnoses among their parents. While this finding has been interpreted as evidence for a possible epigenetic effect of parental PTSD on HPA axis function in the offspring, it may also reflect the direct transmission of a genetic trait that influences cortisol synthesis as well as risk for PTSD, in part through other factors that affect neurotransmission during stress.

When considering the potential for mitigation and potentiation of cortisol effects by other factors at play, as part of the broader neuroendocrine context, it is not surprising at all that one-dimensional comparisons of cortisol levels or responses do not consistently distinguish between individuals with and without PTSD. *Therefore, it is critical that future investigations evaluate the likely roles of cortisol in the pathophysiology of PTSD in the context of its relationships to other relevant neurobiological factors*.

GENETIC CONTRIBUTIONS TO THE RISK OF DEVELOPING PTSD

Genetic vulnerability contributes to the likelihood of developing PTSD upon trauma exposure: a major twin study has shown a significant contribution of inherited factors to PTSD and PTSD symptoms [101]. A reanalyses of the same database [102, 103] reported both specific and additive genetic contribution to PTSD and alcohol and drug dependence and substantial genetic overlap between MDD and PTSD [104]. Despite these reports, PTSD has not been associated with specific polymorphic genes, and the specifics of its eventual inheritance are unknown at this point. Thus, the following discussion mainly addresses the genetics of putative biological risk factors for PTSD.

Gene variants in the *NPY and noradrenergic signaling pathways* have been found to impact physiological processes of relevance to risk for PTSD (e.g. [47,105–107]). Possession of a noradrenergic α_{2C} receptor gene polymorphism ($\alpha_{2C}Del_{322-325}$) has been associated with increases in heart rate, blood pressure, NE release and negative emotional reactions in response to low-dose yohimbine in healthy individuals. These sympathetic system stress reactions would be expected to increase risk for PTSD [108, 109], but whether any of these gene variants do influence risk for PTSD is yet to be examined.

The *BDNF* gene is another compelling candidate for a role in the pathogenesis of PTSD due to its role in synaptic plasticity, neurogenesis and cognition. Soliman *et al*. [109] has shown that the common *BDNF* gene single nucleotide polymorphism (SNP) in which methionine (Met) substitutes for valine (Val) at codon 66 (Val66Met) is associated with slow apprehension of the distinction between neutral and threat cues during conditioning. The human Met carriers also show less activity of the vmPFC and greater activity of the amygdala during extinction.

Numerous other genes have polymorphisms that affect either ACTH or cortisol responses to stress. These include polymorphisms of genes for the μ-opioid receptor, catechol-*O*-methyl-transferase (COMT) and angiotensin I-converting enzyme (ACE-I), the glucocorticoid receptor, the ACTH receptor, and corticotroping releasing factor (CRF) and the CRF receptor.

Gene × environment interactions that affect PTSD risk have been associated with the low-expression allele of the serotonin transporter gene (SLC6A4). In a sample of 589 adult victims of a hurricane, possession of this gene variant increased the risk for PTSD, as well as major depression, by 4.5 times in the context of high hurricane exposure and low social support, after adjusting for sex, age and ancestry [110]. In a group of Rwandan genocide refugees, this SLC6A4 promoter polymorphism was found to increase the risk for PTSD development in the context of relatively low trauma load [111]. In 582 European American and 670 African American individuals, possessing either one or two alleles of the low-expression SLC6A4 promoter polymorphism interacted with adult trauma and childhood adversity to increase the risk for PTSD, especially for those with high rates of both types of trauma exposure [112].

Clearly, the list of genetic polymorphisms with potential influence on the risk for PTSD is incomplete. Nor is it likely that possession of any one of these possible 'fixed' risk factors is determinant. It may take a combination of such factors in the absence of countering protective factors, and in the context of facilitating environmental influences (see below), to increase the risk for development of PTSD. This point is illustrated by work finding an interactive influence on the risk for PTSD in adulthood between childhood trauma and polymorphisms or decreased expression of the FKBP5 gene, which regulates glucocorticoid receptor signaling [113, 114].

EPIGENETIC CONTRIBUTIONS TO THE RISK OF DEVELOPING PTSD

The epigenetic regulation of gene transcription may provide new opportunities for understanding PTSD. Epigenetic effects consist of a coordinated modification of gene promoters and chromatin such that access to the gene by regulatory elements is either enhanced or limited. Methylation of cytosine residues within gene promoters possessing cytosine–guanine dinucleotide repeats (CpG) results in gene silencing. For example, maternal undernutrition has been shown to increase the risk for obesity, insulin resistance, type-2 diabetes and cardiovascular illness, as well as increased defensive behavioural reactivity in adulthood, in part through epigenetically mediated reductions in the expression of the glucocorticoid receptor and 11βHSD-2 genes that promote glucocorticoid hyperreactivity [115]. The NPY gene and genes in the pathway for synthesis of allopregnanolone have promoter-based CpG dinucleotide repeats that may confer susceptibility to transcriptional inactivation by stress, as well as the potential for restoration of function by chromatin remodelling agents such as histone deacetylase inhibitors.

Note that Uddin *et al.* [116] have shown differences between groups of persons with and without PTSD in methylation patterns of DNA in white blood cells. A cluster of unmethylated immune-system function genes characterised PTSD, which otherwise showed a greater number of methylated genes in general. In addition, there were group differences in methylation of the dinucleotide methyl transferase (DNMT) type 3β and 3L genes, which are involved in de novo rather than maintenance methylation, suggesting that specific adaptive epigenetic capacities may themselves be altered in PTSD.

Animal research also supports the potential relevance of epigenetic processes to PTSD. Recent work by Fuchikami *et al.* [117] showed that immobilisation stress in rodents *reduced* expression of *BDNF* gene transcripts I and IV in the hippocampus in association with decreases in the level of histone acetylation of the P1 and P4 promoters. Conversely, Bredy *et al.* [118] showed that extinction of conditioned fear was accompanied by an *increase* in the levels of histone acetylation of the gene promoters for *BDNF* transcripts I and IV in concert with increases in *BDNF* exon I and IV mRNA expression in PFC. *BDNF* gene promoter IV contributes significantly to *activity dependent BDNF* transcription [119]. Together, this work suggests that activation of specific PFC circuits *in combination* with agents that facilitate epigenetic processes which enhance synaptic plasticity and stabilisation of new neuronal circuits may be beneficial in the treatment of PTSD.

This possibility finds support in the work of Bredy *et al.* [120], which showed that valproic acid – a histone deacetylase inhibitor – enhanced fear extinction, but also fear conditioning and reconsolidation, depending on specific adjustments to an otherwise weak extinction paradigm. When seven 'spaced' CS were presented during the extinction session with an intertrial interval (ITI) of 20 minutes, long-term memory for extinction was *enhanced* independent of context. However, when seven 'massed' CS were presented with an ITI of 5 seconds, reconsolidation of the fear memory resulted.

From neurobiology to therapy

We thus suggest that extinction efficiency and recovery from PTSD involve a critical interface between arousal, access to new safety information and coordination of regional brain activity. Characteristics of both external input and internal responses may differentially interact in each trauma-exposed individual. For example, CS intensity and duration can bias extinction in negative and positive directions [120]. Lower glucocorticoid levels enhance LTP in the hippocampus, while higher levels may interfere with it [121].

In line with this view, PTSD patients reporting a moderate, rather than the highest or lowest, level of distress show the greatest reduction in distress in response to prolonged exposure (PE) therapy [122]. In cognitive processing therapy (CPT; [123]) active engagement of PTSD patients in critical evaluation of their trauma-related memories, thoughts and emotions led more rapidly to PTSD symptom reduction than encouraging patients to fully engage the trauma memory and reexperience their peritraumatic emotions before engaging in a critical reappraisal of their traumatic experiences. We submit that frontal lobe-mediated working memory and tonic inhibition of the amygdala may be activated more during critical appraisal, and less so during 'crude' reexperiencing.

Sensitivity to the critical intersection between arousal, access to new information and regional brain activity will also be important when considering new attempts to modulate neuroplasticity pharmacologically or epigenetically in the service of extinction. As reviewed by Pittenger and Duman [124], enhancement of neuroplasticity through any number of pharmacological approaches can have desired antidepressant effects or undesired depressant effects depending on the brain region targeted. On the other hand, the fact that genes that enhance synaptic plasticity and impact arousal, such as promoter 4 of the *BDNF* gene [125] and the Ca^{2+}/ calmodulin-dependent NPY gene promoter [126], are 'activity dependent' suggests that epigenetic and pharmacological interventions could be quite precisely targeted to specific circuits through expert cognitive behaviour interventions.

STRUCTURAL AND FUNCTIONAL NEUROANATOMY

Conceptual framework: ontogenetic and phylogenetic structures

In studying architectonic and stimulation characteristics of the reptilian brain, Dart (1934; cited in [127]) observed a dual-brain structure consisting of a *parapiriform* and a *parahippocampal* subdivision. That duality was later validated in the mammalian neocortex by Abbie (cited in [127]), whose work showed that different cortical cytoarchitectonic fields represent successive evolutionary differentiation waves, independent of either the hippocampus or the piriform cortices. Sanides [128] proposed a similar dual origin of the human neocortex [127].

The piriform and the hippocampal developmental streams share a similar succession of increasing cytoarchitectonic complexity and lamination, starting from allocortex (e.g. in the limbic core) and moving through periallocortical and proisocortical structures to the highly developed six-layered isocortical regions [127,

129, 130]. Figure 3.3 illustrates the two developmental streams and the different cortical types of which they are composed, overlaid on Pandya and Petrides's [131] cytoarchitectonic division.

The *archicortical stream* originates from the hippocampus, passes along the medial aspect of the temporal lobes with periallocortical and proisocortical parahippocampal cortices, then gives rise to structures in the mediodorsal aspects of the parietal and frontal cortex, including the proisocortical posterior cingulate cortex (Brodmann areas (BAs) 31 and 23 posteriorly and 24, 25 and 32 anteriorly), and ultimately to isocortical areas in the dorsomedial and dorsolateral PFC (BA 9, 10, 46 and 8) [130].

The *paleocortical stream* starts in a limbic piriform/amygdala core, and journeys (i) posteriorly along the entire temporal cortex from the proisocortical temporal pole, from where it progressively differentiates as it extends to the caudal section of the temporal gyri, and (ii) anteriorly to the proisocortical regions of the orbital and insular cortices and the isocortical regions of the ventrolateral and lateral orbitofrontal cortex (BAs 8, 10, 11, 12, 14 and 46) [130].

Functionally, the two systems serve two distinct roles in shaping and controlling behaviour. The *dorsal archicortical system* mediates processing of *spatiotemporal and contextual elements in the environment*. The *ventral paleocortical system* mediates the processing of *object identity*, the allocation of *incentive significance* to stimuli and the *motivational components of behaviour*.

Thus, evolutionary brain organisation provides a structural basis for the separate and highly interconnected processing of object identity and contextual information by two cortical systems. Both systems can control behaviour through frontal executive neural networks and both have access to perimotor cortical structures at multiple levels. For example, the dorsal PFC (part of the archicortical system) has extensive connections with supplementary motor/premotor areas and may guide complex behaviours that require temporal structuring and cognitive planning. The ventrolateral motor system may affect behaviour via extensive connections with the amygdala, insular and temporal polar cortices.

Understanding functional neuroanatomy on the basis of phylogenetic and ontogenetic development has great potential for understanding the neural bases of mental disorders. The model has recently been used for understanding schizophrenia and other disorders [132–134]. The following text uses the dual-developmental framework to organise and interpret the abundant neuroimaging literature in PTSD.

Structural brain imaging of PTSD

The first reported structural abnormality in PTSD was a *reduced left hippocampal volume* in Vietnam veterans with PTSD [135]. This finding had been interpreted as reflecting the hippocampus's vulnerability to excessive stress hormone levels

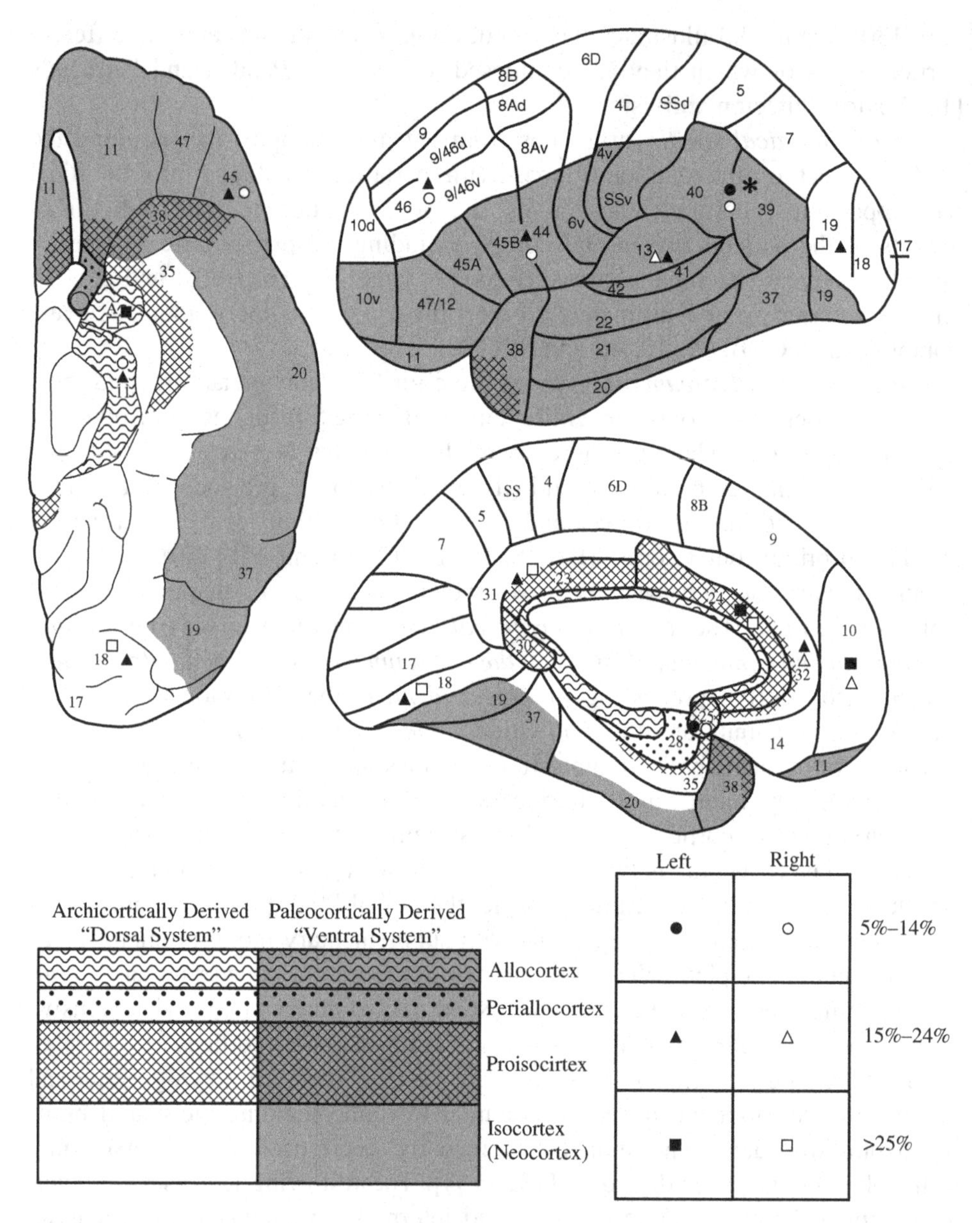

Figure 3.3 Ventral (left), lateral (top right) and medial (bottom right) views of the human brain depicting the evolutionary developmental trends with coding for the archicortical (white) and paleocortical (grey) cortical moieties and the cortical types within each trend (adapted from [134]). Geometrical designs represent the percentage of neuroimaging studies reporting activation differences between PTSD and controls on *emotional/traumatic tasks and stimuli*. Black geometric designs represent left-sided differences and white designs represent right-sided differences. The inferior parietal lobule is marked with * because it is considered a transitional cortex belonging to both developmental trends.

due to prolonged stress [136]. Numerous studies [137–151] subsequently reported either left, right or bilateral hippocampal volume reduction ranging from approximately 5% to a staggering 26%. For comparison, a 40% volume loss reflects a nearly complete loss of hippocampal neurons in adults' acquired amnesia [152], and even lower estimates (20–30%) have been proposed for hippocampal atrophy leading to developmental amnesia [153]. Several studies have failed to replicate this finding [154–159], but recent meta-analyses generally support the existence of reduced hippocampal volume in PTSD [151, 160] – though not its specificity with regard to other mental disorders (e.g. depression and schizophrenia).

The inconsistency between studies may be explained by co-occurring confounders: smaller hippocampal volumes may be related to comorbid depression or alcohol abuse, or may characterise PTSD patients with chronic and severe conditions. For example, in the Gilbertson *et al.* [161] study of monozygotic twins discordant for PTSD, the finding of a smaller hippocampus in PTSD was corroborated when PTSD patients *with the lowest* Clinician Administered PTSD Scale (*CAPS*) symptom *score* (5 out of 17) were removed from the analysis.

Seminal findings of Gilbertson *et al.*'s study were the similarity of hippocampal volumes in PTSD patients and their unaffected co-twins and the significant correlation between hippocampal volumes of unaffected co-twin and PTSD symptom severity in those affected [161]. These findings strongly suggest that smaller hippocampal volume constitutes a vulnerability factor, rather than an acquired attribute of PTSD.

More recent studies report other brain morphometric differences: white matter volume reductions in the corpus callosum [157, 162–165] and grey matter reduction in the amygdale. Studies of reduced grey matter in the insula [166–169] await further confirmation.

The evidence concerning *structural alterations of the amygdala* (e.g. [139, 143, 145, 151, 154–156, 160, 170–178]) is quite weak. Two recent meta-analyses reached somewhat different conclusions. One found that there is overall evidence for smaller left-amygdala volumes in adults with PTSD, but not in paediatric PTSD [160], whereas the other did not find significant volumetric alteration in either population [151].

Several studies have pointed to abnormal structural characteristics in the *anterior cingulate cortex* (*ACC*). PTSD was associated with reduced ACC grey matter volumes compared with controls [168, 177, 179–181] as well as with white matter abnormalities of the cingulum [179]. These reduced volumes may be particularly characteristic of the rostral (BA 32) and subcallosal (BA 25) portions of the ACC, rather than the dorsal ACC [174]. Rostral ACC volume has been found to predict response to cognitive behaviour interventions such that larger volumes were associated with greater symptom reduction [6]. A study of pregenual ACC volumes in monozygotic twins discordant for PTSD suggested that reduced volumes may reflect an acquired trait of PTSD rather than a vulnerability factor [170].

In relation to the dual-developmental trends' frame of reference, structural brain imaging findings in PTSD mainly concern the hippocampus and to some extent the ACC, whereas structural findings in the amygdale and insular cortex are inconsistent. Thus, *there seems to be better evidence for a structural abnormality associated with the dorsal-archicortical than the ventral-paleocortical stream*. The structural deficit affecting the limbic core of the archicortical system (the hippocampus) appears to constitute a risk factor for developing the disorder, whereas further downstream, grey matter reduction in the ACC may represent an acquired trait of PTSD.

Functional brain imaging

Functional neuroimaging studies of PTSD include both resting and activation studies. The latter include symptom provocation, and processing of both emotional and neutral stimuli. Several reviews have been published in recent years [182–189]. For this chapter, we have reviewed 31 neuroimaging studies using emotional stimuli (Table 3.1) and 15 studies that used neutral stimuli or neutral tasks (Table 3.2). We have identified regions that were frequently reported as abnormally activated in PTSD compared with controls and plotted these frequencies on brain cartoons that depict the two developmental trends (Figures 3.3 and 3.4).

Within the limbic core, differences between PTSD and controls have been reported for the amygdala, and less so for the hippocampus. Interestingly, this pattern emerged in both emotional tasks (where one might expect greater differences in amygdale activation) and neutral contrasts.

Outside the limbic core, the vast majority of reported differences in activation between PTSD and controls occur in proisocortical and isocortical territories of the dorsal-archicortical stream. These include regions in the posterior, dorsal and anterior cingulate, occipital and medial prefrontal cortices and dorsolateral PFC. By contrast, relatively few reports exist of differences in activation in ventral-paleocortical regions outside the amygdala. Other regions that seem to be relatively consistently implicated are the bilateral insula and left ventrolateral PFC.

The same overall pattern can be detected for neutral tasks: most abnormal activations appear to occur in the dorsal trend. There are nonetheless several differences: the rostral ACC and subcallosal ACC do not show unique patterns of activity in neutral conditions and only the dorsal ACC appears to be recruited differently in PTSD compared with controls. There is also less consistency across studies, which may reflect the more varied tasks and smaller number of published studies.

Table 3.1 Emotion-related contrasts within studies used for Figure 3.3.

Study	Imaging modality	Contrasts	Brain structures reported to activate differently in PTSD											
			A	H	9/46	40/39	18/19	29/31	Ins 13	44/45	10	25	32	24
Bremner *et al.* [190]	PET	Combat-related slides and sounds vs neutral slides and sounds				RL	R	RL				RL		
Bremner *et al.* [191]	PET	Script-driven imagery of autobiographical events: traumatic vs neutral		R	RL	R	RL	RL		R		R		
[192]	PET	Retrieval of deeply encoded emotional words vs neutral deeply encoded words		L		L	RL	RL			L	RL	RL	
Bremner *et al.* [193]	PET	Emotional stroop vs neutral stroop		R					L				R	
Britton *et al.* [194]	PET	Script-driven imagery of autobiographical events: traumatic vs neutral	L	L					RL				RL	RL
Clark *et al.* [195]	PET	Visuo-verbal target detection: varying vs fixed target conditions			L									
Driessen *et al.* [196]	fMRI	Cued recollection of autobiographical events: traumatic vs negative (nontraumatic)					LR	LR						
Geuze *et al.* [197]	fMRI	Benign temperature vs painful temperatures	R	L					LR					

(*continued overleaf*)

Table 3.1 (*continued*)

Study	Imaging modality	Contrasts	Brain structures reported to activate differently in PTSD											
			A	H	9/46	40/39	18/19	29/31	Ins 13	44/45	10	25	32	24
[198]	PET	Audiotaped script-driven autobiographical imagery: traumatic vs neutral	RL									RL	RL	RL
Hendler *et al.* [199]	fMRI	Backward-masked images of combat vs noncombat content	RL											
Hou *et al.* [200]	fMRI	Traumatic vs neutral pictures								RL				R
Kemp *et al.* [201]	fMRI	Fearful vs neutral faces	RL								RL			
Lanius *et al.* [202]	fMRI	Script-driven imagery of autobiographical traumatic event vs rest					R				RL		RL	
Lanius *et al.* [203]	fMRI	Script-driven imagery of autobiographical traumatic event vs rest					L				R		R	R
Lanius *et al.* [204]	fMRI	1. Script-driven imagery of autobiographical traumatic event vs rest 2. Script-driven imagery of autobiographical sad event vs rest 3. Script-driven imagery of autobiographical anxious event vs rest					RL	L				RL	RL	RL

[205]	fMRI	Script-driven imagery of autobiographical traumatic event vs rest		RL	RL	R	R	L			L	
Lanius *et al*. [206]	fMRI	Script-driven imagery of autobiographical traumatic event vs rest (PTSD with dissociation)				R	R	R	L			
[207]	SPECT	Trauma-related stimuli (combat sounds) vs nonspecific arousing stimuli (white noise)	L									
[208]	PET	Script-driven imagery of autobiographical events: traumatic vs neutral	RL					RL		RL		
[145]	SPECT	Audiotaped script-driven imagery of autobiographical events: traumatic vs neutral								L		
Pardo *et al*. [209]	PET	Script-driven imagery of autobiographical events: fearful vs neutral	R					RL		RL		RL
Protopopescu *et al*. [210]	fMRI	Trauma-related negative words vs neutral words	RL									
Rauch *et al*. [211]	fMRI	Masked fearful faces vs masked happy faces	RL									
Shin *et al*. [212]	PET	Visual mental images of pictures: combat vs neutral	R						L			RL

(*continued overleaf*)

Table 3.1 (*continued*)

Study	Imaging modality	Contrasts	Brain structures reported to activate differently in PTSD											
			A	H	9/46	40/39	18/19	29/31	Ins 13	44/45	10	25	32	24
Shin *et al.* [213]	PET	Audiotaped script-driven autobiographical imagery: traumatic vs neutral			RL		R	RL		L				RL
Shin *et al.* [214]	fMRI	Counting stroop: combat-related vs neutral		L		L	R	R	RL	RL	RL		L	R
[215]	PET	Audiotaped script-driven imagery of autobigraphical events: traumatic vs neutral	L								RL			
[216]	fMRI	Fearful vs happy facial expressions	R					R						RL
Thomaes *et al.* [217]	fMRI	Recognition: false alarms negative vs baseline		L										
[218]	PET	Trauma-related smells vs nontraumatic smells	RL		RL				RL		RL			RL
Whalley *et al.* [219]	fMRI	Emotional vs neutral hits		L				L						
Zubieta *et al.* [220]	SPECT	Combat sounds vs white noise									RL			

Table 3.2 Neutral contrasts within studies used for Figure 3.4.

Study	Imaging modality	Contrasts	Brain structures reported to activate differently in PTSD											
			A	H	9/46	40/39	18/19	29/31	Ins 13	44/45	10	25	32	24
Astur *et al.* [221]	fMRI	Virtual Morris Water Task: cued-navigation to a hidden ball vs navigation to a visible ball		R										
[140]	PET	Encoding of auditory paragraph vs control condition (counting 'd's in the paragraph)		L			R			RL	R			R
Bremner *et al.* [193]	PET	Neutral stroop vs control stimulus				R	R							
Bryant *et al.* [222]	fMRI	Target tones vs nontarget tones (oddball paradigm)	RL		RL	L								RL
Chung *et al.* [223]	SPECT	Rest	L	RL										L
Hendler *et al.* [199]	fMRI	Masked noncombat images	L											
[195]	fMRI	Script-driven imagery of autobiographical neutral event vs rest				L					R			
Lanius *et al.* [206]	fMRI	Script-driven imagery of autobiographical neutral event vs rest. (PTSD with dissociation)											R	RL
Qingling *et al.* [224]	fMRI	Rest	RL				RL		RL		RL			RL

(*continued overleaf*)

Table 3.2 (*continued*)

Study	Imaging modality	Contrasts	Brain structures reported to activate differently in PTSD											
			A	H	9/46	40/39	18/19	29/31	Ins 13	44/45	10	25	32	24
Sachinvala *et al*. [225]	SPECT	Rest		L		L		RL						RL
Semple *et al*. [226]	PET	Auditory continuous performance task (tone volume discrimination) vs rest				RL								
Semple *et al*. [227]	PET	Rest vs auditiory continuous performance task	R											RL
Shaw *et al*. [228]	PET	Neutral target words detection: varying vs fixed target conditions				RL								
[229]	PET	Recollection of neutral deeply vs neutral shallowly encoded words		RL										
Werner *et al*. [230]	fMRI	1. Encoding face-profession pairs (target stimuli) vs watching face stimuli (control stimuli) 2. Retrieval of the matching-face profession vs control task		RL	RL	RL	RL							L
Whalley *et al*. [219]	fMRI	Old vs new items recognition	L				R		RL					
Yehuda *et al*. [100]	PET	HCORT vs placebo	RL	R										

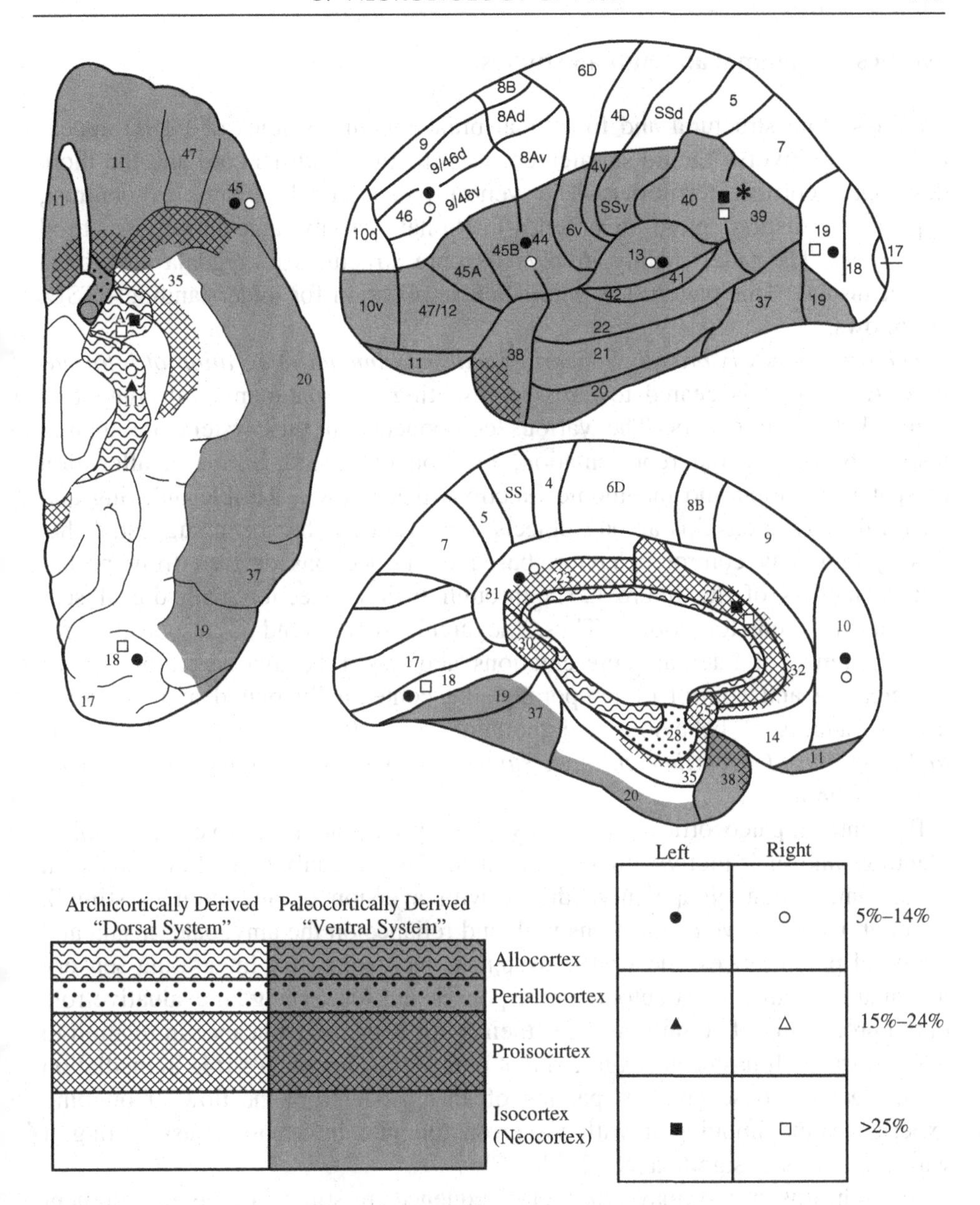

Figure 3.4 Ventral (left), lateral (top right) and medial (bottom right) brain representation identical to Figure 3.3 except that geometrical designs represent the percentage of neuroimaging studies reporting activation differences between PTSD and controls on neutral tasks and stimuli.

Synthesis of animal and human studies

Findings from structural and functional brain imaging studies of PTSD appear to primarily involve the dorsal-archicortical stream – both its core and the more developed cortical territories. The ventral-paleocortical stream, in contrast, appears to display more divergent functional activity and fewer structural alterations. The latter mainly involve its core structures (amygdala and to an extent insula). This pattern has significant implication for understanding PTSD, as follows:

The archicortex is broadly concerned with multimodal integration of information. As such it is geared towards representing the spatiotemporal context in which behaviour occurs. The various components of this system are mainly responsible for spatial representation, location of objects in space, allocation of spatial attention and mnemonic functions that allow a flexible indexing and retrieval of relationships among objects and events. It has been suggested that this system may control behavior, based on projections derived from probabilistic models of the future [231] through their connection with dorsal sectors of the premotor cortex. Thus, the archicortical trend is responsible for the coherence of internal representations and motor behaviours, allowing for the creation and control of temporally and contextually bound and internally driven patterns of behaviour and thought. *They allow for directed behaviour to be organised over time through support of working memory and extended planning processes*.

By contrast, paleocortically derived ventral systems are tuned to external object identities and their motivational significance. They broadly serve functions such as the integration of appetitive drives with aversion or attraction to stimuli. Through its extensive connections with and reliance on the amygdale, insula and temporal pole cortices, the ventral system is well suited for integrating sensory information with viscera-autonomic responses and for serving an evaluative role in the processing of stimuli vis-à-vis their motivational significance in relation to internal states. It has been suggested that part of the amygdala's role in mediation of the fear response involves parsing of an episode from the flow of ongoing experience and imbuing it with viscero-autonomic information, associating it with motivational significance [232].

As such, this system may link motor sequences to stimuli in the environment in a responsive, segmented way [231]. Although such characteristics appear to dominate the behaviour of patients with PTSD, it is interesting to note that aberrations of the ventral system both functionally and structurally are less consistently reported than those associated with the dorsal system. Moreover, there are indications that dorsal-system abnormalities may constitute a risk factor for developing the disorder both structurally, as reflected by hippocampal volume [161], and functionally, as reflected by processing of spatial information [233] and visuospatial memory [234].

Thus, one may cautiously hypothesise that if a primary deficit exists in PTSD, it may be related to decreased ability to organise information and process it in a coherent and contextually bound manner. Observations of hyperactive amygdale may represent the normal function of this structure under conditions in which the archicortical moiety fails to perform its function either during stress or more chronically, but does not constitute a risk factor for developing the disorder [235].

A critical issue for current neurofunctional models of PTSD is the extent and type of involvement of the *prefrontal cortical areas* in the evolution and maintenance of the disorder. As described earlier, the canonical view emphasises the role of medial aspects of the PFC in extinction of conditioned fear. This idea has been inspired by elegant lesion and electrophysiological works in the rat that have demonstrated that the infralimbic cortex in the rat is critical for extinction learning [28, 236]. Findings of hypoactivation of the medial PFC in patients with PTSD have been interpreted as reflecting such failed extinction processes [183, 188, 189, 237, 238]. However, we believe the underlying analogies between animal and human research should be viewed with great caution, as follows:

1. The primate cortical regions that are homologous with the rat infralimbic cortex are obscure. Some have convincingly argued that both subcallosal ACC (BA 25) and rostral ACC (BA 32) in the primate and by extension in humans are homologous to the rat infralimbic cortex [237], whereas others have restricted that homology to the more ventral and orbitofrontal parts of the primate brain [239]. Even if one take the more liberal interpretation of these regions and includes both areas 25 and 32, still fewer than 40% of studies in fact show abnormal activity in these regions, and some of these show hyper rather than hypo activations.
2. Abnormal activations in areas that are considered homologous to the prelimbic region in rats (dorsomedial and dorsolateral PFC) are just as common, if not more so, than that reported for areas 32 and 25. In many studies which report medial prefrontal hypoactivations the centre of activation is more rostral and dorsal, extending well beyond the proisocortical territory of the archicortical stream and into isocortical regions in BAs 9 and 10 [237]. Opposite effects are reported in the rat with regard to prelimbic–amygdala interactions and their effect on extinction.
3. The relationship between imaging and electrophysiological findings in animals is less than straightforward, due to the very different timescale and the unclear relationship between cellular inhibition, excitation and hyper- or hypoactivation in neuroimaging. For example, both inhibitory and excitatory activity at the cellular level might appear as increases in activity in neuroimaging.
4. Most importantly, in human imaging studies, although extinction-related activity has been demonstrated in area 25 [240], it has also been shown that more complex processes associated with emotion regulation (involving dorsal/dorsolateral aspects of the PFC) critically mediate the contribution of these

lower-level mechanisms [241, 242]. Failure of emotional regulation processes, associated with deficient dorsal-stream connectivity, might be as critical a component in the evolution and persistence of PTSD as failed extinction.

Connectivity patterns

One way to understand the inconsistencies in brain imaging findings in PTSD is to think of the different neuroanatomical sites as parts of a functional network. The term 'network' is often used in imaging studies. Most studies, however, explore collections of regions coactivated during a task and compared with baseline or with another task. Often, activity in each region is analysed *independently* of other 'network' components. Consequently, the term 'network' often describes coactivation, rather than mutual relationship between components. More appropriately, studies should investigate interactions between different brain regions by referring to their intrinsic anatomical connections (e.g. by computing differential responses of anatomically related regions). This requires prior knowledge of relevant brain interconnections. Here, we use the abovementioned framework of dual evolutionary trends to examine interactions *within* each neurodevelopmental trend – and *between* them.

Inconsistent connectivity has been generally reported *within the dorsal stream*. Specifically, significantly weaker interactions have been reported between the rostral ACC (BA 32) and posterior dorsal cortices, including retrosplenial cortex (BAs 29/30), lateral parietal cortices (BAs 40 and 7), occipital cortex and anterior dorsolateral PFC (BA 9) [205]. Similarly, reduced connectivity in PTSD has been reported between dorsal/polar prefrontal (BA 10) and occipital cortices (BA 19) during symptom provocation [198], and between retrosplenial (BA 31) and occipital (BA 19) cortices at rest [243].

Conversely, stronger interactions have been reported *between ventral archicortical regions*. These include connections between the rostral ACC (BA 32) and the dorsolateral and medial PFC (BAs 9/10) and the parietal cortex (BA 40) [205], and between rostral ACC and the hippocampus [215]. Only very few differences in connectivity have been reported within the ventral moiety, all associated with interactions between the amygdale and the fusiform gyrus (BA 37) [198, 215] and ventrolateral PFC (BA 45) [198, 215]. Reports of amygdala–insula connectivity include both increases [244] and decreases [245] in PTSD compared with controls.

Connectivity differences between PTSD and control subjects *across paleocortical and archicortical structures* have been extensively reported, primarily involving the amygdala. These include stronger interactions between the amygdale and medial prefrontal cortices (BAs 10/30) [215, 216], BA 24 [198, 244], BA 25 [198], dorsolateral PFC (BAs 9/10) [198] and posterior regions including the precuneus (BAs 18/19) and posterior cingulate (BA 31) [198]. Stronger connectivity in PTSD between the amygdale and hippocampus has also been reported [244].

Two primary patterns are evident from the above: (i) connectivity aberrations in PTSD are most commonly observed within the dorsal-archicortical stream and across paleocortical and archicortical streams, but are relatively infrequent within the ventral stream; and (ii) there is great variability in reports, including reports of reverse patterns of stronger or weaker connectivity in different studies.

The resulting profiles of brain anatomy, brain activation and system-level network interaction are difficult to account for under the currently predominant view of PTSD. If the core and principal process in PTSD involves failed extinction learning coupled with enhanced fear conditioning and mediated by a hyperactive amygdale, one would expect to see more consistent involvement of subcallosal ACC and amygdale in the disorder. However, much more extensive networks of neural structures appear to be involved in the evolution and maintenance of PTSD, and variability appears to be a major characteristic of this involvement.

Considering this variability from a systems perspective might however help us better understand the complex interactions among neurocognitive structures in PTSD, particularly if one considers the different regions not only as foci of primary dysfunction but also as potential sites for adaptive compensatory processes [246].

Archicortical system vulnerability may mediate both failed extinction and deficient contextual conditioning in PTSD, but also other more complex (adjustment) deficits. For example, some patients may use (or attempt to use) a higher level of cognitive structuring and mood-regulation strategies to alter the conditioning extinction network. This may account for the extensive differences in dorsal–dorsal connectivity alterations observed in cohorts of PTSD patients who either use such strategies or don't. Such interactions have been shown to be modulatory during extinction in healthy controls [241].

Moreover, even the imaging data are not completely compatible with the extinction model of PTSD. A failed extinction mechanism of subcallosal or rostral ACC cortex over the amygdala implies that such a process exists for controls but not for patients. Yet the data reflect a reverse pattern in which when significant connectivity patterns are observed, they are observed only or primarily in patient groups. They may therefore reflect *compensatory processes* rather than the absence of a process.

Compensatory responses may include over-recruitment, failed attempted recruitment or no attempt to recruit a particular process. Each of these profiles might induce a different pattern of brain hypo- and hyperactivity as well as different patterns of connectivity. Extensive differences in activation and connectivity patterns during processing of neutral stimuli in PTSD further support the idea that *brain alterations in the disorder are not limited to the processing of fear stimuli*, and that *deficits in the efficient processing of contextual aspects of the environment* may serve as a basis for ineffective processing of fear information. For full characterisation of these complex interactions, more research is needed, which would expand beyond a simple conditioning model of PTSD.

CONCLUSION

Arguably the most intriguing feature of PTSD is its persistence; that is, its nonextinction despite the absence of further stress. Longitudinal studies (reviewed by Peleg and Shalev [247]) have confirmed a frequent pattern of immediate expression of PTSD symptoms followed by recovery in most of those exposed, versus persistence of symptoms, often to a lifetime, in those who 'develop' chronic PTSD. The conditioned fear analogy similarly predicts extinction in the absence of reinforcement. Among risk factors for PTSD, those that follow the traumatic event explain a larger proportion of the variance than either the event itself or preceding risk factors [37]. The latter may interfere with recovery from early PTSD symptoms.

A neurobiological account of PTSD therefore must mainly consider the disorder's maintaining factors: several theoretical models have been used to account for the persistence of PTSD, including a *kindling hypothesis* (e.g. [248]), according to which patterns of pathological neuronal coactivation become 'entrenched' by repeated use; an *allostatic stress hypothesis*, presuming a 'wear and tear' of CNS emotional control systems (e.g. the hippocampus) by chronic stress (e.g. [249]); and what might be referred to as a *subsystem clash* or *truncated response* view, according to which one brain subsystem blocks the other from achieving the full processing of its inherent tasks (e.g. [250]).

To an extent, this review reflects the latter theory. There is something in the redundancy of intrusive recall of PTSD that forcefully evokes an endless and circular repetition of what, in the early aftermath of trauma, is part of the normal healing process: the evocation and elaboration of novel and incongruent recollections. Similarly, in patients who succeed in one of the cognitive behaviour therapies (CBTs), one is often astonished at the quick recovery that follows the resolution of a cognitive emotional block – sometimes after months or years of illness.

Sections of this review have dealt with the reason for 'stalled extinction' in PTSD. Recent studies of extinction recall and reconsolidation [251] have opened new ways to explore and hopefully treat PTSD. Neurobiological studies that address isolated brain components in PTSD must address the following question: do they study a specific aspect of PTSD, or rather a generic fear mechanism? When the control group involves trauma survivors without PTSD – that is, individuals who do not experience fear or perceive the environment as threatening during the experiment – the resulting difference may reflect the presence of fear in one group and not in the other; that is, the activation in the PTSD group of normal – not diseased – fear responses. Having fearful non-PTSD controls in the scanner might answer some of these confounds.

To converge, studies of PTSD must be guided by theory, and a theory of PTSD cannot simply emerge from a summation of findings. This review has offered an attempt to theorise – along with a summary of as large a portion of the literature as possible. Theorising is risky, and admittedly our take on this issue can and should be challenged. By theorising we hope to foster further, clearer and possibly more accurate understanding of PTSD, as new data emerge.

ACKNOWLEDGEMENT

We thank Hila Levinzon and Itamar Berman for their help with developing the figures. AYS work was supported by U.S. Public Health Service Grant #MH086607.

REFERENCES

1. Kardiner, A. (1941) *The Traumatic Neurosis of War*, Hoeber, New York.
2. Kolb, L.C. and Multalipassi, L.R. (1982) The conditioned emotional response: a sub-class of the chronic and delayed post-traumatic stress disorder. *Psychiatry Annals*, **12**, 979–987.
3. Kolb, L.C. (1987) A neuropsychological hypothesis explaining the post-traumatic stress disorder. *American Journal of Psychiatry*, **144**, 989–995.
4. Orr, S.P., Metzger, L.J. and Pitman, R.K. (2002) Psychophysiology of post-traumatic stress disorder. *The Psychiatric Clinics of North America*, **25** (2), 271–293.
5. Shalev, A.Y., Sahar, T., Freedman, S. *et al*. (1998) A prospective study of heart rate responses following trauma and this subsequent development of PTSD. *Archives of General Psychiatry*, **55**, 553–559.
6. Bryant, R.A., Felmingham, K., Whitford, T.J. *et al*. (2008) Rostral anterior cingulate volume predicts treatment response to cognitive-behavioural therapy for posttraumatic stress disorder. *Journal of Psychiatry and Neuroscience*, **33** (2), 142–146.
7. American Psychiatric Association (1994) *American Psychiatric Association Diagnostic and Statistical Manual of Mental Disorders*, 4th edn, APA, Washington, DC.
8. Rasmusson, A.M., Pinna, G., Paliwal, P. *et al*. (2006) Decreased cerebrospinal fluid allopregnanolone levels in women with PTSD. *Biological Psychiatry*, **60**, 704–713.
9. Gill, J., Vythilingam, M. and Page, G.G. (2008) Low cortisol, high DHEA, and high levels of stimulated TNF-alpha, and IL-6 in women with PTSD. *Journal of Traumatic Stress*, **21**, 530–539.
10. Rosenkranz, J.A., Buffalari, D.M. and Grace, A.A. (2006) Opposing influence of basolateral amygdala and footshock stimulation on neurons of the central amygdala. *Biological Psychiatry*, **59** (9), 801–811.

11. Jhamandas, J.H., Petrov, T., Harris, K.H. *et al*. (1996) Parabrachial nucleus projection to the amygdala in the rat: electrophysiological and anatomical observations. *Brain Research Bulletin*, **39** (2), 115–126.
12. Rogan, M.T., Staubli, U.V. and LeDoux, J.E. (1997) Fear conditioning induces associative long-term potentiation in the amygdala. *Nature*, **390** (6660), 604–607. [Erratum appears in (1998) *Nature*, **391** (6669), 818].
13. Rosenkranz, J.A. and Grace, A.A. (2001) Dopamine attenuates prefrontal cortical suppression of sensory inputs to the basolateral amygdala of rats. *Journal of Neuroscience*, **21**, 4090–4103.
14. Davis, M. (2000) The role of the amygdala in conditioned and unconditioned fear and anxiety, in *The Amygdala: A Functional Analysis* (ed. J.P. Aggleton), Oxford University Press, New York, pp. 213–287.
15. LeDoux, J.E. (2000) Emotion circuits in the brain. *Annual Review of Neuroscience*, **23**, 155–184.
16. Goldstein, L.E., Rasmusson, A.M., Bunney, B.S. *et al*. (1996) Role of the amygdala in the coordination of behavioral, neuroendocrine, and prefrontal cortical monoamine responses to psychological stress in the rat. *Journal of Neuroscience*, **16**, 4787–4798.
17. Morrow, B.A., Elsworth, J.D., Rasmusson, A.M. *et al*. (1999) The role of mesoprefrontal dopamine neurons in the acquisition and expression of conditioned fear in the rat. *Neuroscience*, **92**, 553–564.
18. Robbins, T.W. and Arnsten, A.F. (2009) The neuropsychopharmacology of fronto-executive function: monoaminergic modulation. *Annual Review of Neuroscience*, **32**, 267–287.
19. Rosenkranz, J.A. and Grace, A.A. (2002) Cellular mechanisms of infralimbic and prelimbic prefrontal cortical inhibition and dopaminergic modulation of basolateral amygdala neurons in vivo. *Journal of Neuroscience*, **22** (1), 324–337.
20. Ameli, R., Ip, C. and Grillon, C. (2001) Contextual fear-potentiated startle conditioning in humans: replication and extension. *Psychophysiology*, **38**, 383–390.
21. DeBock, F., Kurz, J., Azad, S.C. *et al*. (2003) Alpha2-adrenoreceptor activation inhibits LTP and LTD in the basolateral amygdala: involvement of Gi/o-protein-mediated modulation of Ca2+-channels and inwardly rectifying K+-channels in LTD. *European Journal of Neuroscience*, **17**, 1411–1424.
22. Buffalari, D.M. and Grace, A.A. (2007) Noradrenergic modulation of basolateral amygdala neuronal activity: opposing influences of α-2 and β receptor activation. *Journal of Neuroscience*, **27** (45), 12358–12366.
23. Braga, M.F., Aroniadou-Anderjaska, V., Manion, S.T. *et al*. (2004) Stress impairs alpha(1A) adrenoceptor-mediated noradrenergic facilitation of GABAergic transmission in the basolateral amygdala. *Neuropsychopharmacology*, **29** (1), 45–58.
24. Martijena, I.D., Rodriguez Manzanares, P.A., Lacerra, C. and Molina, V.A. (2002) Gabaergic modulation of the stress response in frontal cortex and amygdala. *Synapse*, **45** (2), 86–94.

25. Chhatwal, J.P., Myers, K.M., Ressler, K.J. and Davis, M. (2005) Regulation of gephyrin and GABAA receptor binding within the amygdala after fear acquisition and extinction. *Journal of Neuroscience*, **25** (2), 502–506.
26. Heldt, S.A. and Ressler, K.J. (2007) Training-induced changes in the expression of GABAA-associated genes in the amygdala after the acquisition and extinction of Pavlovian fear. *European Journal of Neuroscience*, **26**, 3631–3644.
27. Chhatwal, J.P., Myers, K.M., Ressler, K.J. and Davis, M. (2005) Regulation of gephyrin and GABAA receptor binding within the amygdala after fear acquisition and extinction. *Journal of Neuroscience*, **25**, 502–506.
28. Milad, M.R. and Quirk, G.J. (2002) Neurons in medial prefrontal cortex signal memory for fear extinction. *Nature*, **420** (6911), 70–74.
29. Santini, E., Ge, H., Ren, K. *et al*. (2004) Consolidation of fear extinction requires protein synthesis in the medial prefrontal cortex. *Journal of Neuroscience*, **24**, 5704–5710.
30. Burgos-Robles, A., Vidal-Gonzalez, I., Santini, E. and Quirk, G.J. (2007) Consolidation of fear extinction requires NMDA receptor-dependent bursting in the ventromedial prefrontal cortex. *Neuron*, **53** (6), 871–880.
31. Laviolette, S.R., Lipski, W.J. and Grace, A.A. (2005) A subpopulation of neurons in the medial prefrontal cortex encodes emotional learning with burst and frequency codes through a dopamine D4 receptor-dependent basolateral amygdala input. *Journal of Neuroscience*, **25**, 6066–6075.
32. Mueller, D., Porter, J.T. and Quirk, G.J. (2008) Noradrenergic signaling in infralimbic cortex increases cell excitability and strengthens memory for fear extinction. *Journal of Neuroscience*, **28**, 369–375.
33. Corcoran, K.A. and Quirk, G.J. (2007) Recalling safety: cooperative functions of the ventromedial prefrontal cortex and the hippocampus in extinction. *CNS Spectrums*, **12**, 200–206.
34. Correl, C.M., Rosenkranz, J.A. and Grace, A.A. (2005) Chronic cold stress alters prefrontal cortical modulation of amygdala neuronal activity in rats. *Biological Psychiatry*, **58**, 382–391.
35. Arnsten, A.F. (2009) Stress signalling pathways that impair prefrontal cortex structure and function. *Nature Reviews Neuroscience*, **10**, 410–422.
36. Cerqueira, J.J., Mailliet, F., Almeida, O.F. *et al*. (2007) The prefrontal cortex as a key target of the maladaptive response to stress. *Journal of Neuroscience*, **27** (11), 2781–2787.
37. Brewin, C., Andrews, B. and Valentine, J. (2000) Meta-analysis of risk factors for posttraumatic stress disorder in trauma exposed adults. *Journal of Consulting and Clinical Psychology*, **68**, 748–766.
38. Isoardi, N.A., Bertotto, M.E., Martijena, I.D. *et al*. (2007) Lack of feedback inhibition on rat basolateral amygdala following stress or withdrawal from sedative-hypnotic drugs. *European Journal of Neuroscience*, **26**, 1036–1044.
39. Britton, K.T., Southerland, S., Van Uden, E. *et al*. (1997) Anxiolytic activity of NPY receptor agonists in the conflict test. *Psychopharmacology*, **132**, 6–13.

40. Britton, K.T., Akwa, Y., Southerland, S. *et al.* (2000) Neuropeptide Y blocks the 'anxiogenic-like' behavioral action of corticotropin-releasing factor. *Peptides*, **21**, 37–44.
41. Heilig, M., Soderpalm, B., Engel, J. *et al.* (1989) Centrally administered neuropeptide Y (NPY) produces anxiolytic-like effects in animal anxiety models. *Psychopharmacology*, **98**, 524–529.
42. Heilig, M., McLeod, S., Brot, M. *et al.* (1993) Anxiolytic-like action of neuropeptide Y: mediation by Y1 receptors in amygdala, and dissociation from food intake effects. *Neuropsychopharmacology*, **8**, 357–363.
43. Kask, A., Rago, L. and Harro, J. (1996) Anxiogenic-like effect of the neuropeptide Y Y1 receptor antagonist BIBP3226: antagonism with diazepam. *European Journal of Pharmacology*, **317**, R3–R4.
44. Kask, A., Rago, L. and Harro, J. (1997) Alpha-helical CRF9-41 prevents anxiogenic-like effect of NPY Y_1 receptor antagonist BIBP3226 in rats. *NeuroReport*, **8**, 3645–3647.
45. Howell, O.W., Silva, S., Scharfman, H.E. *et al.* (2007) Neuropeptide Y is important for basal and seizure-induced precursor cell proliferation in the hippocampus. *Neurobiology of Disease*, **26**, 174–188.
46. Hansel, D.E., Eipper, B.A. and Ronnett, G.V. (2001) Neuropeptide Y functions as a neuroproliferative factor. *Nature*, **410**, 940–944.
47. Zhou, Z., Zhu, G., Hariri, A.R. *et al.* (2008) Genetic variation in human NPY expression affects stress response and emotion. *Nature*, **452**, 997–1001.
48. Morgan, C.A., Wang, S., Southwick, S.M. *et al.* (2000) Plasma neuropeptide-Y concentrations in humans exposed to military survival training. *Biological Psychiatry*, **47**, 902–909.
49. Morgan, C.A. III, Rasmusson, A.M., Wang, S. *et al.* (2002) Neuroeptide Y and subjective distress in humans exposed to acute stress: replication and extension of previous report. *Biological Psychiatry*, **52**, 136–142.
50. Rasmusson, A.M., Southwick, S.M., Hauger, R.L. *et al.* (1998) Plasma neuropeptide Y (NPY) increases in response to the α_2 antagonist yohimbine. *Neuropsychopharmacology*, **19**, 95–98.
51. Rasmusson, A.M., Hauger, R.L., Morgan, C.A. III *et al.* (2000) Low baseline and yohimbine-stimulated plasma neuropeptide Y (NPY) in combat-related posttraumatic stress disorder. *Biological Psychiatry*, **47**, 526–539.
52. Yehuda, R., Brand, S. and Yank, R.K. (2005) Plasma neuropeptide Y concentrations in combat exposed veterans: relationship to trauma exposure, recovery from PTSD and coping. *Biological Psychiatry*, **59**, 660–663.
53. Shih, C-D., Chan, J.Y.H. and Chan, S.H.H. (1992) Tonic suppression of baroreceptor reflex response by endogenous neuropeptide Y at the nucleus tractus solitarius of the rat. *Neuroscience Letters*, **148**, 169–172.
54. Ergene, E., Dunbar, J.C. and Barraco, R.A. (1993) Visceroendocrine responses elicited by neuropeptide Y in the nucleus tractus solitarius. *Brain Research Bulletin*, **32**, 461–465.
55. Potter, E.K. and Ulman, L.G. (1994) Neuropeptides in sympathetic nerves affect vagal regulation of the heart. *News in Physiological Sciences*, **9**, 174–177.

56. Shine, J., Potter, E.K., Biden, T. *et al.* (1994) Neuropeptide Y and regulation of the cardiovascular system. *Journal of Hypertension*, **12** (Suppl. 10), S41–S45.
57. Zukowska-Grojec, Z. (1995) Neuropeptide Y. A novel sympathetic stress hormone and more. *Annals of the New York Academy of Science*, **771**, 219–233.
58. Yang, L., Scott, K.A., Hyun, J. *et al.* (2009) Role of dorsomedial hypothalamic neuropeptide Y in modulating food intake and energy balance. *Journal of Neuroscience*, **29**, 179–190.
59. Kuo, L.E., Kitlinska, J.B., Tilan, J.U. *et al.* (2007) Neuropeptide Y acts directly in the periphery on fat tissue and mediates stress-induced obesity and metabolic syndrome. *Nature Medicine*, **13**, 803–811.
60. Antonijevic, I.A., Murck, H., Bohlhalter, S. *et al.* (2000) Neuropeptide Y promotes sleep and inhibits ACTH and cortisol release in young men. *Neuropharmacology*, **39**, 1474–1481.
61. Held, K., Antonijevic, I., Murck, H. *et al.* (2006) Neuropeptide Y (NPY) shortens sleep latency but does not suppress ACTH and cortisol in depressed patients and normal controls. *Psychoneuroendocrinology*, **31**, 100–107.
62. Morgan, C.A., Rasmusson, A.M., Winters, B. *et al.* (2003) Trauma exposure rather than PTSD is associated with reduced baseline plasma neuropeptide-Y levels. *Biological Psychiatry*, **54**, 1087–1091.
63. Southwick, S.M., Krystal, J.H., Morgan, C.A. *et al.* (1993) Abnormal noradrenergic function in posttraumatic stress disorder. *Archives of General Psychiatry*, **50**, 266–274.
64. Southwick, S.M., Rasmusson, A.M., Barron, J. *et al.* (2005) Neurobiological and neurocognitive alterations in PTSD: a focus on norepinephrine, serotonin, and the HPA axis, in *Neuropsychology of PTSD* (eds J. Vasterling and C. Brewin), Guilford Publications, New York.
65. Lambert, J.J., Belelli, D., Peden, D.R. *et al.* (2003) Neurosteroid modulation of $GABA_A$ receptors. *Progress in Neurobiology*, **71**, 67–80.
66. Puia, G., Mienville, J.-M., Matsumoto, K. *et al.* (2003) On the putative physiological role of allopregnanolone on $GABA_A$ receptor function. *Neuropharmacology*, **44**, 49–55.
67. Mitchell, S.J. and Silver, R.A. (2003) Shunting inhibition modulates neuronal gain during synaptic excitation. *Neuron*, **38**, 433–445.
68. Mody, I. and Pearce, R.A. (2004) Diversity of inhibitory neurotransmission through $GABA_A$ receptors. *Trends in Neuroscience*, **27**, 569–575.
69. Semyanov, A., Walker, M.C., Kullmann, D.M. *et al.* (2004) Tonically active GABAA receptors: modulating gain and maintaining the tone. *Trends in Neuroscience*, **27**, 262–269.
70. Purdy, R.H., Morrow, A.L., Moore, P.H. Jr *et al.* (1991) Stress-induced elevations of gamma-aminobutyric acid type A receptor-active steroids in the rat brain. *Proceedings of the National Academy of Science*, **88**, 4553–4557.
71. Barbaccia, M.L., Serra, M., Purdy, R.H. and Biggio, G. (2001) Stress and neuroactive steroids. *International Review of Neurobiology*, **46**, 243–272.
72. Paul, S.M. and Purdy, R.H. (1992) Neuroactive steroids. *FASEB Journal*, **6**, 2311–2322.

73. Genazzani, A.R., Petraglia, F. and Bernardi, F. (1998) Circulating levels of allopregnanolone in humans: gender, age, and endocrine influences. *Journal of Clinical Endocrinology and Metabolism*, **83**, 2099–2103.
74. Ghoumari, A.M., Ibanez, C., El-Etr, M. *et al*. (2003) Schumacher M. Progesterone and its metabolites increase myelin basic protein expression in organotypic slice cultures of rat cerebellum. *Journal of Neurochemistry*, **86**, 848–859.
75. VanLandingham, J.W., Cekic, M., Cutler, S. *et al*. (2007) Neurosteroids reduce inflammation after TBI through CD55 induction. *Neuroscience Letters*, **425**, 94–98.
76. Guidotti, A., Dong, E., Matsumoto, K. *et al*. (2001) The socially-isolated mouse: a model to study the putative role of allopregnanolone and 5?-dihydroprogesterone in psychiatric disorders. *Brain Research Reviews*, **37**, 110–115.
77. Pibiri, F., Nelson, M., Guidotti, A. *et al*. (2008) Decreased corticolimbic allopregnanolone expression during social isolation enhances contextual fear: a model relevant for posttraumatic stress disorder. *Proceedings of the National Academy of Sciences*, **105**, 5567–5572.
78. Pinna, G., Costa, E. and Guidotti, A. (2009) SSRIs act as selective brain steroidogenic stimulants (SBSSs) at low doses that are inactive on 5-HT reuptake. *Current Opinion in Pharmacology*, **9**, 24–30.
79. Rosenfeld, R.S., Hellman, L. and Roffwarg, H. (1971) Dehydroisoandrosterone is secreted episodically and synchronously with cortisol by normal man. *Journal of Clinical Endocrinology*, **33**, 87–92.
80. Compagnone, N.A. and Mellon, S.H. (2000) Neurosteroids: Biosynthesis and function of these novel neuromodulators. *Frontiers in Neuroendocrinology*, **21**, 1–56.
81. Rasmusson, A.M., Vythilingam, M. and Morgan, C.A.I.I.I. (2003) The neuroendocrinology of PTSD – new directions. *CNS Spectrums*, **8**, 651–667.
82. Balazs, Z., Schweizer, R.A., Frey, F.J. *et al*. (2008) DHEA induces 11α-HSD2 by acting on CCAAT/enhancer-binding proteins. *Journal of the American Society of Nephrology*, **19**, 92–101.
83. Sondergaard, H.P., Hansson, L.O. and Theorell, T. (2002) Elevated blood levels of dehydroepiandrosterone sulphate vary with symptom load in posttraumaticstress disorder: findings from a longitudinal study of refugees in Sweden. *Psychotherapy and Psychosomatics*, **71**, 298–303.
84. Spivak, B., Maayan, R., Kotler, M. *et al*. (2000) Elevated circulatory level of GABA A-antagonistic neurosteroids in patients with combat-related post-traumatic stress disorder. *Psychological Medicine*, **30**, 1227–1231.
85. Yehuda, R., Brand, S.R., Golier, J.A. *et al*. (2006) Clinical correlates of DHEA associated with post-traumatic stress disorder. *Acta Psychiatrica Scandinavica*, **114**, 187–193.
86. Morgan, C.A. III, Southwick, S., Hazlett, G. *et al*. (2004) Relationships among plasma DHEA(S), cortisol, symptoms of dissociation and objective performance in humans exposed to acute stress. *Archives of General Psychiatry*, **61**, 819–812.
87. Morgan, C.A., Rasmusson, A., Pietrzak, R.H. *et al*. (2009) Relationships among plasma dehydroepiandrosterone and dehydroepiandrosterone sulfate, cortisol, symptoms of dissociation and objective performance in humans exposed to underwater navigation stress. *Biological Psychiatry*, **66** (44), 334–340.

88. Kudielka, B.M., Hellhammer, J., Hellhammer, D.H. *et al.* (1998) Sex differences in endocrine and psychological responses to psychosocial stress in healthy elderly subjects and the impact of a two-week DHEA treatment. *Journal of Clinical Endocrinology and Metabolism*, **83**, 1756–1761.
89. Deuster, P.A., Faraday, M.M., Chrousos, G.P. and Poth, M.A. (2005) Effects of dehydroepiandrosterone and alprazolam on hypothalamic-pituitary responses to exercise. *Journal of Clinical Endocrinology and Metabolism*, **90**, 4777–4783.
90. Kroboth, P.D., Amico, J.A., Stone, R.A. *et al.* (2003) Influence of DHEA administration on 24-hour cortisol concentrations. *Journal of Clinical Psychopharmacology*, **23**, 96–99.
91. Genazzani, A.D., Stomati, M., Bernardi, F. *et al.* (2003) Long-term low-dose dehydroepiandrosterone oral supplementation in early and late postmenopausal women modulates endocrine parameters and synthesis of neuroactive steroids. *Fertility & Sterility*, **80**, 1495–1501.
92. Wolkowitz, O.M., Reus, V.I., Keebler, A. (2009) Double-blind treatment of major depression with dehydroepiandrosterone. *American Journal of Psychiatry*, **156**, 646–649.
93. Schmidt, P.J., Daly, R.C., Bloch, M. *et al.* (2005) Dehydroepiandrosterone monotherapy in midlife-onset major and minor depression. *Archives of General Psychiatry*, **62**, 154–162.
94. Yehuda, R. (2002) Current status of cortisol findings in post-traumatic stress disorder. *Psychiatric Clinics of North America*, **25** (2), 341–368.
95. Young, E.A. and Breslau, N. (2004) Saliva cortisol in posttraumatic stress disorder: a community epidemiologic study. *Biological Psychiatry*, **56** (3), 205–209.
96. Meewisse, M.L., Reitsma, J.B., de Vries, G.J. *et al.* (2007) Cortisol and post-traumatic stress disorder in adults: systematic review and meta-analysis. *British Journal of Psychiatry*, **191**, 387–392.
97. Handwerger, K. (2009) Differential patterns of HPA activity and reactivity in adult posttraumatic stress disorder and major depressive disorder. *Harvard Review of Psychiatry*, **17**, 184–205.
98. Shalev, A.Y., Videlock, E.J. and Peleg, T. (2008) Stress hormones and post-traumatic stress disorder in civilian trauma victims: a longitudinal study. Part I: HPA axis responses. *International Journal of Neuropsychopharmacology*, **11**, 365–372.
99. Hou, Y.T., Lin, H.K. and Penning, T.M. (1998) Dexamethasone regulation of the rat 3?-hydroxysteroid/dihydrodiol dihydrogenase (3?-HSD/DD) gene. *Molecular Pharmacology*, **53**, 459–466.
100. Yehuda, R. and Bierer, L.M. (2008) Transgenerational transmission of cortisol and PTSD risk. *Progress in Brain Research*, **167**, 121–135.
101. True, W.R., Rice, J., Eisen, S.A. *et al.* (1993) A twin study of genetic and environmental contributions to liability for posttraumatic stress symptoms. *Archives of General Psychiatry*, **50**, 257–264.
102. Xian, H., Chantarujikapong, S.I., Scherrer, J.F. *et al.* (2000) Genetic and environmental influences on posttraumatic stress disorder, alcohol and drug dependence in twin pairs. *Drug and Alcohol Dependence*, **22**, 95–102.

103. McLeod, D.S., Koenen, K.C., Meyer, J.M. *et al*. (2001) Genetic and environmental influences on the relationship among combat exposure, posttraumatic stress disorder symptoms, and alcohol use. *Journal of Traumatic Stress*, **14**, 259–275.
104. Koenen, K.C., Fu, Q.J., Ertel, K. *et al*. (2008) Common genetic liability to major depression and posttraumatic stress disorder in men. *Journal of Affective Disorders*, **105**, 109–115.
105. Kallio, J., Pesonen, U., Kaipio, K. *et al*. (2001) Altered intracellular processing and release of neuropeptide Y due to leucine 7 to proline 7 polymorphism in the signal peptide of preproneuropeptide Y in humans. *FASEB Journal*, **15** (7), 1242–1244.
106. Lavebratt, C., Alpman, A., Persson, B. *et al*. (2006) Common neuropeptide Y2 receptor gene variant is protective against obesity among Swedish men. *International Journal of Obesity*, **30**, 453–459.
107. Neumeister, A., Charney, D.S., Belfer, I. *et al*. (2005) Sympathoneural and adrenomedullary functional effects of alpha$_{2C}$-adrenoreceptor gene polymorphism in healthy humans. *Pharmacogenetic Genomics*, **15**, 143–149.
108. Neumeister, A., Drevets, W.C., Belfer, I. *et al*. (2006) Effects of a alpha 2C-adrenoreceptor gene polymorphism on neural responses to facial expressions in depression. *Neuropsychopharmacology*, **31**, 1750–1756.
109. Soliman, F., Glatt, C.E., Bath, K.G. *et al*. (2010) A genetic variant BDNF polymorphism alters extinction learning in both mouse and human. *Science*, **327**, 863–866.
110. Kilpatrick, D.G., Koenen, K.C., Ruggeiero, K.J. *et al*. The serotonin transporter genotype and social support and moderation of posttraumatic stress disorder and depression in hurricane-exposed adults. *American Journal of Psychiatry*, **164**, 1693–1699.
111. Kolassa, I.T., Ertl, V., Eckart, C. *et al*. (2010) Association study of trauma load and SLC6A4 promoter polymorphism in posttraumatic stress disorder: evidence from survivors of the Rwandan genocide. *Journal of Clinical Psychiatry*, **71**, 543–547.
112. Xie, P., Kranzler, H.R., Poling, J. *et al*. (2009) Interactive effect of stressful life events and the serotonin transporter 5-HTTLPR genotype on posttraumatic stress disorder diagnosis in 2 independent populations. *Archives of General Psychiatry*, **66**, 1201–1209.
113. Binder, E.B., Bradley, R.G., Liu, W. *et al*. (2008) Association of FKBP5 polymorphisms and childhood abuse with risk of posttraumatic stress disorder symptoms in adults. *Journal ofAmerican Medical Association*, **299**, 1291–1305.
114. Yehuda, R., Cai, G., Golier, J.A. *et al*. (2009) Gene expression patterns associated with posttraumatic stress disorder following exposure to the World Trade Center attacks. *Biological Psychiatry*, **66**, 708–711.
115. Seckl, J.R. and Meaney, M.J. (2006) Glucocorticoid "programming" and PTSD risk. *Annals of the New York Academy of Sciences*, **1071**, 351–378.
116. Uddin, M., Aiello, A.E., Wildman, D.E. *et al*. (2010) Epigenetic and immune function profiles associated with posttraumatic stress disorder. *Proceedings of the National Academy of Sciences*, **107**, 9470–9475.
117. Fuchikami, M., Morinobu, S., Kurata, A. *et al*. (2009) Single immobilization stress differentially alters the expression profile of transcripts of the brain-derived

neurotrophic factor (BDNF) gene and histone acetylation at its promoters in the rat hippocampus. *International Journal of Neuropsychopharmacology*, **12** (1), 73–82.

118. Bredy, T.W., Wu, H., Crego, C. *et al*. (2007) Histone modifications around individual BDNF gene promoters in prefrontal cortex are associated with extinction of conditioned fear. *Learning Memory*, **14**, 268–276.
119. Lewin, G.R. and Barde, Y.-A. (1996) Physiology of the neurotrophins. *Annual Review of Neuroscience*, **19**, 289–317.
120. Bredy, T.W. and Barad, M. (2008) The histone deacetylase inhibitor valproic acid enhances acquisition, extinction, and reconsolidation of conditioned fear. *Learning & Memory*, **15** (1), 39–45.
121. De Kloet, E.R. (2004) Hormones and the stressed brain. *Annals of the New York Academy of Science*, **1018**, 1–15.
122. Jaycox, L.H., Foa, E.B. and Morral, A.R. (1998) Influence of emotional engagement and habituation on exposure therapy for PTSD. *Annals of the New York Academy of Science*, **66**, 185–192.
123. Resick, P.A., Galovski, T.E., O'Brien Uhlmansiek, M. *et al*. (2008) A randomized clinical trial to dismantle components of cognitive processing therapy for post-traumatic stress disorder in female victims of interpersonal violence. *Journal of Consulting Clinical Psychology*, **76**, 243–258.
124. Pittenger, C. and Duman, R.S. (2008) Stress, depression, and neuroplasticity: a convergence of mechanisms. *Neuropsychopharmacology*, **33**, 88–109.
125. Sakata, K., Woo, N.H., Martinowich, K. *et al*. (2009) Critical role of promoter IV-driven BDNF transcription in GABAergic transmission and synaptic plasticity in the prefrontal cortex. *Proceedings of the National Academy of Sciences*, **106**, 5942–5947.
126. Higuchi, H., Nakano, K., Kim, C.H. *et al*. (1996) Ca2+/calmodulin-dependent transcriptional activation of neuropeptide Y gene induced by membrane depolarization: determination of Ca(2+)- and cyclic AMP/phorbol 12-myristate 13-acetate-responsive elements. *Journa lof Neurochemistry*, **66**, 1802–1809.
127. Sanides, F. (1970) Functional architecture of motor and sensory cortices in primates in the light of a new concept of neocortex evolution, in *Advances in Primatology*, The Primate Brain, Vol. **1** (eds C.R. Noback and W. Montagna), Appleton-Century-Crofts, Meredith Corporation, New-York, pp. 137–208.
128. Sanides, F. (1962) Structure and function of the human frontal lobe. *Neuropsychologia*, **2** (3), 209–219.
129. Mega, M.S., Cummings, J.L., Salloway, S. and Malloy, P. (1997) The limbic system: an anatomic, phylogenetic, and clinical perspective. *Journal of Neuropsychiatry*, **9**, 315–330.
130. Pandya, D.N., Seltzer, B. and Barbas, H. (1988) Input-output organization of the primate cerebral cortex, in *Comparative Primate Biology*, Neuroscience, Vol. **4** (eds H.D. Steklis and J. Erwin), Alan R. Liss Inc., New York, pp. 39–80.
131. Petrides, M. and Pandya, D.N. (1994) Comparative architectonic analysis of the human and the macaque frontal cortex, in *Handbook of Neuropsychology*, Vol. **9**, (eds F. Boller and J. Grafman), Elsevier, Amsterdam, pp. 17–58.

132. Antonova, E., Sharma, T., Morris, R. and Kumari, V. (2004) The relationship between brain structure and neurocognition in schizophrenia: a selective review. *Schizophrenia Research*, **70** (2-3), 117–145.
133. Christensen, B.K. and Bilder, R.M. (2000) Dual cytoarchitectonic trends: an evolutionary model of frontal lobe functioning and its application to psychopathology. *Canadian Journal of Psychiatry*, **45** (3), 247–256.
134. Giaccio, R.G. (2006) The dual origin hypothesis: an evolutionary brain-behavior framework for analyzing psychiatric disorders. *Neuroscience and Biobehavioral Reviews*, **30** (4), 526–550.
135. Bremner, J.D., Randall, P., Scott, T.M. *et al*. (1995) MRI-based measurement of hippocampal volume in patients with combat-related posttraumatic stress disorder. *American Journal of Psychiatry*, **152** (7), 973–981.
136. Sapolsky, R.M., Krey, L.C. and McEwen, B.S. (1986) The neuroendocrinology of stress and aging: the glucocorticoid cascade hypothesis. *Endocrine Reviews*, **7** (3), 284–301.
137. Bonne, O., Vythilingam, M., Inagaki, M. *et al*. (2008) Reduced posterior hippocampal volume in posttraumatic stress disorder. *Journal of Clinical Psychiatry*, **69** (7), 1087–1091.
138. Bossini, L., Tavanti, M., Calossi, S. *et al*. (2008) Magnetic resonance imaging volumes of the hippocampus in drug-naive patients with post-traumatic stress disorder without comorbidity conditions. *Journal of Psychiatric Research*, **42** (9), 752–762.
139. Bremner, J.D., Randall, P., Vermetten, E. *et al*. (1997) Magnetic resonance imaging-based measurement of hippocampal volume in posttraumatic stress disorder related to childhood physical and sexual abuse – a preliminary report. *Biological Psychiatry*, **41** (1), 23–32.
140. Bremner, J.D., Vythilingam, M., Vermetten, E. *et al*. (2003) MRI and PET study of deficits in hippocampal structure and function in women with childhood sexual abuse and posttraumatic stress disorder. *American Journal of Psychiatry*, **160** (5), 924–932.
141. Emdad, R., Bonekamp, D., Sondergaard, H.P. *et al*. (2006) Morphometric and psychometric comparisons between non-substance-abusing patients with posttraumatic stress disorder and normal controls. *Psychotherapy and Psychosomatics*, **75** (2), 122–132.
142. Felmingham, K., Williams, L.M., Whitford, T.J. *et al*. (2009) Duration of posttraumatic stress disorder predicts hippocampal grey matter loss. *Neuroreport*, **20** (16), 1402–1406.
143. Gurvits, T.V., Shenton, M.E., Hokama, H. *et al*. (1996) Magnetic resonance imaging study of hippocampal volume in chronic, combat-related posttraumatic stress disorder. *Biological Psychiatry*, **40** (11), 1091–1099.
144. Hedges, D.W., Allen, S., Tate, D.F. *et al*. (2003) Reduced hippocampal volume in alcohol and substance naive Vietnam combat veterans with posttraumatic stress disorder. *Cognitive and Behavioral Neurology*, **16** (4), 219–224.
145. Lindauer, R.J., Vlieger, E.J., Jalink, M. *et al*. (2004) Smaller hippocampal volume in Dutch police officers with posttraumatic stress disorder. *Biological Psychiatry*, **56** (5), 356–363.

146. Shin, L.M., Shin, P.S., Heckers, S. *et al*. (2004) Hippocampal function in posttraumatic stress disorder. *Hippocampus*, **14** (3), 292–300.
147. Stein, M.B., Koverola, C., Hanna, C. *et al*. (1997) Hippocampal volume in women victimized by childhood sexual abuse. *Psychological Medicine*, **27** (4), 951–959.
148. Vermetten, E., Vythilingam, M., Southwick, S.M. *et al*. (2003) Long-term treatment with paroxetine increases verbal declarative memory and hippocampal volume in posttraumatic stress disorder. *Biological Psychiatry*, **54** (7), 693–702.
149. Villarreal, G., Hamilton, D.A., Petropoulos, H. *et al*. (2002) Reduced hippocampal volume and total white matter volume in posttraumatic stress disorder. *Biological Psychiatry*, **52** (2), 119–125.
150. Vythilingam, M., Luckenbaugh, D.A., Lam, T. *et al*. (2005) Smaller head of the hippocampus in Gulf War-related posttraumatic stress disorder. *Psychiatry Research*, **139** (2), 89–99.
151. Woon, F.L. and Hedges, D.W. (2008) Hippocampal and amygdala volumes in children and adults with childhood maltreatment-related posttraumatic stress disorder: a meta-analysis. *Hippocampus*, **18** (8), 729–736.
152. Gold, J.J. and Squire, L.R. (2005) Quantifying medial temporal lobe damage in memory-impaired patients. *Hippocampus*, **15** (1), 79–85.
153. Isaacs, E.B., Vargha-Khadem, F., Watkins, K.E. *et al*. (2003) Developmental amnesia and its relationship to degree of hippocampal atrophy. *Proceedings of the National Academy of Sciences of United States of America*, **100** (22), 13060–13063.
154. Bonne, O., Brandes, D., Gilboa, A. *et al*. (2001) Longitudinal MRI study of hippocampal volume in trauma survivors with PTSD. *American Journal of Psychiatry*, **158** (8), 1248–1251.
155. Carrion, V.G., Weems, C.F., Eliez, S. *et al*. (2001) Attenuation of frontal asymmetry in pediatric posttraumatic stress disorder. *Biological Psychiatry*, **50** (12), 943–951.
156. De Bellis, M.D., Hall, J., Boring, A.M. *et al*. (2001) A pilot longitudinal study of hippocampal volumes in pediatric maltreatment-related posttraumatic stress disorder. *Biological Psychiatry*, **50** (4), 305–309.
157. De Bellis, M.D., Keshavan, M.S., Shifflett, H. *et al*. (2002) Brain structures in pediatric maltreatment-related posttraumatic stress disorder: a sociodemographically matched study. *Biologicla Psychiatry*, **52** (11), 1066–1078.
158. Golier, J.A., Yehuda, R., De Santi, S. *et al*. (2005) Absence of hippocampal volume differences in survivors of the Nazi Holocaust with and without posttraumatic stress disorder. *Psychiatry Research*, **139** (1), 53–64.
159. Jatzko, A., Rothenhofer, S., Schmitt, A. *et al*. (2006) Hippocampal volume in chronic posttraumatic stress disorder (PTSD): MRI study using two different evaluation methods. *Journal of Affective Disorders*, **94** (1–3), 121–126.
160. Karl, A., Schaefer, M., Malta, L.S. *et al*. (2006) A meta-analysis of structural brain abnormalities in PTSD. *Neuroscience and Biobehavioral Reviews*, **30** (7), 1004–1031.
161. Gilbertson, M.W., Shenton, M.E., Ciszewski, A. *et al*. (2002) Smaller hippocampal volume predicts pathologic vulnerability to psychological trauma. *Nature Neuroscience*, **5** (11), 1242–1247.

162. De Bellis, M.D. and Keshavan, M.S. (2003) Sex differences in brain maturation in maltreatment-related pediatric posttraumatic stress disorder. *Neuroscience and Biobehavioral Reviews*, **27** (1–2), 103–117.

163. Jackowski, A.P., Douglas-Palumberi, H., Jackowski, M. *et al.* (2008) Corpus callosum in maltreated children with posttraumatic stress disorder: a diffusion tensor imaging study. *Psychiatry Research*, **162** (3), 256–261.

164. Kitayama, N., Brummer, M., Hertz, L. *et al.* (2007) Morphologic alterations in the corpus callosum in abuse-related posttraumatic stress disorder: a preliminary study. *Journal of Nervous and Mental Disease*, **195** (12), 1027–1029.

165. Villarreal, G., Hamilton, D.A., Graham, D.P. *et al.* (2004) Reduced area of the corpus callosum in posttraumatic stress disorder. *Psychiatry Research*, **131** (3), 227–235.

166. Chen, S., Li, L., Xu, B. and Liu, J. (2009) Insular cortex involvement in declarative memory deficits in patients with post-traumatic stress disorder. *BMC Psychiatry*, **9**, 39.

167. Chen, S., Xia, W., Li, L. *et al.* (2006) Gray matter density reduction in the insula in fire survivors with posttraumatic stress disorder: a voxel-based morphometric study. *Psychiatry Research*, **146** (1), 65–72.

168. Corbo, V., Clement, M.H., Armony, J.L. *et al.* (2005) Size versus shape differences: contrasting voxel-based and volumetric analyses of the anterior cingulate cortex in individuals with acute posttraumatic stress disorder. *Biological Psychiatry*, **58** (2), 119–124.

169. Kasai, K., Yamasue, H., Gilbertson, M.W. *et al.* (2008) Evidence for acquired pregenual anterior cingulate gray matter loss from a twin study of combat-related posttraumatic stress disorder. *Biological Psychiatry*, **63** (6), 550–556.

170. Cohen, R.A., Grieve, S., Hoth, K.F. *et al.* (2006) Early life stress and morphometry of the adult anterior cingulate cortex and caudate nuclei. *Biological Psychiatry*, **59** (10), 975–982.

171. Fennema-Notestine, C., Stein, M.B., Kennedy, C.M. *et al.* (2002) Brain morphometry in female victims of intimate partner violence with and without posttraumatic stress disorder. *Biological Psychiatry*, **52** (11), 1089–1101.

172. Hara, E., Matsuoka, Y., Hakamata, Y. *et al.* (2008) Hippocampal and amygdalar volumes in breast cancer survivors with posttraumatic stress disorder. *Journal of Neuropsychiatry and Clinical Neurosciences*, **20** (3), 302–308.

173. Matsuoka, Y., Yamawaki, S., Inagaki, M. *et al.* (2003) A volumetric study of amygdala in cancer survivors with intrusive recollections. *Biological Psychiatry*, **54** (7), 736–743.

174. Rauch, S.L., Shin, L.M., Segal, E. *et al.* (2003) Selectively reduced regional cortical volumes in post-traumatic stress disorder. *Neuroreport*, **14** (7), 913–916.

175. Rogers, M.A., Yamasue, H., Abe, O. *et al.* (2009) Smaller amygdala volume and reduced anterior cingulate gray matter density associated with history of post-traumatic stress disorder. *Psychiatry Research*, **174** (3), 210–216.

176. Wignall, E.L., Dickson, J.M., Vaughan, P. *et al*. (2004) Smaller hippocampal volume in patients with recent-onset posttraumatic stress disorder. *Biological Psychiatry*, **56** (11), 832–836.

177. Woodward, S.H., Kaloupek, D.G., Streeter, C.C. *et al*. (2006) Decreased anterior cingulate volume in combat-related PTSD. *Biological Psychiatry*, **59** (7), 582–587.

178. Woon, F.L. and Hedges, D.W. (2009) Amygdala volume in adults with posttraumatic stress disorder: a meta-analysis. *Journal of Neuropsychiatry and Clinical Neurosciences*, **21** (1), 5–12.

179. Abe, O., Yamasue, H., Kasai, K. *et al*. (2006) Voxel-based diffusion tensor analysis reveals aberrant anterior cingulum integrity in posttraumatic stress disorder due to terrorism. *Psychiatry Research*, **146** (3), 231–242.

180. Kitayama, N., Quinn, S. and Bremner, J.D. (2006) Smaller volume of anterior cingulate cortex in abuse-related posttraumatic stress disorder. *Journal of Affective Disorders*, **90** (2–3), 171–174.

181. Yamasue, H., Kasai, K., Iwanami, A. *et al*. (2003) Voxel-based analysis of MRI reveals anterior cingulate gray-matter volume reduction in posttraumatic stress disorder due to terrorism. *Proceedings of the National Academy of Sciences of the United States of America*, **100** (15), 9039–9043.

182. Bremner, J.D. (2006) The relationship between cognitive and brain changes in posttraumatic stress disorder. *Annals of the New York Academy of Science*, **1071**, 80–86.

183. Bremner, J.D. (2007) Neuroimaging in posttraumatic stress disorder and other stress-related disorders. *Neuroimaging Clinics of North America*, **17** (4), 523–538, ix.

184. Cannistraro, P.A. and Rauch, S.L. (2003) Neural circuitry of anxiety: evidence from structural and functional neuroimaging studies. *Psychopharmacology Bulletin*, **37** (4), 8–25.

185. Deckersbach, T., Dougherty, D.D. and Rauch, S.L. (2006) Functional imaging of mood and anxiety disorders. *Journal of Neuroimaging*, **16** (1), 1–10.

186. Francati, V., Vermetten, E. and Bremner, J.D. (2007) Functional neuroimaging studies in posttraumatic stress disorder: review of current methods and findings. *Depression and Anxiety*, **24** (3), 202–218.

187. Lanius, R.A., Bluhm, R., Lanius, U. and Pain, C. (2006) A review of neuroimaging studies in PTSD: heterogeneity of response to symptom provocation. *Journal of Psychiatric Research*, **40** (8), 709–729.

188. Liberzon, I. and Sripada, C.S. (2008) The functional neuroanatomy of PTSD: a critical review. *Progress in Brain Research*, **167**, 151–169.

189. Shin, L.M., Rauch, S.L. and Pitman, R.K. (2006) Amygdala, medial prefrontal cortex, and hippocampal function in PTSD. *Annals of the New York Academy of Science*, **1071**, 67–79.

190. Bremner, J.D., Staib, L.H., Kaloupek, D. *et al*. (1999) Neural correlates of exposure to traumatic pictures and sound in Vietnam combat veterans with and without

posttraumatic stress disorder: a positron emission tomography study. *Biological Psychiatry*, **45** (7), 806–816.

191. Bremner, J.D., Narayan, M., Staib, L.H. *et al*. (1999) Neural correlates of memories of childhood sexual abuse in women with and without posttraumatic stress disorder. *The American Journal of Psychiatry*, **156** (11), 1787–1795.
192. Bremner, J.D., Vythilingam, M., Vermetten, E. *et al*. (2003) Neural correlates of declarative memory for emotionally valenced words in women with posttraumatic stress disorder related to early childhood sexual abuse. *Biological Psychiatry*, **53** (10), 879–889.
193. Bremner, J.D., Vermetten, E., Vythilingam, M. *et al*. (2004) Neural correlates of the classic color and emotional stroop in women with abuse-related posttraumatic stress disorder. *Biological Psychiatry*, **55** (6), 612–620.
194. Britton, J.C., Phan, K.L., Taylor, S.F. *et al*. (2005) Corticolimbic blood flow in posttraumatic stress disorder during script-driven imagery. *Biological Psychiatry*, **57** (8), 832–840.
195. Clark, C.R., McFarlane, A.C., Morris, P. *et al*. (2003) Cerebral function in posttraumatic stress disorder during verbal working memory updating: a positron emission tomography study. *Biological Psychiatry*, **53** (6), 474–481.
196. Driessen, M., Beblo, T., Mertens, M. *et al*. (2004) Posttraumatic stress disorder and fMRI activation patterns of traumatic memory in patients with borderline personality disorder. *Biological Psychiatry*, **55** (6), 603–611.
197. Geuze, E., Westenberg, H.G., Jochims, A. *et al*. (2007) Altered pain processing in veterans with posttraumatic stress disorder. *Archives of General Psychiatry*, **64** (1), 76–85.
198. Gilboa, A., Shalev, A.Y., Laor, L. *et al*. (2004) Functional connectivity of the prefrontal cortex and the amygdala in posttraumatic stress disorder. *Biological Psychiatry*, **55** (3), 263–272.
199. Hendler, T., Rotshtein, P., Yeshuron, Y. *et al*. (2003) Sensing the invisible: differential sensitivity of visual cortex and amygdala to traumatic context. *Neuroimage*, **19** (3), 587–600.
200. Hou, C., Liu, J., Wang, K. *et al*. (2007) Brain responses to symptom provocation and trauma-related short-term memory recall in coal mining accident survivors with acute severe PTSD. *Brain Research*, **1144**, 165–174.
201. Kemp, A.H., Felmingham, K.L., Falconer, E. *et al*. (2009) Heterogeneity of non-conscious fear perception in posttraumatic stress disorder as a function of physiological arousal: an fMRI study. *Psychiatry Research*, **174** (2), 158–161.
202. Lanius, R.A., Williamson, P.C., Densmore, M. *et al*. (2001) Neural correlates of traumatic memories in posttraumatic stress disorder: a functional MRI investigation. *The American Journal of Psychiatry*, **158** (11), 1920–1922.
203. Lanius, R.A., Williamson, P.C., Boksman, K. *et al*. (2002) Brain activation during script-driven imagery induced dissociative responses in PTSD: a functional magnetic resonance imaging investigation. *Biological Psychiatry*, **52** (4), 305–311.

204. Lanius, R.A., Williamson, P.C., Hopper, J. *et al*. (2003) Recall of emotional states in posttraumatic stress disorder: an fMRI investigation. *Biological Psychiatry*, **53** (3), 204–210.
205. Lanius, R.A., Williamson, P.C., Densmore, M. *et al*. (2004) The nature of traumatic memories: a 4-T FMRI functional connectivity analysis. *American Journal of Psychiatry*, **161** (1), 36–44.
206. Lanius, R.A., Williamson, P.C., Bluhm, R.L. *et al*. (2005) Functional connectivity of dissociative responses in posttraumatic stress disorder: a functional magnetic resonance imaging investigation. *Biological Psychiatry*, **57** (8), 873–884.
207. Liberzon, I., Taylor, S.F., Amdur, R. *et al*. (1999) Brain activation in PTSD in response to trauma-related stimuli. *Biological Psychiatry*, **45** (7), 817–826.
208. Liberzon, I., Britton, J.C., Phan, K.L. *et al*. (2003) Neural correlates of traumatic recall in posttraumatic stress disorder. *Stress*, **6** (3), 151–156.
209. Pardo, J., Fahnhorst, S., Lee, J.T. *et al*. (2009) PET Study of Script-Driven Fear Imagery: Combat Veterans with Active vs. Remitted PTSD. *Neuroimage*, **47**, S70–S70.
210. Protopopescu, X., Pan, H., Tuescher, O. *et al*. (2005) Differential time courses and specificity of amygdala activity in posttraumatic stress disorder subjects and normal control subjects. *Biological Psychiatry*, **57** (5), 464–473.
211. Rauch, S.L., Whalen, P.J., Shin, L.M. *et al*. (2000) Exaggerated amygdala response to masked facial stimuli in posttraumatic stress disorder: a functional MRI study. *Biological Psychiatry*, **47** (9), 769–776.
212. Shin, L.M., Kosslyn, S.M., McNally, R.J. *et al*. (1997) Visual imagery and perception in posttraumatic stress disorder. A positron emission tomographic investigation. *Archives of General Psychiatry*, **54** (3), 233–241.
213. Shin, L.M., McNally, R.J., Kosslyn, S.M. *et al*. (1999) Regional cerebral blood flow during script-driven imagery in childhood sexual abuse-related PTSD: A PET investigation. *The American Journal of Psychiatry*, **156** (4), 575–584.
214. Shin, L.M., Whalen, P.J., Pitman, R.K. *et al*. (2001) An fMRI study of anterior cingulate function in posttraumatic stress disorder. *Biological Psychiatry*, **50** (12), 932–942.
215. Shin, L.M., Orr, S.P., Carson, M.A. *et al*. (2004) Regional cerebral blood flow in the amygdala and medial prefrontal cortex during traumatic imagery in male and female Vietnam veterans with PTSD. *Archives of General Psychiatry*, **61** (2), 168–176.
216. Shin, L.M., Wright, C.I., Cannistraro, P.A. *et al*. (2005) A functional magnetic resonance imaging study of amygdala and medial prefrontal cortex responses to overtly presented fearful faces in posttraumatic stress disorder. *Archives of General Psychiatry*, **62** (3), 273–281.
217. Thomaes, K., Dorrepaal, E., Draijer, N.P. *et al*. (2009) Increased activation of the left hippocampus region in Complex PTSD during encoding and recognition of emotional words: a pilot study. *Psychiatry Research*, **171** (1), 44–53.
218. Vermetten, E., Schmahl, C., Southwick, S.M. *et al*. (2007) Positron tomographic emission study of olfactory induced emotional recall in veterans with and

without combat-related posttraumatic stress disorder. *Psychopharmacological Bulletin*, **40** (1), 8–30.

219. Whalley, M.G., Rugg, M.D., Smith, A.P. *et al*. (2009) Incidental retrieval of emotional contexts in post-traumatic stress disorder and depression: an fMRI study. *Brain and Cognition*, **69** (1), 98–107.
220. Zubieta, J.K., Chinitz, J.A., Lombardi, U. *et al*. (1999) Medial frontal cortex involvement in PTSD symptoms: a SPECT study. *Journal of Psychiatric Research*, **33** (3), 259–264.
221. Astur, R.S., St Germain, S.A., Tolin, D. *et al*. (2006) Hippocampus function predicts severity of post-traumatic stress disorder. *Cyberpsychology & Behavior*, **9** (2), 234–240.
222. Bryant, R.A., Felmingham, K.L., Kemp, A.H. *et al*. (2005) Neural networks of information processing in posttraumatic stress disorder: a functional magnetic resonance imaging study. *Biological Psychiatry*, **58** (2), 111–118.
223. Chung, Y.A., Kim, S.H., Chung, S.K. *et al*. (2006) Alterations in cerebral perfusion in posttraumatic stress disorder patients without re-exposure to accident-related stimuli. *Clinical Neurophysiology*, **117** (3), 637–642.
224. Qingling, H., Guangming, L. and Zhiqiang, Z. (2009) Resting-state fMRI Study of Posttraumatic Stress Disorder. *Journal of Clinical Radiology*, **06**, 2009.
225. Sachinvala, N., Kling, A., Suffin, S. *et al*. (2000) Increased regional cerebral perfusion by 99mTc hexamethyl propylene amine oxime single photon emission computed tomography in post-traumatic stress disorder. *Military Medicine*, **165** (6), 473–479.
226. Semple, W.E., Goyer, P.F., McCormick, R. *et al*. (1996) Attention and regional cerebral blood flow in posttraumatic stress disorder patients with substance abuse histories. *Psychiatry Research*, **67** (1), 17–28.
227. Semple, W.E., Goyer, P.F., McCormick, R. *et al*. (2000) Higher brain blood flow at amygdala and lower frontal cortex blood flow in PTSD patients with comorbid cocaine and alcohol abuse compared with normals. *Psychiatry*, **63** (1), 65–74.
228. Shaw, M.E., Strother, S.C., McFarlane, A.C. *et al*. (2002) Abnormal functional connectivity in posttraumatic stress disorder. *Neuroimage*, **15** (3), 661–674.
229. Shin, L.M., Shin, P.S., Heckers, S. *et al*. (2004) Hippocampal function in posttraumatic stress disorder. *Hippocampus*, **14** (3), 292–300.
230. Werner, N.S., Meindl, T., Engel, R.R. *et al*. (2009) Hippocampal function during associative learning in patients with posttraumatic stress disorder. *Journal of Psychiatric Research*, **43** (3), 309–318.
231. Goldberg, G. (1985) Supplementary motor area structure and function: review and hypotheses. *Behavioral and Brain Sciences*, **8**, 567–616.
232. Pribram, K.H. (1991) *Brain and Perception: Holonomy and Structure in Figural Processing*, Erlbaum, Hillsdale, NJ.
233. Gilbertson, M.W., Williston, S.K., Paulus, L.A. *et al*. (2007) Configural cue performance in identical twins discordant for posttraumatic stress disorder: theoretical implications for the role of hippocampal function. *Biological Psychiatry*, **62** (5), 513–520.

234. Marx, B.P., Doron-Lamarca, S., Proctor, S.P. and Vasterling, J.J. (2009) The influence of pre-deployment neurocognitive functioning on post-deployment PTSD symptom outcomes among Iraq-deployed Army soldiers. *Journal of the International Neuropsychological Society*, **15** (6), 840–852.

235. Milad, M.R., Orr, S.P., Lasko, N.B. *et al*. (2008) Presence and acquired origin of reduced recall for fear extinction in PTSD: results of a twin study. *Journal of Psychiatric Research*, **42** (7), 515–520.

236. Lebron, K., Milad, M.R. and Quirk, G.J. (2004) Delayed recall of fear extinction in rats with lesions of ventral medial prefrontal cortex. *Learning and Memory*, **11** (5), 544–548.

237. Milad, M.R., Rauch, S.L., Pitman, R.K. and Quirk, G.J. (2006) Fear extinction in rats: implications for human brain imaging and anxiety disorders. *Biological Psychology*, **73** (1), 61–71.

238. Rauch, S.L., Shin, L.M. and Phelps, E.A. (2006) Neurocircuitry models of posttraumatic stress disorder and extinction: human neuroimaging research–past, present, and future. *Biological Psychiatry*, **60** (4), 376–382.

239. Vertes, R.P. (2004) Differential projections of the infralimbic and prelimbic cortex in the rat. *Synapse*, **51** (1), 32–58.

240. Phelps, E.A., Delgado, M.R., Nearing, K.I. and LeDoux, J.E. (2004) Extinction learning in humans: role of the amygdala and vmPFC. *Neuron*, **43** (6), 897–905.

241. Delgado, M.R., Nearing, K.I., Ledoux, J.E. and Phelps, E.A. (2008) Neural circuitry underlying the regulation of conditioned fear and its relation to extinction. *Neuron*, **59** (5), 829–838.

242. Schiller, D. and Delgado, M.R. (2011) Overlapping neural systems mediating extinction, reversal and regulation of fear. *Trends in Cognitive Sciences*, **14** (6), 268–276

243. Bluhm, R.L., Williamson, P.C., Osuch, E.A. *et al*. (2009) Alterations in default network connectivity in posttraumatic stress disorder related to early-life trauma. *Journal of Psychiatry and Neuroscience*, **34** (3), 187–194.

244. Osuch, E.A., Willis, M.W., Bluhm, R. *et al*. (2008) Neurophysiological responses to traumatic reminders in the acute aftermath of serious motor vehicle collisions using [15O]-H2O positron emission tomography. *Biological Psychiatry*, **64** (4), 327–335.

245. Simmons, A.N., Paulus, M.P., Thorp, S.R. *et al*. (2008) Functional activation and neural networks in women with posttraumatic stress disorder related to intimate partner violence. *Biological Psychiatry*, **64** (8), 681–690.

246. Ressler, K.J. and Mayberg, H.S. (2007) Targeting abnormal neural circuits in mood and anxiety disorders: from the laboratory to the clinic. *Nature Neuroscience*, **10** (9), 1116–1124.

247. Peleg, T. and Shalev, A.Y. (2006) Longitudinal studies of PTSD: overview of findings and methods. *CNS Spectrums*, **11**, 589–602.

248. Post, R.M., Weiss, S.R.B. and Smith, M. (1995) Sensitization and kindling: implications for the evolving neural substrates of post-traumatic stress disorder, in *Neurobiological and Clinical Consequences of Stress* (eds J.M. Friedman, D.S. Charney and A.Y. Deutch), Lipnicott-Raven, Philadelphia, pp. 203–224.

249. McEwen, B.S. (2002) The neurobiology and neuroendocrinology of stress. Implications for post-traumatic stress disorder from a basic science perspective. *Psychiatric Clinics of North America*, **25**, 469–494.

250. Brewin, C.R., Gregory, J.D., Lipton, M. and Burgess, N. (2010) Intrusive images in psychological disorders: characteristics, neural mechanisms, and treatment implications. *Psychological Review*, **117**, 210–232.

251. Pitman, R.K., Gilbertson, M.W., Gurvits, T.V. *et al*. (2006) Clarifying the origin of biological abnormalities in PTSD through the study of identical twins discordant for combat exposure. *Annals of the New York Academy of Science*, **1071**, 242–254.

COMMENTARY

3.1 Translational Theory-Driven Hypotheses and Testing Are Enhancing Our Understanding of PTSD and its Treatment

Brian H. Harvey

Division of Pharmacology, Unit for Drug Research and Development, School of Pharmacy, North-West University (Potchefstroom campus), Potchefstroom, South Africa

Hans Selye [1] first explained the importance of the stress response in health and disease. This seminal work would later lead to the concepts of stress vulnerability and resilience. The stress response can be conceptualised as a set of coping mechanisms that initially resists a stressor and later improves response to the same stressor, a process that requires behavioural, psychological and physiological adaptation and is vital for survival (allostasis; [2]). However, allostasis is challenged by repeated physical/psychosocial stressors that may overwhelm these coping mechanisms, leading to maladaptive behavioural and neuroendocrine responses, structural brain changes and the development of a mental illness (allostatic load; [2]). Stress-related mental illnesses are therefore dependent on genetic predisposition but also on the nature and duration of the stressor. Basic animal research has advanced our understanding of the importance of stressor type [3] and individual susceptibility to trauma [4].

When considering the nature of the stressor and how it influences the biobehavioural stress response, a distinction can be made between limbic-sensitive and limbic-insensitive (physiological) stressors [5]. The former are more sensitive to

Post-traumatic Stress Disorder, First Edition. Edited by Dan Stein, Matthew Friedman, and Carlos Blanco.

stressors involving high-order sensory processing by the prefrontal cortex, hippocampus or amygdala before the stress response is initiated. Limbic-insensitive stressors, however, become stressful only after comparison with prior experience, although if survival is immediately compromised they gain direct access to the paraventricular nucleus in the hypothalamus to rapidly initiate the stress response and regain cardiovascular and respiratory homeostasis [5]. Thus, how a stressor is presented and managed will ultimately determine progression to the diseased state or predict recovery.

Although first conceptualised as a normal reaction to an abnormal event, post-traumatic stress disorder (PTSD) is a psychiatric disorder characterised by a unique psychobiological basis [6]. A range of normative symptoms occur post-trauma, and typically gradually diminish. In PTSD, however, such symptoms persist, leading to chronicity of symptoms and significant comorbidity and disability [7]. Indeed, only 20–30% of trauma survivors will go on to develop PTSD [8]. Analogous findings are apparent in some animal models [4]. Thus environmental adversity separates stress-sensitive from stress-resilient populations [9]. As Dr Shalev and colleagues point out, a disabling of critical cortical processes necessary to correctly process extinction of trauma memory is less functional in susceptible individuals, so perpetuating a vicious cycle of trauma recollection and reexperiencing. The neurobiology of resilience is therefore critical to our understanding of the neurobiology of psychological trauma.

If we are to obtain a deeper understanding of PTSD, we need to fully understand how the development of PTSD is linked to risk factors associated with the illness, including demographic features (e.g. female gender), clinical variables (e.g. dissociation during the trauma, exposure to multiple traumas) and biological and genetic factors [10, 11]. Animal models play a vital role in this process. The roles of monoamines, neurostereroids, decreased dehydroepiandrosterone (DHEA), decreased neuropeptide Y (NPY), hypo- versus hypercortisolism and the presence of particular genetic variants are addressed in this chapter, while there is increasing evidence for the role of glutamate and its subcellular messengers in PTSD and also in the neurobiology of resilience [12–14]. Screening populations after trauma will aid in optimising the early detection of psychiatric morbidity [15]. Just as certain symptoms of acute stress disorder may help determine those at high risk for developing PTSD [16], new knowledge of the neurobiology of stress may identify biological substrates (markers) that predict long-term outcome, as well as aid in selecting more appropriate post-trauma pharmacotherapy to prevent fear-memory consolidation and/or hasten its extinction.

This chapter presents a conceptual framework of PTSD which informatively helps optimise our understanding of its neurobiology and treatment. For example, the authors describe how the frontal cortical-amygdala adrenergic system facilitates the encoding of emotional memories responsible for propagating post-traumatic symptoms, where adrenergic α_1 and α_2 receptors are important in expressing the intensity of the adverse experience. This knowledge has in turn prompted investigation into the use of α-1 and β-adrenergic blockers to treat sleep disturbances and nightmares in PTSD patients, and to prevent the onset of PTSD in traumatised subjects, respectively [17, 18]. Studies in animal models have found that acute trauma and re-experience differently affect the hypothalamic-pituitary-adrenal axis, evoking regional-specific brain changes in serotonin, dopamine and noradrenalin that will ultimately lead to certain maladaptive behaviors [19]. Prior knowledge of the specific monoaminergic imbalance may thus have great value in selecting the correct and appropriate drug treatment for a patient with PTSD, i.e. rationalised pharmacotherapy targeting either serotonin, noradrenalin or dopamine. For example, although 5-HT is involved in the regulation of stress and anxiety [19–21], and that drug treatment of PTSD invariably involves using selective serotonin reuptake inhibitors (see Stein and Ipser, this volume), there is evidence that serotonin may actually play a bidirectional role in the development of PTSD [22]. Another illustration of the importance and benefits of fully understanding the underlying neurobiology of stress concerns kindling and the role of γ-amino butyric acid (GABA), which also occupies a central role in fear-memory circuitry. However, while bolstering GABA mechanisms with acute benzodiazepine treatment is effective in treating some anxiety disorders, these drugs may actually exacerbate PTSD symptoms [23]. Clearly, we need to understand these mechanisms in order to improve drug treatment for PTSD.

Theory-driven hypotheses need to be formulated and tested at both a pre-clinical and a clinical level to further develop our understanding of PTSD and to improve its treatment. This chapter, and indeed this volume, contributes to this process.

COMMENTARY

3.2 Precipitating and design approaches to PTSD

Eric Vermetten
Military Mental Health, Department of Defence; Department of Psychiatry, University Medical Center, Utrecht, The Netherlands

INTRODUCTION

The study of the biological, psychological and emotional consequences of traumatic stress has become a burgeoning and important field in psychiatric research and treatment. In fact, the diagnosis of PTSD is now so frequently made that one wonders how we once got by without it. PTSD is of particular interest in the twenty-first century, when the entire world is filled with the spectre of terrorism – a stressor of great magnitude that can strike anytime and anywhere.

The field of PTSD is fuelled with intriguing findings and paradoxes, as illustrated by Shalev *et al.*'s impressive review describing a conceptual framework for its neurobiology. This commentary focuses on two elementary requirements for advancing our knowledge in PTSD: a model of PTSD beyond fear conditioning and extinction, and true prospective studies. As Shalev *et al.* stipulate, studies of PTSD must be guided by theory, but this cannot simply emerge from a summation of findings. As they argue, theorising is risky, and this commentary will challenge some parts of their work.

FROM FEAR CONDITIONING TO EMOTION REGULATION

Since the conceptualisation of PTSD in the Diagnostic and Statistical Manual III (DSM-III), several models of PTSD have been entertained. Currently, the dominant paradigm in PTSD informing research and treatment is the fear conditioning and extinction model (as reviewed by Shalev *et al.*; see also [24]), which has been supported and validated by a wealth of research. The newly recognised

Post-traumatic Stress Disorder, First Edition. Edited by Dan Stein, Matthew Friedman, and Carlos Blanco.

criteria for PTSD in DSM-5, however, are moving beyond a conceptualisation of PTSD as predominantly a fear response and include dysregulation of a variety of emotional states (see also [25]). A model that describes the relationship between fear and other emotional symptoms in PTSD has thus far been lacking. Recently, two models of emotion dysregulation in PTSD were postulated in which fear is not the prevailing emotion but only one of several components that are implicated in a neural system that also mediates dysregulation of anger, guilt, shame, dissociation and numbing [26]. The term 'emotion dysregulation' can be used to collectively refer to disturbances in a variety of emotional responses [27].

The first model describes emotion dysregulation as an outcome of fear conditioning through stress sensitisation and kindling. As Shalev *et al*. have reviewed, the major support for the process of fear leading to general emotion dysregulation comes from the literature on the biological mechanisms underlying sensitisation. There is ample evidence to support the notion that fear reactions experienced during the acute aftermath of a traumatic event followed by repeated reexperiencing of the traumatic memory can lead to a process of sensitisation to subtle reminders of traumatic and related memories. Sensitisation of the fear and stress response has been hypothesised to involve complex interactions between the individual's distress, psychophysiological reactivity and related neurotransmitter and neurohormonal responses (Shalev *et al*.; see also [28, 31]). It can result in a progressive augmentation and kindling of the reactivity of an individual and lead to an associated emergence of general emotion dysregulation, including anger, grief, numbing and dissociation, as well as a generalisation of the fear response. In PTSD, in a similar way to the kindling of seizures, the progressive augmentation and expansion of symptoms occurs over time and may be related to the neural circuitry associated with the emotional memory response becoming increasingly strengthened and expanding into neighbouring neural circuits [32, 33].

In contrast to the first model, where fear is central to the origin of PTSD, the second model has a broader approach that includes one or more events that occurred before the traumatic event [26, 34]. It constitutes a classical stress-diathesis model. Specifically, this pathway proposes that an early childhood environment, which is generally impoverished due to the unavailability of a responsive attachment figure, or which specifically involves instances of childhood maltreatment and abuse, leads to inadequate neurodevelopment of the emotional and arousal regulatory systems and associated emotion dysregulation. The latter in turn results in an inability to regulate physiological arousal to threatening events, including traumatic experiences, thereby leading to exacerbation of emotion dysregulation after exposure to traumatic event(s) later in life. There is increasing evidence from the animal literature that early-life adverse experience has significant and long-lasting effects on the development of neurobiological systems and may lead to 'programming' of later increased morbidity and susceptibility to stress-related disorders (e.g. [35, 36]). This may explain some of the 'noise' in biological studies, for example in relation to hippocampal volume in depressed patients [37], the response on the combined Dexamethasone/CRH test in Borderline personality disorder (BPD) patients [38] or in healthy subjects [39], and even prediction of adult personality [40].

THE VALUE OF TRUE PROSPECTIVE STUDIES

There is a need for prospectively designed studies in this field. The three decades since the inclusion of PTSD in DSM-III have been characterised by the urge to seek acknowledgement for those suffering from the consequences of psychotrauma through biological validation of the disorder. Yet cross-sectional studies do not allow for determination of causal relationships, no matter how carefully the control populations are matched. The field has also received some criticism for weak study designs that do not control for trauma exposure, and the unreliability of memory recollections about exposure and symptoms.

One of the major and earliest postulates in PTSD was that of hypersensitivity of the hypothalamic–pituitary–adrenal (HPA) axis: that in patients who suffer from PTSD, there was a failure to mount sufficient levels of circulating cortisol at the time of the traumatic event. Essentially, no studies have looked at this proposition in a true prospective design. To test this, our group prospectively investigated whether expression of glucocorticoid receptor could be a risk factor for the development of PTSD symptoms [41]. We measured glucocorticoid receptor binding capacity in peripheral blood mononuclear cells in soldiers pre-deployment, then compared this with the presence of PTSD symptoms after deployment to a combat zone. Interestingly, we found that soldiers who reported high levels of PTSD symptoms six months after deployment had shown significantly higher expression of glucocorticoid receptors pre-deployment compared to matched controls. Thus, increased glucocorticoid receptor binding capacity of peripheral blood mononuclear cells is a vulnerability factor for subsequent development of PTSD symptoms.

As Shalev *et al.* acknowledge, threat appraisal is another important factor that needs to be taken into account when examining biological responses. We have been looking into this. In another prospective study with functional magnetic resonance imaging (fMRI), we investigated central processes in soldiers before and after deployment to a combat zone. As expected, combat stress increased amygdala and insula reactivity to biologically salient stimuli across the group of combat-exposed individuals. Intriguingly, the influence of combat stress on amygdala coupling with the insula and dorsal anterior cingulate cortex was dependent on perceived threat, rather than actual exposure. This suggests that (threat) appraisal affects interoceptive awareness and amygdala regulation. Interestingly, combat stress had sustained consequences on neural responsivity, suggesting a key role for the appraisal of threat in an amygdala-centred neural network in the aftermath of severe stress [42]. Subsequent follow-up study will determine whether these stress-induced neural changes indeed represent resilience or vulnerability factors.

CONCLUSION

The models of PTSD described above are not necessarily mutually exclusive. They show that longitudinal studies are required to examine the underlying biology of PTSD in a prospective manner in order to capture the dynamic nature of the biological alterations that manifest in the disorder. Moreover, it will become increasingly important not only to examine how stress, psychophysiological and neural responses underlying PTSD can change with exposure to stressors or progression of the illness, but also to look at early life trauma as well as different pre-trauma biological risk factors. Such studies have the potential to provide empirical support for our theoretical approaches to PTSD, allow different phenotypes of the disorder to be identified, and inform the nosology, phenomenology and treatment of this complex disorder.

REFERENCES

1. Selye, H. (1936) A syndrome produced by diverse nocuous agents. *Nature*, **138**, 32.
2. McEwen, B.S. (1998) Protective and damaging effects of stress mediators. *New England Journal of Medicine*, **338**, 171–179.
3. Uys, J.D., Stein, D.J., Daniels, W.M. and Harvey, B.H. (2003) Animal models of anxiety disorders. *Current Psychiatry Reports*, **5**, 274–281.
4. Cohen, H., Zohar, J., Matar, M.A. *et al*. (2004) Setting apart the affected: the use of behavioral criteria in animal models of post traumatic stress disorder. *Neuropsychopharmacology*, **29**, 1962–1970.
5. Herman, J.P. and Cullinan, W.E. (1997) Neurocircuitry of stress: central control of the hypothalamo-pituitary-adrenocortical axis. *Trends in Neurosciences*, **20**, 78–84.
6. Yehuda, R. and McFarlane, A.C. (1995) Conflict between current knowledge about posttraumatic stress disorder and its original conceptual basis. *American Journal of Psychiatry*, **152**, 1705–1713.
7. Kessler, R.C. (2002) Posttraumatic stress disorder: the burden to the individual and to society. *Journal of Clinical Psychiatry*, **61** (Suppl. 5), 4–12.
8. Breslau, N., Davis, G.C., Andreski, P. and Peterson, E. (1991) Traumatic events and posttraumatic stress disorder in an urban population of young adults. *Archives of General Psychiatry*, **48**, 216–222.
9. Connor, K.M. and Zhang, W. (2006) Recent advances in the understanding and treatment of anxiety disorders. Resilience: determinants, measurement, and treatment responsiveness. *CNS Spectrums*, **11** (Suppl. 12), 5–12.

10. Yehuda, R. (2004) Risk and resilience in posttraumatic stress disorder. *Journal of Clinical Psychiatry*, **65** (Suppl. 1), 29–36.
11. Brewin, C.R., Andrews, B. and Valentine, J.D. (2000) Meta-analysis of risk factors for posttraumatic stress disorder in trauma-exposed adults. *Journal of Consulting and Clinical Psychology*, **68**, 748–766.
12. Harvey, B.H., Oosthuizen, F., Brand, L. *et al*. (2004) Stress-restress evokes sustained iNOS activity and altered GABA levels and NMDA receptors in rat hippocampus. *Psychopharmacology (Berlin)*, **175** (4), 494–502.
13. Nair, J. and Singh Ajit, S. (2008) The role of the glutamatergic system in posttraumatic stress disorder. *CNS Spectrums*, **13** (7), 585–591.
14. Wegener, G. Harvey, B.H., Bonefeld, B. *et al*. (2010) Increased stress-evoked nitric oxide signalling in the Flinders sensitive line (FSL) rat: a genetic animal model of depression. *The International Journal of Neuropsychopharmacology*, **13** (4), 461–473.
15. Silove, D., Blaszczynski, A., Manicavasager, V. *et al*. (2003) Capacity of screening questionnaires to predict psychiatric morbidity 18 months after motor vehicle accidents. *Journal of Nervous and Mental Disease*, **191**, 604–610.
16. Brewin, C.R., Rose, S., Andrews, B. *et al*. (2002) Brief screening instrument for post-traumatic stress disorder. *British Journal of Psychiatry*, **181**, 158–162.
17. Vaiva, G., Ducrocq, F., Jezequel, K. *et al*. (2003) Immediate treatment with propranolol decreases posttraumatic stress disorder two months after trauma. *Biological Psychiatry*, **54**, 947–949.
18. Raskind, M.A., Peskind, E.R., Hoff, D.J. *et al*. (2007) A parallel group placebo controlled study of prazosin for trauma nightmares and sleep disturbance in combat veterans with post-traumatic stress disorder. *Biological Psychiatry*, **61**, 928–934.
19. Harvey, B.H., Brand, L., Jeeva, Z. and Stein, D.J. (2006) Cortical/hippocampal monoamines, HPA-axis changes and aversive behavior following stress and restress in an animal model of post-traumatic stress disorder. *Physiology and Behavior*, **87** (5), 881–890.
20. Harvey, B.H., Naciti, C. and Stein, D.J. (2003) Endocrine, cognitive and hippocampal/cortical 5HT 1A/2A receptor changes evoked by a time-dependent sensitisation (TDS) stress model in rats. *Brain Research*, **983** (1–2), 97–107.
21. Krystal, J.H. and Neumeister, A., (2009) Noradrenergic and serotonergic mechanisms in the neurobiology of posttraumatic stress disorder and resilience. *Brain Research*, **1293**, 13–23.
22. Harvey, B.H., Naciti, C., Brand, L. and Stein, D.J. (2004) Serotonin and stress: protective or malevolent actions in the biobehavioral response to repeated trauma? *Annals of the New York Academy of Sciences*, **1032**, 267–272.
23. Gelpin, E., Bonne, E., Peri, T. *et al*. (1996) Treatment of recent trauma survivors with benzodiazepines: a prospective study. *Journal of Clinical Psychiatry*, **57**, 390–394.
24. Shin, L.M. and Handwerger, K. (2009) Is posttraumatic stress disorder a stress-induced fear circuitry disorder? *Journal of Traumatic Stress*, **22** (5), 409–415.
25. Resick, P.A. and Miller, M.W. (2009) Posttraumatic stress disorder: anxiety or traumatic stress disorder? *Journal of Traumatic Stress*, **22** (5), 384–390.

26. Lanius, R.A., Frewin, P.A., Vermetten, E. and Yehuda, R. Fear conditioning and early life vulnerabilities: two distinct pathways of emotional dysregulation and brain dysfunction in PTSD. *European Journal of Psychotraumatology*, 1,5467, doi:10.3402/ejpt.vlio.5467.
27. Lanius, R.A., Vermetten, E., Loewenstein, R.J. *et al*. (2010) Emotion modulation in PTSD: clinical and neurobiological evidence for a dissociative subtype. *American Journal of Psychiatry*, **167** (6), 640–647.
28. Yehuda, R. and Antelman, S.M. (1993) Criteria for rationally evaluating animal models of posttraumatic stress disorder. *Biological Psychiatry*, **33** (7), 479–486.
29. Charney, D.S., Deutch, A.Y., Krystal, J.H. *et al*. (1993) Psychobiologic mechanisms of posttraumatic stress disorder. *Archives of General Psychiatry*, **50** (4), 295–305.
30. Post, R.M., Weiss, S.R., Smith, M. *et al*. (1997) Kindling versus quenching. Implications for the evolution and treatment of posttraumatic stress disorder. *Annals of the New York Academy of Sciences*, **821**, 285–295.
31. Yehuda, R. (2006) Advances in understanding neuroendocrine alterations in PTSD and their therapeutic implications. *Annals of the New York Academy of Sciences*, **1071**, 137–166.
32. McFarlane, A.C., Yehuda, R. and Clark, C.R. (2002) Biologic models of traumatic memories and post-traumatic stress disorder. The role of neural networks. *The Psychiatric Clinics of North America*, **25**, 253–270.
33. McFarlane, A.C. (2010) The long-term costs of traumatic stress: intertwined physical and psychological consequences. *World Psychiatry*, **9**, 3–10.
34. Yehuda, R., Flory, J., Pratchett, L.C. *et al*. (2010) Putative biological mechanisms for the association between early life adversity and the subsequent development of PTSD. *Psychopharmacology (Berlin)* **212**, (3), 405–417.
35. Seckl, J.R. and Meany, M.J. (2006) Glucocorticoid 'programming' and PTSD risk. *Annals of the New York Academy of Sciences*, **1071**, 351–378.
36. Felitti, V.J., Anda, R.F., Nordenberg, D. *et al*. (1998) Relationship of childhood abuse and household dysfunction to many of the leading causes of death in adults. The Adverse Childhood Experiences (ACE) Study. *American Journal of Preventive Medicine*, **14** (4), 245–258.
37. Vythilingam, M., Heim, C., Newport, J. *et al*. (2002) Childhood trauma associated with smaller hippocampal volume in women with major depression. *American Journal of Psychiatry*, **159** (12), 2072–2080.
38. Rinne, T., de Kloet, E.R., Wouters, L. *et al*. (2002) Hyperresponsiveness of hypothalamic-pituitary-adrenal axis to combined dexamethasone/corticotropin-releasing hormone challenge in female borderline personality disorder subjects with a history of sustained childhood abuse. *Biological Psychiatry*, **52** (11), 1102–1112.
39. Klaassens, E.R., Giltay, E.J., van Veen, T. *et al*. (2010) Trauma exposure in relation to basal salivary cortisol and the hormone response to the dexamethasone/CRH test in male railway employees without lifetime psychopathology. *Psychoneuroendocrinology*, **35** (6), 878–886.

40. Rademaker, A.R., Vermetten, E., Geuze, E. *et al*. (2008) Self-reported early trauma as a predictor of adult personality: a study in a military sample. *Journal of Clinical Psychology*, **64** (7), 863–875.
41. van Zuiden, M., Geuze, E., Willemen, H.L. *et al*. (2010) Pre-existing high glucocorticoid receptor number predicting development of posttraumatic stress symptoms after military deployment. *American Journal of Psychiatry*.
42. van Wingen, G.A., Geuze, E., Vermetten, E. and Fernendez, G. Perceived threat predicts the neural sequelae of combat stress. *Molecular Psychiatry*, Jan 18.
43. Raskind, M.A., Peskind, E.R., Hoff, D.J., Hart, K.L., Holmes, H.A., Warren, D., Shofer, J., O'Connell, J., Taylor, F., Gross, C., Rohde, K., McFall, M.E. (2007) A parallel group placebo controlled study of prazosin for trauma nightmares and sleep disturbance in combat veterans with post-traumatic stress disorder. *Biol Psychiatry* **61**, 928–34.
44. Nair, J., Singh, Ajit S. (2008) The role of the glutamatergic system in posttraumatic stress disorder. *CNS Spectr*, Jul; **13** (7), 585–91.
45. Wegener, G., Harvey, B.H., Bonefeld, B., Müller, H.K., Volke, V., Overstreet, D.H., Elfving, B. (2010) Increased stress-evoked nitric oxide signalling in the Flinders sensitive line (FSL) rat: a genetic animal model of depression. *Int J Neuropsychopharmacol*., Oct; **175** (4), 461–73.
46. Harvey B.H., Oosthuizen, F., Brand L., Wegener, G., Stein, D.J. (2004) Stress-restress evokes sustained iNOS activity and altered GABA levels and NMDA receptors in rat hippocampus. *Psychopharmacology (Berl)*., **175** (4), 494–502.
47. Krystal, J.H., Neumeister, A. (2009) Noradrenergic and serotonergic mechanisms in the neurobiology of posttraumatic stress disorder and resilience. *Brain Res*., Oct 13; **1293**, 13–23.
48. Harvey, B.H., Brand, L., Jeeva, Z., Stein, D.J. (2006) Cortical/hippocampal monoamines, HPA-axis changes and aversive behavior following stress and restress in an animal model of post-traumatic stress disorder. *Physiol Behav*., May 30; **87** (5), 881–90.
49. Harvey, B.H., Naciti, C., Brand, L., Stein, D.J. (2004) Serotonin and stress: protective or malevolent actions in the biobehavioral response to repeated trauma?. *Ann N Y Acad Sci*., Dec; **1032**, 267–72.
50. Harvey, B.H., Naciti, C., Brand, L., Stein, D.J. (2003) Endocrine, cognitive and hippocampal/cortical 5HT 1A/2A receptor changes evoked by a time-dependent sensitisation (TDS) stress model in rats., *Brain Res*., Sep 5; **983** (1–2), 97–107.

CHAPTER 4

Pharmacotherapy of PTSD

Dan J. Stein[1] and Jonathan C. Ipser[2]

[1] *Department of Psychiatry, University of Cape Town, Cape Town, South Africa; Mount Sinai School of Medicine, New York, NY, USA*

[2] *Department of Psychiatry, University of Cape Town, Cape Town, South Africa*

INTRODUCTION

Important advances have been made in the pharmacotherapy of post-traumatic stress disorder (PTSD). At the same time, this area of clinical practice and research continues to be a subject of some dispute. In this chapter we summarise the development of the field, and outline various ongoing controversies. We aim to make explicit the theoretical positions underlying different approaches to these controversies, in order to try and achieve some resolution.

DEVELOPMENT

An early controversy in the field was the question of whether pharmacotherapy should even be considered for PTSD at all. After all, if PTSD was a normal response to an abnormal event, then there would be no theoretical basis for attempting to disrupt such a stress response. At least three counterarguments to this view exist, and many in the field are now quite comfortable with the idea that pharmacotherapy may be an appropriate option for some patients with PTSD.

First, it is now well accepted that trauma is a common experience, and that PTSD is not simply a normal stress response [1]. Epidemiological data (see Chapter 1) have demonstrated that the majority of the population are exposed to traumatic stress, and that only a minority go on to develop PTSD. While it is true that relatively unusual and severe traumas (e.g. rape, combat) are more likely to be associated with PTSD, the majority of PTSD cases are a consequence of relatively common ‘everyday’ kinds of trauma (e.g. motor-vehicle accidents) [2]. Clinical data have shown that although post-traumatic stress symptoms are

Post-traumatic Stress Disorder, First Edition. Edited by Dan Stein, Matthew Friedman, and Carlos Blanco.

common in the immediate aftermath of a traumatic experience, in the majority of cases they decrease over time [3]. Various risk factors, including prior exposure to trauma, predict who will go on to develop PTSD [4, 5]. Psychobiological data (see Chapter 2) have shown that PTSD is accompanied by a range of abnormalities, including alterations in neurocircuitry and neurochemistry and in associated cognitive and affective function [6, 7]. Pharmacotherapy may be able to reverse some of these abnormalities [8].

A second response to the question of whether it is appropriate to treat a stress response emerges from the growing literature on evolutionary medicine [9]. Although this literature has perhaps not yet had a wide influence on clinicians, it provides a sophisticated conceptual and empirical foundation for thinking about pharmacotherapy of physiological defences. Evolutionary medicine emphasises that many evolved responses can cause symptoms: in response to infection, for example, organisms have developed complex physiological defences, including pyrexia. It turns out that medical interference with such responses may be somewhat detrimental; for example, the use of antipyretics may be associated with a slightly longer course of infection. At the same time, there is no reason for clinicians not to use such interventions; antipyretics are widely and appropriately used, on the basis of an analysis of the relevant risks and benefits.

Indeed, a third response is to insist on rigorous empirical trials, which allow the relative risks and benefits of pharmacotherapeutic intervention to be examined. As different psychotropic agents have been introduced into the market, typically for the treatment of mood or anxiety disorders, they have been studied in double-blind trials for PTSD. Thus, there is now a relatively large evidence base on the pharmacotherapy of PTSD, including work on various antidepressants (tricyclic antidepressants, monoamine oxidase inhibitors, selective serotonin reuptake inhibitors (SSRIs), serotonin noradrenaline reuptake inhibitors (SNRIs)), benzodiazepines, antipsychotics, anticonvulsants and other agents [10].

The earliest work on the pharmacotherapy of PTSD, therefore, was with early antidepressants, namely the tricyclic antidepressants and the monoamine oxidase inhibitors [11, 12]. This work arguably suffered from a number of methodological flaws, including small samples, relatively short duration of treatment and the lack of well-validated symptom measures as primary outcome measures. Nevertheless, it was rigorous insofar as it used placebo controls, and it was important insofar as it provided an important proof of principle that the benefits of pharmacotherapy might outweigh its risks, so that psychotropic intervention for PTSD could be considered a potential treatment option.

The introduction of the SSRIs was a particularly important advance as these agents, with their good safety profile, had the potential to move the risk : benefit ratio in an even more favourable direction [13]. Furthermore, large trials on these agents were sponsored by the pharmaceutical industry, in the hope of obtaining regulatory approval for the specific indication of PTSD. Sertraline was the first molecule to obtain such approval (from the US Food and Drug Administration (FDA), and it was followed relatively quickly by paroxetine. The

Table 4.1 Selected SSRI trials in PTSD.

Authors	Intervention vs Placebo	Subjects	Outcome
Brady *et al.* [14]	Sertraline (50-200 mg/d) × 12 weeks	187 DSM-III-R PTSD	Sertraline > Placebo
Brady *et al.* [45]	Sertraline (50-150 mg/d) × 12 weeks	94 DSM-IV PSTD with alcoholism	Alcohol use decreased in both groups
Conner *et al.* [15]	Fluoxetine (20-60 mg/d) × 12 weeks	53 DSM-III PTSD	Fluoxetine > Placebo
Davidson *et al.* [41]	Sertraline (25-200 mg/d) × 12 weeks	208 DSM-III-R PTSD	Sertraline > Placebo
Marshall *et al.* [36]	Paroxetine (25-50 mg/d) × 12 weeks	563 DSM-IV PTSD	Paroxetine > Placebo
Martenyi *et al.* [16]	Fluoxetine (20-80 mg/d) × 12 weeks	301 DSM-IV PTSD	Fluoxetine > Placebo
Martenyi *et al.* [37]	Fluoxetine (20-40 mg/d) × 12 weeks	411 DSM-IV PTSD	Fluoxetine = Placebo
Tucker *et al.* [17]	Paroxetine (20-50 mg/d) × 12 weeks	323 DSM-IV PTSD	Paroxetine > Placebo

pharmaceutical industry also sponsored a series of trials on other antidepressants, including fluoxetine and venlafaxine, although a marketing decision was made not to submit these agents for approval. The bulk of the evidence on the pharmacotherapy of PTSD derives from these trials (Table 4.1).

A range of additional pharmacotherapy trials have been undertaken on PTSD. Neurobiological advances in PTSD have given impetus to the study of particular molecules, looking for example at evidence that PTSD might involve the dopaminergic system, adrenergic system or sensitisation effects encouraged trials on antipsychotic, alpha-adrenergic and anticonvulsant agents. Ongoing clinical issues in the area of PTSD have also encouraged various trials, for example to determine the effects of pharmacotherapy in particular populations (e.g. patients with comorbid substance use, paediatric PTSD), to test the effectiveness of medications in addressing specific PTSD symptoms (e.g. prazosin for disrupted sleep), to assess the longer-term effects of pharmacotherapy, to address the value of combining pharmacotherapy with psychotherapy and to determine the effects of combinations of different agents in treatment-refractory PTSD [10, 18].

At the same time, it is important to acknowledge a key concern underlying much of the early debate about whether medication should be considered in PTSD. This has to do with the explanatory models used by both clinicians and therapists to address trauma and its response, and the worry that if PTSD is conceptualised as a biological disruption, requiring pharmacotherapeutic intervention, then an important aspect of many potentially useful models, namely a focus on resilience and recovery, might be lost. With this in mind, we would certainly advise clinicians to carefully address patients' explanatory models of

PTSD and to emphasise that the use of pharmacotherapy does not at all contradict the possibility that facing trauma also presents the patient with an opportunity to grow and to become more resilient [19].

ASSESSING THE EVIDENCE

A second controversy has emerged, however, from the assessment of this evidence base. As the knowledge base in psychopharmacology in general has grown, so have professional bodies and regulatory agencies been increasingly interested in assessing the relevant data in order to promote evidence-based practice. Reviews include those undertaken by the American Psychiatric Association [20], the British Psychopharmacology Association [21], the Canadian Psychiatric Association [22], the International Society for Traumatic Stress Studies [23], the Institute of Medicine (IOM) [24], the UK National Institute of Clinical Excellence (NICE) [25], the World Federation of Societies of Biological Psychiatry [26] and a range of other expert consensus groups [7, 27, 28].

It is notable that these different guidelines have reached quite different conclusions. In general, professional bodies have typically concluded that the SSRIs constitute the first-line pharmacotherapy of choice for PTSD. However, NICE concluded that mirtazepine was the pharmacotherapy of choice, and the IOM concluded that the evidence for most interventions for PTSD was inadequate. It is important to establish the different underlying theoretical positions which led to these conclusions, and to provide clinicians with a rational basis for drawing their own conclusions.

From the perspective of many professional bodies, there have now been a relatively large number of randomised controlled trials on the pharmacotherapy of PTSD. There is a particularly large body of evidence on the SSRIs, with several of these agents having accumulated sufficient data to convince regulatory bodies of their approvability for the PTSD indication (Table 4.1). They are also effective for disorders that are often comorbid with PTSD, especially depression, and have a more acceptable side-effect profile than many other classes of psychotropic agents. Such considerations have proven persuasive to expert clinicians.

NICE took a particular approach to their meta-analysis that led to a somewhat different conclusion [25]. They decided that trials had to have an effect size of at least 0.5 in order to qualify as clinically significant. Whereas regulatory bodies may allow approval of a particular drug even when negative trials exist, NICE also placed emphasis on meta-analytic results that included both positive and negative trials. Thus, none of the SSRIs were viewed as clinically significant. Sertraline was emphasised as not effective in a trial of US veterans with chronic PTSD, despite the fact that this population might differ in several respects both from civilian populations in the USA, from more recent VA cohorts [29] and from veteran populations elsewhere [30]; the data were therefore viewed as negative.

Although PTSD is a relatively difficult disorder to treat, and one in which placebo response may be relatively high, the effect size in the paroxetine trials was also interpreted by NICE as not clinically significant.

Similar considerations were also emphasised by the IOM [24], which thus noted that most studies on PTSD, whether pharmacotherapeutic or psychotherapeutic, had important methodological limitations. These included the inclusion of patients with comorbidity (especially depression), high dropout rates and weak handling of missing data. The report also put a great deal of emphasis on the lack of available research data, noting that there was simply an absence of evidence on a range of PTSD populations, including ethnic and cultural minorities. The IOM reviewers argued that they were not tasked with the development of clinical guidelines, and therefore did not need to address the practical question of what treatments to offer when there was an absence of evidence (no evidence of efficacy is of course not the same as evidence of lack of efficacy).

From an advocacy perspective, it is of course key to emphasise the relative paucity of data on interventions for PTSD. Given the burden of disease attributable to trauma in general and to PTSD in particular, and the possibility that efficacious and cost-effective treatments exist, there is every reason to support additional research in this area. At the same time, when making clinical treatment recommendations it is important to (i) use similar criteria to those used in other disorders and (ii) take into account the particularities of the relevant condition. Thus, in many areas of psychiatry, trials are not uniformly positive; this issue has often been addressed in the depression literature, where there is some acceptance that effect sizes are higher in more severe patients and in academic settings, and lower in patients with milder symptoms and in 'real-world' settings. Similarly, in PTSD, from a clinical perspective, it seems reasonable to put particular emphasis on the data from multisite trials that have focused on civilians (which are often positive), while noting that trials done in USA veterans have a particular bias (and are often negative).

Our conclusion that the evidence base for the pharmacotherapy of PTSD is strong enough to support a recommendation that SSRIs (and perhaps venlafaxine) be used as a first-line pharmacotherapy for PTSD may reflect a clinical bias. At the same time, we would argue that such a clinical bias is not unreasonable; PTSD is a highly prevalent disorder, often requiring treatment, and at the current point in time we are fortunate that a number of SSRIs have been appropriately approved for the management of this disorder on the basis of a convincing risk : benefit ratio. This does not, of course, diminish the facts that treatment outcomes remain far from optimal, that we lack good data on a whole range of important clinical questions and that significantly more research is required in order to optimise future outcomes.

From a clinical perspective it is also important to emphasise that we would not recommend other classes of medication, such as the benzodiazepines, antipsychotics or anticonvulsants, as a first line of treatment for PTSD. Again, although the clinical trials database is very limited, what data do exist are not entirely persuasive that these agents are helpful as monotherapy. Nevertheless, some studies of antipsychotic, anticonvulsant and alpha-adrenergic agents have been promising, particularly in certain PTSD subpopulations [31, 32–34, 35], encouraging further research in this area.

KEY ISSUES

The next set of controversies are those that emerge once it has been decided that psychotropics may be worth considering, and that there is sufficient evidence that SSRIs are the first-line choice for pharmacotherapy. In this section we will address several key issues concerning the optimal pharmacotherapy of PTSD, including the optimal SSRI for PTSD, the dose and duration of pharmacotherapy, PTSD subtypes and spectrums, the relative merits of pharmacotherapy and psychotherapy, treatment-refractory PTSD and PTSD prophylaxis.

The optimal SSRI for PTSD

What is the optimal SSRI (or SNRI) for the pharmacotherapy of PTSD? Several considerations are relevant.

First, each of the SSRIs may have a slightly different efficacy and tolerability profile, based in part on its particular affinity for various neuroreceptors. Thus, paroxetine has increased affinity for cholinergic receptors, and may potentially therefore be associated with more sedating effects as well as with greater weight gain. A number of guidelines have argued that the adverse event profile of venlafaxine is somewhat less acceptable than that of the SSRIs in general, although there is some inconsistency on this issue.

Second, individual responses to each particular SSRI may vary somewhat, depending on genetic variability in neuroreceptors and other relevant genes. Thus, for example, some patients may have particular variants in their cytochrome P450 system, leading to variations in the metabolism of certain SSRIs. When patients are on multiple medications, and there is scope for drug–drug interactions, SSRIs with less susceptibility to such interactions will be advantageous.

Third, not all SSRIs have been well studied in PTSD, and there is a paucity of head-to-head studies comparing different SSRIs in the treatment of PTSD. Although it has been claimed that certain SSRIs are associated with earlier and more robust response in disorders such as depression, or that SNRIs are associated with greater remission of symptoms in these conditions, in general the field has yet to conclude that any particular one of these agents is generally more efficacious than the others [10].

Dose and duration of pharmacotherapy

If one is going to use an SSRI for the pharmacotherapy of PTSD, what is the optimal dose, how long should an initial trial of pharmacotherapy be, and how long should pharmacotherapy be maintained if there is a response? Once again, there are relatively few data on which to base answers.

First, there are few fixed-dose comparative studies of SSRIs in PTSD. Those which do exist do not indicate that there is a robust dose–response relationship [36, 37], consistent with data from a range of other disorders, such as depression. Nevertheless, the expert consensus recommendation, when considering both PTSD and conditions such as depression, often advises clinicians that some individuals may respond more robustly to a higher dose of medication. Thus clinicians are often provided with the dose range for each SSRI (Table 4.1) and advised to use as low a dose as possible, but to consider higher doses when there is not a maximal response.

Second, relatively few studies have examined the question of what proportion of nonresponders at, say, week 8, go on to become responders at, say, week 12. Data from studies of major depression and of other anxiety disorders indicate that in general, early response is a predictor of those patients who will respond by the end of the trial. At the same time, a significant proportion of nonresponders at week 8 do go on to become responders at week 12. For this reason, expert-consensus recommendations often indicate the advisability of an initial trial of at least 12 weeks for PTSD.

Third, there are only a few maintenance and/or discontinuation studies of pharmacotherapy in PTSD [38]. The data from these studies indicate that during the course of treatment there is continuous improvement on medication for several months, and that discontinuation of medication within the first 12 months of treatment is associated with a greater risk of relapse. For this reason, expert-consensus recommendations typically recommend that pharmacotherapy be continued for at least 12 months before discontinuation is considered, and that the dose of SSRIs should be decreased only gradually.

PTSD subtypes and spectrums

It has long been speculated that different PTSD subtypes are mediated by different psychobiological mechanisms. It is possible, for example, that different PTSD symptoms reflect the involvement of different neurotransmitter systems [39, 40]. Although there are some suggestions that different agents may be associated with different symptom-response profiles [41], treatment studies are typically not powered to determine whether there are significant differences between medication and placebo for particular symptom clusters. Furthermore, treatment studies have in general indicated that although certain symptoms may improve at different rates [7], given treatment of sufficient duration most symptoms will demonstrate a response. At the same time, a number of trials have now indicated that prazosin may be particularly effective in PTSD and insomnia [31, 42].

It is possible that a range of other PTSD subtypes and spectrums have a somewhat different pharmacotherapeutic response. For example, it is possible that delayed PTSD has a specific neurobiology that requires targeting by a particular pharmacotherapy. Similarly, it is conceivable that various symptoms that begin in the immediate aftermath of traumatic stress, including dissociative symptoms, can be distinguished by specific neurobiological anomalies and associated responses to pharmacotherapy. Once again, however, there is a relative dearth of relevant data from randomised controlled trials. It is notable that patients with a history of early trauma and PTSD do not appear to be more refractory to standard pharmacotherapy intervention [43]. There is also evidence that some combat-exposed patients do respond to pharmacotherapy [30]. In general we would advise clinicians to begin with the most evidence-based pharmacotherapy intervention (i.e. SSRIs) for PTSD, but to consider and document alternative rationales where cases differ from those included in most PTSD trials.

A similar logic applies to PTSD populations that differ on a variety of demographic and clinical variables that are not well sampled in the trial base, including those that vary in terms of age (e.g. paediatric and geriatric populations), ethnicity and comorbidity [44]. In general, one would consider applying the lessons from the general database, albeit with appropriate adjustments. Thus, for example, there is some evidence from both open-label trials in PTSD and controlled trials in mood and anxiety disorders that certain SSRIs are effective in paediatric patients with these conditions. At the same time, the clinician needs to bear in mind age-related adverse events (e.g. the possibility of medication-related increases in suicidal ideation) and circumstances (e.g. the possibility that developmental issues need to be addressed by a more comprehensive set of interventions). Unfortunately, patients with PTSD and comorbid substance abuse appear to respond less well to SSRIs [45]. Furthermore, the clinician needs to bear in mind particular clinical issues of relevance (e.g. the possible need for interventions focused specifically on substance-use disorder, such as detoxification).

Pharmacotherapy and psychotherapy

There is a relatively small evidence base directly addressing pharmacotherapy versus psychotherapy in the treatment of PTSD [46]. Further, there is a growing awareness of the importance of studies that do not simply contrast these modalities, but which also address the optimal sequencing of intervention. A few general comments can perhaps be made.

First, it is often problematic to compare effect sizes from the pharmacotherapy and psychotherapy literature. Many psychotherapy trials do not have an active comparison arm, leading to an inflated estimate of effect size. Second, there is surprisingly little evidence that pharmacotherapy is effective in psychotherapy nonresponders [47, 48] and only some evidence that psychotherapy is effective in pharmacotherapy nonresponders [49]. Third, there is a clinical tradition of combining pharmacotherapy and psychotherapy in PTSD [5-], which has recently been informed by translational research on fear extinction [51] and thus more rigorously examined [52].

Treatment-refractory PTSD

A first question is the definition of treatment-refractory PTSD. Possible options are to define treatment resistance in terms of percentage reduction on a gold-standard symptom measure such as the clinician administered PTSD scale (CAPS), in terms of a clinician-rated scale that is used in a range of anxiety and mood disorders such as the clinical global impressions (CGI) scale, or in terms of scales that assess impairment and quality of life. In addition, different definitions might emphasise the failure to respond to one or more pharmacotherapy trials, at specific doses and durations. It is reasonable to recommend that a clinician should use different measures during a trial of treatment, in order to make an accurate and comprehensive evaluation of treatment response. There has also been recent interest in assessing resilience during the treatment of PTSD [53].

A second question is whether to switch medications or whether to augment. There is a dearth of effectiveness trials addressing the sequencing of pharmacotherapy treatments in PTSD. Expert consensus therefore tends to follow the work in disorders such as depression and makes the very preliminary suggestion that a switch can perhaps be considered in patients with no response, while augmentation is perhaps a reasonable option in patients with partial response. There is some support from the depression literature for the idea that where one medication is not effective, a different entity from the same class, or a medication from a different class, may be useful.

A third question addresses augmenting the agent of choice. A number of trials have now been undertaken in this area. Basic studies on the role of the dopamine system in stress responses, and clinical studies on its role in PTSD, have given impetus to studies of antipsychotic augmentation [14]. The evidence to date is promising, but it is important to carefully consider the risk : benefit ratio, given the propensity of these agents for a range of metabolic side effects [14]. Similarly, there are good reasons for considering whether anticonvulsant augmentation might be useful in patients refractory to antidepressant medication. Here there have been fewer rigorous trials, and the data are not yet persuasive [54].

PTSD prophylaxis

There is growing interest in the question of whether pharmacotherapy might be effective in the prophylaxis of PTSD. Animal studies have been useful in suggesting that particular psychopharmacological interventions, administered immediately after trauma exposure, may lead to a decrease in the expected stress response [55, 56]. A series of studies on beta-blockers, given in the acute trauma setting, have provided proof-of-principle evidence that similar interventions might be useful for humans. However, subsequent evidence has not been as persuasive [7]. For now, although this remains an extremely interesting area for research, psychopharmacological intervention cannot be clinically recommended at the time of trauma.

CONCLUSION

Although there are a series of controversies in the area of PTSD pharmacotherapy, a close examination of one's theoretical assumptions, and of the empirical evidence, perhaps allows some resolution of these issues. We have argued for a number of conclusions, as follows.

First, there is a good rationale and substantial evidence for the notion that PTSD pharmacotherapy may be a valuable part of the treatment of this condition. Certainly, there is a growing understanding of the neurobiology of PTSD, and a number of agents have been registered for the treatment of this condition. Additional work is needed to document fully the cost-effectiveness of pharmacotherapy interventions in different clinical settings.

Second, although the clinical trials database for the pharmacotherapy of PTSD has significant limitations and deserves considerable expansion, there is a reasonable evidence base showing the value of SSRIs in its treatment. For this reason, many clinical treatment guidelines have concluded that the SSRIs are the first-line pharmacotherapy intervention of choice in PTSD. Additional work is needed to explicate fully the predictors of response to SSRIs; currently there are very few of these (although chronic PTSD in US VA settings is a negative predictor of response).

Third, given the limitations of the clinical base, in real-world clinical settings the clinician must use his or her judgement in selecting and using a particular medication. Issues such as age and comorbidity should be taken into consideration. Despite the limitations of the PTSD database, principles of treatment do emerge from the related literature on pharmacotherapy of depression and anxiety disorders, and it behooves the clinician to carefully document the rationale underlying their decision-making.

Fourth, there are a number of areas in which additional research is clearly needed. One area of particular importance is patients with treatment-refractory

PTSD; findings from antipsychotic augmentation studies give impetus to additional work. There have been several promising developments in PTSD pharmacotherapy, including the use of a translational approach to justify particular combinations of medication or of medication with pharmacotherapy, and the potential incorporation of genetic [57] and imaging [8] data into clinical trials. At the same time, the field is at an early stage and much additional efficacy and effectiveness work remains to be done.

REFERENCES

1. Yehuda, R. and McFarlane, A.C. (1995) Conflict between current knowledge about posttraumatic stress disorder and its original conceptual basis. *American Journal of Psychiatry*, **152**, 1705–1713.
2. Kessler, R.C. (2002) Posttraumatic stress disorder: the burden to the individual and to society. *The Journal of Clinical Psychiatry*, **61S5**, 4–12.
3. Foa, E.B., Stein, D.J., McFarlane, A.C. *et al*. (2006) Symptomatology and psychopathology of mental health problems after disaster. *Journal of Clinical Psychiatry*, **67**, 15–25.
4. Brewin, C.R., Andrews, B. and Valentine, J.D. (2000) Meta-analysis of risk factors for posttraumatic stress disorder in trauma-exposed adults. *Journal of Consulting and Clinical Psychology*, **68**, 748–766.
5. Yehuda, R. (1999) *Risk Factors for Posttraumatic Stress Disorder*, American Psychiatric Press, Washington, DC.
6. Nemeroff, C.B., Bremner, J.D. and Foa, E.B. (2006) Posttraumatic stress disorder: a state-of-the-science review. *Journal of Psychiatric Research*, **40**, 1–21.
7. Stein, D.J., Cloitre, M., Nemeroff, C.B. *et al*. (2009) Cape Town consensus on posttraumatic stress disorder. *CNS Spectrums*, **14S1**, 52–58.
8. Seedat, S., Warwick, J., van Heerden, B. *et al*. (2003) Single photon emission computed tomography in posttraumatic stress disorder before and after treatment with a selective serotonin reuptake inhibitor. *Journal of Affective Disorders*, **80**, 45–53.
9. Nesse, R.M. and Williams, G.C. (1994) *Why We Get Sick: the New Science of Darwinian Medicine*, Vintage Books, New York.
10. Stein, D.J., Ipser, J.C. and Seedat, S. (2006) Pharmacotherapy for post traumatic stress disorder (PTSD). *Cochrane Database of Systematic Reviews* (1:CD002795).
11. Frank, J.B., Kosten, T.R., Giller, E.L. and Dan, E. (1988) A randomized clinical-trial of phenelzine and imipramine for posttraumatic stress disorder. *American Journal of Psychiatry*, **145**, 1289–1291.
12. Davidson, J., Kudler, H., Smith, R. *et al*. (1990) Treatment of posttraumatic-stress-disorder with amitriptyline and placebo. *Archives of General Psychiatry*, **47**, 259–266.
13. Connor, K.M. and Davidson, J.R.T. (1998) The role of serotonin in posttraumatic stress disorder: Neurobiology and pharmacotherapy. *CNS Spectrums*, **3S2**, 43–51.

14. Brady, K., Pearlstein, T., Asnis, G. M. *et al*. (2000) Efficacy and safety of sertraline treatment of posttraumatic stress disorder: A randomized controlled trial. *JAMA*, **283**, 1837–1844.
15. Connor, K. M., Sutherland, S.M., Tupler, L.A. *et al*. (1999) Fluoxetine in post-traumatic stress disorder - Randomised, double-blind study. *British Journal of Psychiatry*, **175**, 17–22.
16. Martenyi, F., Brown, E.B., Zhang, H. *et al*. (2002) Fluoxetine versus placebo in posttraumatic stress disorder. *Journal of Clinical Psychiatry*, **63**, 199–206.
17. Tucker, P., Zaninelli, R., Yehuda, R. *et al*. (2001) Paroxetine in the treatment of chronic posttraumatic stress disorder: Results of a placebo-controlled, flexible-dosage trial. *Journal of Clinical Psychiatry*, **62**, 860–868.
18. Ipser, J.C., Carey, P., Dhansay, Y. *et al*. (2006) Pharmacotherapy augmentation strategies in treatment-resistant anxiety disorders. *Cochrane Database of Systematic Reviews* (4: CD005473).
19. Tedeschi, R.G., Park, C.L. and Calhoun, L.G. (1998) *Posttraumatic Growth: Positive Changes in the Aftermath of Crisis*, Lawrence Erlbaum Associates.
20. Ursano, R.J., Bell, C., Eth, S. *et al*. (2004) Practice guideline for the treatment of patients with acute stress disorder and posttraumatic stress disorder. *The American Journal of Psychiatry*, **161**, 3–31.
21. Baldwin, D.S., Anderson, I.M., Nutt, D.J. *et al*. (2005) Evidence-based guidelines for the pharmacological treatment of anxiety disorders: recommendations from the British Association for Psychopharmacology. *Journal of Psychopharmacology*, **19**, 567–596.
22. Swinson, R.P., Antony, M.M., Bleau, P.B. *et al*. (2006) Clinical practice guidelines: management of anxiety disorders. *Canadian Journal of Psychiatry*, **51S2**, 1–92.
23. Foa, E.B., Keane, T.M., Friedman, M.J. and Cohen, J.A. (2009) *Effective Treatments for PTSD: Practice Guidelines from the International Society for Traumatic Stress Studies*, 2nd edn, Guilford Press, New York.
24. Institute of Medicine (2008) *Treatment of PTSD: An Assessment of the Evidence*, National Academies Press, Washington, DC.
25. National Institute for Clinical Excellence (2005) *The Management of Post Traumatic Stress Disorder in Primary and Secondary Care*, NICE, London.
26. Bandelow, B., Zohar, J. and Hollander, E. (2008) World Federation of Societies of Biological Psychiatry (WFSBP) guidelines for the pharmacological treatment of anxiety, obsessive-compulsive and post-traumatic stress disorders – first revision. *World Journal of Biological Psychiatry*, **9**, 248–312.
27. Ballenger, J.C., Davidson, J.R., Lecrubier, Y. *et al*. (2004) Consensus statement update on posttraumatic stress disorder from the international consensus group on depression and anxiety. *Journal of Clinical Psychiatry*, **65** (Suppl. 1), 55–62.
28. Davidson, J., Bernik, M., Connor, K.M. *et al*. (2005) A new treatment algorithm for posttraumatic stress disorder. *Psychiatric Annals*, **35**, 887–898.
29. Friedman, M., Davidson, J. and Stein, D.J. (2008) Pharmacotherapy for posttraumatic stress disorder, in *Effective Treatments for PTSD: Practice Guidelines from the*

International Society for Traumatic Stress Studies, 2nd edn (eds E. Foa, T.M. Keane, M.J. Friedman and J.D. Cohen), Guilford, New York.

30. Zohar, J., Amital, D., Miodownik, C. *et al*. (2002) Double-blind placebo-controlled pilot study of sertraline in military veterans with posttraumatic stress disorder. *Journal of Clinical Psychopharmacology*, **22**, 190–195.
31. Taylor, F.B., Martin, P., Thompson, C. *et al*. (2008) Prazosin effects on objective sleep measures and clinical symptoms in civilian trauma posttraumatic stress disorder: a placebo-controlled study. *Biological Psychiatry*, **63**, 629–632.
32. Reich, D.B., Winternitz, S., Hennen, J. *et al*. (2004) A preliminary study of risperidone in the treatment of posttraumatic stress disorder related to childhood abuse in women. *Journal of Clinical Psychiatry*, **65**, 1601–1606.
33. Padala, P.R., Madison, J., Monnahan, M. *et al*. (2006) Risperidone monotherapy for post-traumatic stress disorder related to sexual assault and domestic abuse in women. *International Journal of Clinical Psychopharmacology*, **21**, 275–280.
34. Tucker, P., Trautman, R.P., Wyatt, D.B. *et al*. (2007) Efficacy and safety of topiramate monotherapy in civilian posttraumatic stress disorder: a randomized, double-blind, placebo-controlled study. *Journal of Clinical Psychiatry*, **68**, 201–206.
35. Berger, W., Mendlowicz, M.V., Marques-Portella, C. *et al*. (2009) Pharmacologic alternatives to antidepressants in posttraumatic stress disorder: a systematic review. *Progress in Neuropsychopharmacology & Biological Psychiatry*, **33**, 169–180.
36. Marshall, R.D., Beebe, K.L., Oldham, M. *et al*. (2001) Efficacy and safety of paroxetine treatment for chronic PTSD: a fixed-dose, placebo-controlled study. *American Journal of Psychiatry*, **158**, 1982–1988.
37. Martenyi, F., Brown, E.B., Caldwell, C.D. (2007) Failed efficacy of fluoxetine in the treatment of posttraumatic stress disorder: results of a fixed-dose, placebo-controlled study. *Journal of Clinical Psychopharmacology*, **27**, 166–170.
38. Stein, D.J., Bandelow, B., Hollander, E. *et al*. (2003) WCA recommendations for the long-term treatment of posttraumatic stress disorder. *CNS Spectrums*, **8**, 31–39.
39. Lanius, R.A., Vermetten, E., Loewenstein, R.J. *et al*. (2010) Emotion modulation in PTSD: clinical and neurobiological evidence for a dissociative subtype. *American Journal of Psychiatry*, **167**, 640–647.
40. Charney, D.S., Deutch, A.Y. and Krystal, J.H. (1993) Psychobiologic mechanisms of posttraumatic stress disorder. *Archives of General Psychiatry*, **50**, 295–305.
41. Davidson, J.R.T., Rothbaum, B.O., van der Kolk, B.A. *et al*. (2001) Multicenter, double-blind comparison of sertraline and placebo in the treatment of posttraumatic stress disorder. *Archives of General Psychiatry*, **58**, 485–492.
42. Taylor, F. and Raskind, M.A. (2002) The alpha 1-adrenergic antagonist prazosin improves sleep and nightmares in civilian trauma posttraumatic stress disorder. *Journal of Clinical Psychopharmacology*, **22**, 82–85.
43. Stein, D.J., Van der Kolk, B. and Austin, C. (2003) Efficacy of sertraline in posttraumatic stress disorder secondary to interpersonal trauma or childhood abuse. *European Neuropsychopharmacology*, **13**, S363–S364.

44. Marshall, R.D., Lewis-Fernandez, R., Blanco, C. *et al*. (2007) A controlled trial of paroxetine for chronic PTSD, dissociation, and interpersonal problems in mostly minority adults. *Depression and Anxiety*, **24**, 77–84.
45. Brady, K.T., Sonne, S., Anton, R.F. *et al*. (2005) Sertraline in the treatment of co-occurring alcohol dependence and posttraumatic stress disorder. *Alcoholism: Clinical & Experimental Research*, **29**, 395–401.
46. van der Kolk, B.A., Spinazzola, J., Blaustein, M.E. *et al*. (2007) A randomized clinical trial of eye movement desensitization and reprocessing (EMDR), fluoxetine, and pill placebo in the treatment of posttraumatic stress disorder: treatment effects and long-term maintenance. *Journal of Clinical Psychiatry*, **68**, 37–46.
47. Simon, N.M., Connor, K.M., Lang, A.J. *et al*. (2008) Paroxetine CR augmentation for posttraumatic stress disorder refractory to prolonged exposure therapy. *Journal of Clinical Psychiatry*, **69**, 400–405.
48. Hofmann, S.G., Sawyer, A.T, Korte, K.J. *et al*. (2009) Is it Beneficial to Add Pharmacotherapy to Cognitive-Behavioral Therapy when Treating Anxiety Disorders? A Meta-Analytic Review. *International Journal of Cognitive Therapy*, **2**, 160–175.
49. Rothbaum, B.O., Cahill, S.P., Foa, E.B. *et al*. (2006) Augmentation of sertraline with prolonged exposure in the treatment of posttraumatic stress disorder. *Journal of Traumatic Stress*, **19**, 625–638.
50. Southwick, S.M., Yehuda, R. (1993) The interaction between pharmacotherapy and psychotherapy in the treatment of posttraumatic stress disorder. *American Journal of Psychotherapy*, **47**, 404–410.
51. Davis, M., Ressler, K., Rothbaum, B.O. *et al*. (2006) Effects of D-cycloserine on extinction: translation from preclinical to clinical work. *Biological Psychiatry*, **60**, 369–375.
52. Choi, D.C., Rothbaum, B.O., Gerardi, M. *et al*. (2010) Pharmacological enhancement of behavioral therapy: focus on posttraumatic stress disorder. *Current Topics in Behavioral Neurosciences*, **2**, 279–299.
53. Davidson, J., Baldwin, D.S., Stein, D.J. *et al*. (2008) Effects of venlafaxine extended release on resilience in posttraumatic stress disorder: an item analysis of the Connor-Davidson Resilience Scale. *International Clinical Psychopharmacology*, **23**, 299–303.
54. Lindley, S.E., Carlson, E.B., Hill, K. (2007) A randomized, double-blind, placebo-controlled trial of augmentation topiramate for chronic combat-related posttraumatic stress disorder. *Journal of Clinical Psychopharmacology*, **27**, 677–681.
55. Cohen, H., Matar, M.A., Buskila, D. *et al*. (2008) Early post-stressor intervention with high-dose corticosterone attenuates posttraumatic stress response in an animal model of posttraumatic stress disorder. *Biological Psychiatry*, **64**, 708–717.
56. Kaplan, G.B., Moore, K.A. (2011) The use of cognitive enhancers in animal models of fear extinction. *Pharmacology Biochemistry & Behavior*, Jan 20. [Epub ahead of print]
57. Amstadter, A.B., Nugent, N.R., Koenen, K.C. (2009) Genetics of PTSD: Fear Conditioning as a Model for Future Research. *Psychiatr Ann.*, **39**, 358–367.

COMMENTARY

4.1 Critical View of the Pharmacological Treatment of Trauma

Marcelo F. Mello
Department of Psychiatry, Universidade Federal de São Paulo, São Paulo, Brazil

The chapter 'Pharmacotherapy of PTSD' written by Stein and Ipser is an important contribution to our knowledge of post-traumatic stress disorder (PTSD) treatment.

The authors contextualise the evolution of the diagnosis of PTSD, noting how it has been criticised since it entered the official nomenclature. Despite the fact that the psychopathological consequences of violence have been described for thousands of years, scepticism about the validity of the diagnosis of PTSD remains in many quarters.

Perhaps as a result of this scepticism, and also as a consequence of the late entry of PTSD into the diagnostic system, advances in pharmacological treatment have not received great attention from pharmaceutical companies, the only entities able to finance the development of new molecules and test them for clinical use. However, partly in response to criticism of the validity of the diagnosis of PTSD, biological studies focused on human responses to trauma have flourished and created support for PTSD as a disorder, and have encouraged the search for potential specific targets for drug development.

The authors' contextualisation allows readers to understand how the field advanced to its current status, and to think through the next steps in its future. They emphasise that the available scientific literature has been differently interpreted by various medical organisations and associations around the globe. At the same time, they detail currently available pharmacological treatments, and provide a set of reflections and opinions this is valuable for clinicians who are required to manage patients with PTSD.

Post-traumatic Stress Disorder, First Edition. Edited by Dan Stein, Matthew Friedman, and Carlos Blanco.

COMMENTARY

4.2 Shortcomings and Future Directions of the Pharmacotherapy of PTSD

Michael Van Ameringen and Beth Patterson
Department of Psychiatry and Behavioural Neurosciences, McMaster University, Hamilton, Ontario, Canada

Drs Stein and Ipser have written a thoughtful and concise review of the pharmacotherapy of PTSD. This chapter will be a useful tool to help clinicians understand the controversies, and their underlying theoretical positions, surrounding the treatment of patients with PTSD. The chapter aptly underscores the holes in our current knowledge base, while providing an evidence-based treatment approach with treatment recommendations. The chapter begins with the examination of the rationale for treating PTSD with medication. The authors present key arguments for and against this treatment modality and ultimately conclude that there is more evidence to support using pharmacotherapy than not. The history of using medications to treat PTSD is briefly reviewed, with the strengths and shortcomings of these foundational studies being highlighted. Summarising the investigations of selective serotonin reuptake inhibitors (SSRIs) in table format is a helpful mode of presentation. Key issues in using SSRIs are addressed, including which agent to choose, dose, duration of treatment and relapse. The authors are clear in their support of using SSRIs as first-line agents (without suggesting efficacy of one over another), but acknowledge that there is some current evidence to support the additional use of antipsychotics, anticonvulsants or alpha-adrenergic agents. The review presents more tentative recommendations regarding specific medication options. The authors point out that several treatment guidelines have come to very different conclusions as to the best approach to use. The section on treatment resistance aptly identifies the paucity of literature

Post-traumatic Stress Disorder, First Edition. Edited by Dan Stein, Matthew Friedman, and Carlos Blanco.

in this area. Clinicians are encouraged to switch to an alternative first-line agent in cases of nonresponse and to consider augmentation in cases of partial response. Antipsychotic agents currently have the most evidence to support their use as augmentation agents.

The authors highlight some of the key gaps in our current knowledge of the pharmacological treatment of PTSD, but there are a few further issues that should be raised. The treatment effects (or lack thereof) seen in pharmacological studies of PTSD may be the result of either the efficacy of the particular drug treatment, the characteristics of the sample population or issues related to study design [1]. Although there is a reasonably large treatment literature, the populations used in the studies are heterogeneous with respect to type of trauma. There is evidence to suggest that individuals with combat-related traumas are less responsive to treatment than patients with noncombat PTSD [2, 3], however many of the study samples include a wide range of combat-related traumas. This may be a significant contributor to the inconsistent treatment results and low effect sizes found in some studies. Furthermore, sexual traumas appear to make up a large percentage of civilian PTSD treatment study populations and these individuals may respond differently to treatment. Unfortunately, most individual studies have not been powered enough to ascertain differences in types of trauma by treatment response. However, in a pooled analysis of brofaromine studies, sexual traumas were found to be predictive of placebo response [4]. This is further supported by an early review of response characteristics [1], where a relatively equal efficacy to treatment was found in combat and civilian PTSD (although civilian PTSD had a higher placebo response than combat-related trauma). Other studies have examined predictors of pharmacological treatment response, including duration of time after trauma, age, gender and type of trauma, but no consistent predictors have emerged.

Some authors have raised concerns about the high rates of placebo response in the pharmacotherapy of PTSD. It has been suggested that this may be a factor of study methodology. Davidson *et al.* [1] observed a difference in the quality of drug and placebo response in some studies of civilian PTSD with high placebo response rates. They found that the magnitude of response was much greater for drug over placebo when the endpoint criteria was set at a higher bar; that is, a Clinical Global Impression-Improvement (CGI-I) score of 1 (very much improved), which yielded impressive effect sizes in the range of 0.85.

As Drs Stein and Ipser point out in this chapter, current knowledge of the pharmacotherapy of PTSD has significant limitations and requires considerable expansion. However, despite the limitations, there are some promising new directions for the use of pharmacotherapy in the treatment of PTSD. D-cycloserine (DCS), a broad-spectrum antibiotic previously used in the treatment of tuberculosis, is a partial agonist of the N-methyl-D-aspartate (NMDA) receptor. It has been used in several trials of anxiety disorders as a cognitive enhancer, where it is administered prior to exposure-therapy sessions. It has been shown to enhance fear extinction in both human and animal models and has demonstrated efficacy in conjunction with cognitive behaviour therapy (CBT) for social phobia and for specific phobia. To date, there is no published evidence to support its use with CBT for PTSD, but trials examining the use of DCS to enhance imaginal exposure or virtual-reality enhanced exposure are currently in progress. The prophylaxis of PTSD using β-blockers was noted in the chapter as a very interesting area of the literature, although it currently lacks consistent evidence to support its use. The β-blocker, propranolol is also being used as an adjunctive agent with CBT for PTSD, in a treatment known as memory reconsolidation blockade. Propranolol appears to erase the emotional and physiologic reaction to the traumatic memory. Although the literature is in its early stages, there is very encouraging evidence from one randomised controlled trial [5] and several open-label studies [6] that propranolol affects traumatic memory retrieval. Brunet *et al.* [5] asked 19 subjects with chronic PTSD (average duration of symptoms: 10 years) to describe their traumatic event during a script-preparation session. Subjects were then randomised to receive a one-day dose of propranolol (n = 9) or placebo (n = 10), in double-blind fashion. One week later, subjects engaged in script-driven mental imagery of their traumatic event while heart rate, skin conductance and left-corrugator electromyogram were measured. The authors found that physiological responses were significantly decreased in the subjects who had received post-reactivation propranolol one week earlier. These researchers also conducted three open-label studies (n = 70) using six-weekly doses of propranolol in PTSD patients with a wide range of traumatic experiences. Subjects were given initial doses of propranolol immediately after memory recall, followed by another dose 90 minutes later. Subjects received concomitant doses of propranolol at five subsequent sessions. PTSD symptoms were reduced by more than 50% at post-test and at follow-up [6, 7]. According to Brunet *et al*., these studies have enhanced our knowledge by providing evidence that old fear memories can be updated with nonfearful information when it is provided during the reconsolidation window. Fear responses appear to no be longer expressed, an effect that has lasted at least a year and is selective only to reactivated memories without affecting others [7].

There have been significant gains in the pharmacological treatment of PTSD, particularly in the demonstration of the efficacy of SSRIs and their use as first-line treatments. Medications present an efficacious and readily available treatment option for those suffering from the disorder. Recent work with propranolol and DCS presents promising new ways of using medication in concert with psychotherapy to treat PTSD. Several unanswered questions remain, however, and warrant further investigation, including predictors of treatment response as well as an evidence-based approach to treatment-refractory PTSD.

COMMENTARY

4.3 Dire Need for New PTSD Pharmacotherapeutics

Murray B. Stein
Department of Psychiatry and Family and Preventive Medicine, University of California San Diego, CA, USA

Drs Stein and Ipser have been integral contributors to, and commentators on, the pharmacotherapy literature in PTSD. They succinctly summarise the literature in this chapter and supplement it with their own expert view of the state of the art, including clinical management. There is very little to disagree with in this authoritative review. Consequently, I will use this opportunity to cover some broader aspects of PTSD pharmacotherapy, which will include taking a look at some sociopolitical considerations that influence PTSD drug development and approval.

As Drs Stein and Ipser note in their chapter, PTSD has for the most part been an afterthought in the minds of psychotropic drug developers. None of the medications with current regulatory approval for PTSD were developed specifically with an understanding of the psychobiology of PTSD, nor of the particular needs of PTSD patients. Rather, PTSD has been a 'me, too' indication, studied in medications that already had market approval (e.g. SSRIs, SNRIs), where the added cost to obtain a regulatory approval for PTSD was thought to be relatively small. As the authors note, in some instances, even when a well-planned series of clinical trials proved positive (e.g. for venlafaxine extended-release), market economic considerations contributed to the company's decision not to seek a specific regulatory approval for PTSD. It is unclear what data the pharmaceutical companies have that would dissuade them from seeking approval for treatment of a disorder that is thought to affect upwards of 3% of the general population [8]. It is possible that there lingers the perception, aided and abetted by the Institute of Medicine (IOM) report [9], that PTSD is not especially responsive to pharmacotherapy. But, as Drs Stein and Ipser point out, other reviews of the

Post-traumatic Stress Disorder, First Edition. Edited by Dan Stein, Matthew Friedman, and Carlos Blanco.

same data have reached different conclusions. Moreover, as stock-market pundits like to say, 'Past performance is no guarantee of future success'. New drugs, particularly those with new mechanisms of action, may turn out be remarkably successful in the treatment of PTSD. But the IOM report, which of course could only comment on a handful of past studies and was not meant to damn all PTSD pharmacotherapies in a single breath, has had a chilling effect on the willingness of drug developers to seriously go after a PTSD indication. The IOM report alone, of course, is not to blame. The economic downturn which began in 2008 has resulted in the dissolution of many pharmaceutical research programmes and of entire companies. Those remaining are necessarily more risk averse than ever and more focused on high-profile (i.e. potential high-dollar) indications, which for the most part do not include PTSD or other anxiety and depressive disorders. This scenario does not bode well for PTSD pharmacotherapeutics.

Yet the demand for new and better PTSD medicines is higher now than it has ever been. In the USA alone, the recent conflicts in Iraq and Afghanistan have resulted in the development of a new cohort of well over 1 million military veterans, one in four of whom have PTSD and/or another combat-related disorder such as depression or substance abuse [10, 11]. Clinicians are doing the best they can to manage these problems, but polypharmacy is rampant [12], a sure sign that the medicines we do have are insufficiently robust to result in broad therapeutic improvement for most patients. When word of new PTSD pharmacological treatments has become available, even when that information has yet to be confirmed in large randomised controlled trials, uptake has been quick [13], again indicating the desperation of practitioners to adopt treatments that might work.

Though we may not be able to count on the traditional pharmaceutical industry ('big pharma') to deliver us new treatments for PTSD in the foreseeable future, this is not to say that new treatments may not emerge. There are too many inspiring observational (e.g. post-traumatic administration of opiates possibly reducing incidence of PTSD [14, 15]) and translational (e.g. use of drugs such as DCS, a partial NMDA agonist, to enhance extinction learning [16]) leads to ignore. There is thus every reason to believe that psychopharmacological clinician-researchers will rise to the challenge, and that new PTSD medicines (or new ways of using old medicines) will become available in the near future. Let's hope so, because they are sorely needed.

REFERENCES

1. Davidson, J.R.T., Malik, M.L. and Sutherland, S.L. (1997) Response characteristics to antidepressants and placebo in post-traumatic stress disorder. *International Clinical Psychopharmacology*, **12**, 291–296.

2. Rothbaum, B.O., Davidson, J.R.T., Stein, D.J. *et al*. (2008) A pooled analysis of gender and trauma-type effects on responsiveness to treatment of PTSD with venlafaxine extended release or placebo. *Journal of Clinical Psychiatry*, **69**, 1529–1539.
3. Ipser, J., Seedat, S. and Stein, D.J. (2006) Pharmacotherapy for post-traumatic stress disorder – a systematic review and meta-analysis. *South African Medical Journal*, **96**, 1088–1096.
4. Connor, K.M., Hidalgo, R.B., Crocket, B. *et al*. (2001) Predictors of response in patients with posttraumatic stress disorder. *Progress in Neuro-Psychopharmacology and Biological Psychiatry*, **25**, 337–345.
5. Brunet, A., Orr, S.P., Tremblay, J. *et al*. (2008) Effect of post-retrieval propranolol on psychophysiologica responding during subsequent script-driven traumatic imagery in post-traumatic stress disorder. *Journal of Psychiatric Research*, **42**, 503–506.
6. Brunet, A. (2010) Advances in PTSD treatment: novel approaches in the modulation of the human fear memory. Presented at the Annual Meeting of the International Society for Traumatic Stress Studies, Montreal, Quebec, Canada, November 4–6, 2010.
7. Johnson, K. (2010) *Propranolol Shows Early Promise for PTSD*. Internal Medicine News Digital Network, http://www.internalmedicinenews.com/news/mental-health/single-article/propranolol-shows-early-promise-for-ptsd/58b8ef7c3b.html (accessed 2 December 2010).
8. Kessler, R.C. and Wang, P.S. (2008) The descriptive epidemiology of commonly occurring mental disorders in the United States. *Annual Review of Public Health*, **29**, 115–129.
9. Committee on Treatment of Posttraumatic Stress Disorder (Institute of Medicine) (2007) *Treatment of Posttraumatic Stress Disorder: An Assessment of the Evidence*, The National Academies Press, Washington, DC.
10. Seal, K.H., Metzler, T.J., Gima, K.S. *et al*. (2009) Trends and risk factors for mental health diagnoses among Iraq and Afghanistan veterans using Department of Veterans Affairs health care, 2002–2008. *American Journal of Public Health*, **99**, 1651–1658.
11. Thomas, J.L., Wilk, J.E., Riviere, L.A. *et al*. (2010) Prevalence of mental health problems and functional impairment among active component and National Guard soldiers 3 and 12 months following combat in Iraq. *Archives of General Psychiatry*, **67**, 614–623.
12. Mohamed, S. and Rosenheck, R.A. (2008) Pharmacotherapy of PTSD in the U.S. Department of Veterans Affairs: diagnostic- and symptom-guided drug selection. *Journal of Clinical Psychiatry*, **69**, 959–965.
13. Harpaz-Rotem, I. and Rosenheck, R.A. (2009) Tracing the flow of knowledge: geographic variability in the diffusion of prazosin use for the treatment of posttraumatic stress disorder nationally in the Department of Veterans Affairs. *Archives of General Psychiatry*, **66**, 417–421.

14. Bryant, R.A., Creamer, M., O'Donnell, M. *et al*. (2009) A study of the protective function of acute morphine administration on subsequent posttraumatic stress disorder. *Biological Psychiatry*, **65**, 438–440.
15. Holbrook, T.L., Galarneau, M.R., Dye, J.L. *et al*. (2010) Morphine use after combat injury in Iraq and post-traumatic stress disorder. *New England Journal of Medicine*, **362**, 110–117.
16. Cukor, J., Spitalnick, J., Difede, J. *et al*. (2009) Emerging treatments for PTSD. *Clinical Psychology Review*, **29**, 715–726.

CHAPTER 5

Psychological Interventions for Trauma Exposure and PTSD

Richard A. Bryant
University of New South Wales, Sydney, Australia

INTRODUCTION

Psychological interventions are a first-line treatment for post-traumatic stress disorder (PTSD). Most international treatment guidelines, including those in the UK [1], the USA [2] and Australia [3], converge on the conclusion that trauma-focused psychotherapy is the treatment of choice relative to other modalities. This chapter reviews the background and rationale for trauma-focused psychotherapy, outlines the evidence for the major variants of psychological interventions and discusses clinical guidelines for implementing these interventions with patients suffering PTSD.

HISTORICAL OVERVIEW

The major form of trauma-focused therapy involves cognitive behaviour therapy (CBT). This has its historical roots in learning principles that emerged in the 1920s. Beginning with the famous case study of 'Little Albert', Watson and Raynor demonstrated that pairing an aversive noise with a toy white rat to a baby boy resulted in him fearing a wide range of white furry objects. This principle of classical conditioning laid the basis for behaviour therapy, which gained momentum in the 1950s, and led to a range of behaviour therapy techniques, including systematic desensitisation [4] and stress-inoculation training [5]. Through the 1970s, exposure therapy was applied to the treatment of a range of anxiety disorders, including phobias, social anxiety and obsessive compulsive disorder [6–8]. In these therapies, anxious patients were typically exposed to a feared situation (e.g. social interactions, heights) until they

Post-traumatic Stress Disorder, First Edition. Edited by Dan Stein, Matthew Friedman, and Carlos Blanco.

learned that these situations did not result in the feared outcomes. In the 1970s behaviour therapy was extended to incorporate the role of thoughts, in which CBT recognised that correcting irrational thoughts could alleviate anxiety and mood problems [9].

In the 1980s more attention was given to traumatic stress disorders, partly because of the introduction of PTSD into the Diagnostic and Statistical Manual III (DSM-III) [10]. Although some initial evidence indicated the efficacy of CBT for PTSD [4], other reports suggested that the effects were only modest [11]. This cautious support for CBT was probably due to the emphasis placed on systematic desensitisation, which involves brief pairings of trauma reminders with calming exercises – conceptualised as a form of 'counter-conditioning'. More successful trials emerged when greater emphasis was placed on exposure therapy. A series of small studies reported promising effects with prolonged exposure to trauma memories in Vietnam veterans [12, 13]. In 1991 a seminal study was conducted by Edna Foa, who reported the first properly controlled trial of CBT, which randomly assigned female rape survivors with PTSD to either prolonged exposure (imaginal and in vivo), stress-inoculation training, supportive counselling or a wait-list control group [14]. Stress-inoculation training comprised education, breathing retraining and muscle relaxation, thought-stopping, cognitive restructuring, modelling and role-plays. This study provided participants with nine twice-weekly sessions, and included blind assessments at both post-treatment and three-month follow-up. Whereas stress-inoculation training resulted in greater gains than supportive counselling or wait-list control at post-treatment, the prolonged exposure condition led to greater reduction in PTSD symptoms at follow-up. This study marked the beginning of many controlled trials that evaluated the efficacy of CBT in treating people with PTSD.

MAJOR PSYCHOLOGICAL INTERVENTIONS

Cognitive behaviour therapy

CBT for PTSD typically includes psychoeducation, exposure, cognitive restructuring and anxiety management. Psychoeducation informs the patient about common symptoms following a traumatic event and discusses the way in which the core symptoms will be treated during the course of therapy. The aim is to legitimise the trauma reactions, to help the patient develop a formulation of their symptoms and to establish a rationale for treatment. Exposure usually involves both imaginal and in vivo exposure.

Imaginal exposure requires the individual with PTSD to vividly imagine the trauma for prolonged periods, usually for at least 30 minutes. The therapist assists the patient in providing a narrative of their traumatic experience in a way that emphasises all relevant details, including sensory cues and affective responses.

There have been variants of imaginal exposure, such as requiring the patient to write down detailed descriptions of the experience (known as 'cognitive processing therapy' (CPT)) [15] and implementing exposure with the assistance of virtual-reality paradigms implemented via computer-generated imagery [16]. Most exposure treatments supplement imaginal exposure with in vivo exposure, which involves live graded exposure to the feared trauma-related stimuli. Cognitive restructuring involves teaching patients to identify and evaluate the evidence for negative automatic thoughts, as well as helping them to evaluate their beliefs about the trauma, their self, the world and the future [17]. Anxiety management techniques aim to provide individuals with coping skills to assist them in gaining a sense of mastery over their fear, reduce arousal levels and assist them when engaging in exposure to the traumatic memories. Anxiety management approaches have included stress-inoculation training that incorporates psychoeducation, relaxation skills, thought-stopping and self-talk [5].

The duration of CBT for chronic PTSD is typically 8–12 sessions. Therapy typically occurs on an individual basis because exposure-based therapies are often not conducive to group-therapy format. The treatment components are described above as distinct entities but in reality there is much overlap from one component to another. Therapy sessions usually occur over a period of 60–90 minutes, although sessions including imaginal or in vivo exposure often need 90 or more minutes.

Mechanisms of CBT

In terms of the mechanisms underpinning CBT techniques, there are two major models that can account for this treatment. Fear-conditioning models posit that a traumatic event (unconditioned stimulus) leads to a strong fear reaction (unconditioned response), which becomes conditioned to many stimuli associated with the traumatic event. Accordingly, when people are exposed to reminders of the trauma (conditioned stimuli), they experience a strong fear reaction (conditioned response) [18]. This perspective is supported by much evidence that patients with PTSD have strong conditioned responses to trauma reminders [19–21]. The fear-conditioning model proposes that successful recovery from trauma involves extinction learning, in which repeated exposure to trauma reminders or memories results in new learning that these reminders no longer signal threat [22]. This model is further supported by findings that impaired extinction learning prior to trauma is a strong predictor of those who will suffer persistent post-traumatic stress [23]. As exposure therapy involves repeated exposures to memories and reminders until the patient masters their anxiety, CBT is conceptualised as a form of extinction learning in which conditioned fear responses are inhibited by new learning of safe associations [24].

The other major perspective driving CBT is cognitive models of PTSD [25, 26]. Current models posit that psychopathological trauma responses may be mediated by two core factors: (i) maladaptive appraisals of the trauma and its aftermath and (ii) disturbances in autobiographical memory that involve impaired retrieval and strong associative memory [25]. It is proposed that mental representations of the traumatic experience are laid down at the time of trauma under conditions of extreme stress, and accordingly are often encoded in fragmented, often perceptually focused, ways [27]. This results in these memories not being adequately integrated into the patient's normal autobiographical memory base, which contributes to intrusive memories and ongoing disorder. It is argued that these memories need to be integrated into normal autobiographical memory because this permits mastery of the memory and associated anxiety (similar to extinction learning). It is for this reason that many cognitive models advocate the use of exposure-based therapy, since this facilitates the integration of trauma memories into a coherent narrative of the event.

Cognitive models also posit that it is essential to correct catastrophic or extreme appraisals of the traumatic experience because these highlight the patient's perceptions of guilt, potential future harm or hopelessness about the future. There is much evidence that catastrophic appraisals about the patient's self or their future in the period after trauma exposure predict subsequent PTSD [28–30]. Further, people with acute stress disorder (ASD) exaggerate both the probability of future negative events occurring and the adverse effects of these events [31, 32].

There is ongoing debate concerning the specific change mechanisms operating in CBT, and particularly exposure [33, 34]. It is postulated that exposure may benefit patients because it: (i) promotes habituation to feared stimuli and therefore reduces anxiety; (ii) promotes correction of the belief that anxiety remains unless avoidance occurs; (iii) impedes the negative reinforcement associated with fear reduction that leads to cognitive avoidance; (iv) promotes the incorporation of corrective information in to the trauma memory; (v) establishes the trauma as a discrete event that is not indicative of the world being globally threatening; and (vi) enhances self-mastery through management of the exposure exercise. Cognitive therapy is also regarded as being beneficial for multiple reasons, because whereas it primarily aims to correct unrealistic appraisals, the discussion of trauma necessarily involves activation of trauma memories and in this sense some of the mechanisms purported to underpin exposure are likely to function in cognitive therapy.

Eye-movement desensitisation and reprocessing (EMDR)

A variant of CBT is eye-movement desensitisation and reprocessing (EMDR). EMDR differs from CBT insofar as it requires the patient to focus their attention on a traumatic memory while simultaneously visually tracking the therapist's finger as it is moved across their visual field, and then to engage in restructuring of the memory [35]. More specifically, after moving their eyes for approximately

20 seconds and focusing on a traumatic memory, the patient is asked to 'blank it out', to let go of the memory. After this process, the patient is asked to identify more adaptive or positive thoughts related to the memory or traumatic experience and to again track the therapist's fingers. EMDR often also includes other coping techniques, such as relaxation skills or positive visualisation. The exact mechanisms by which eye movements are purported to enhance treatment gains are not well specified. In short, moving one's eyes is intended to facilitate information processing [36].

SUMMARY OF THE EVIDENCE

In recent years numerous treatment guidelines have been published that are based on systematic reviews of the published literature. These include guidelines from the UK National Institute for Clinical Excellence (NICE) [1], the US Department of Veterans Affairs/Department of Defence [2], the US Institute of Medicine [37], the Australian National Health and Medical Research Council (NHMRC) [38] and the International Society of Traumatic Stress Studies [39]. Each of these provides detailed summaries of systematic reviews. Additionally, there have been several comprehensive meta-analyses of trials of psychological interventions [40–45]. In this section we review the major findings of these systematic reviews, focusing particularly on CBT and EMDR because these interventions are currently the major variants of psychological therapy with the strongest evidence for treating PTSD.

CBT for adults

Table 5.1 presents a summary of the major findings of systematic reviews for adults with PTSD. Limiting the reviews to those published in recent years (because they encompass the results of prior reviews), it is apparent from Table 5.1 that trauma-focused therapies that incorporate CBT and EMDR are the treatment of choice for PTSD. Different reviews have reported more specific outcomes of various studies, however many of these attempts to dismantle trauma-focused therapies have not been sufficiently replicated to represent an adequate body of work. The majority of studies indicate that treatments that incorporate prolonged exposure to either trauma memories or situations that remind the individual of trauma are beneficial. There is debate concerning the role of other CBT techniques, such as cognitive restructuring, in relation to exposure. Several studies suggest that exposure and cognitive restructuring provide comparable treatment gains [17, 46–48], while others indicate that combining cognitive restructuring with exposure does not provide additive effects above exposure alone [17, 46–48]. There is tentative evidence from one study that combination

Table 5.1 Summary of systematic reviews of cognitive behaviour therapy for PTSD.

Study	Number of studies	Major finding	Conclusion
Bradley *et al.* [40]	26	CBT vs control: effect size = 1.26 EMDR vs control: effect size = 0.75	Both CBT and EMDR more effective than control conditions
NICE [1]	13	CBT vs wait-list: SMD = −1.36	CBT more effective than wait-list
NHMRC [57]	3	CBT vs wait-list: SMD = −1.32	CBT more effective than wait-list
Mendes *et al.* [58]	6	CBT vs supportive therapy: RR = 0.30	CBT more effective than supportive counselling

SMD, standard mean difference; RR, relative risk.

with cognitive restructuring may enhance the effect of exposure, but this study only used imaginal exposure and did not permit any discussion of the trauma memory in the exposure condition [49]. This latter point is important because proponents of exposure emphasise that optimal implementation of exposure does involve a subsequent discussion of the experience in which the therapist clarifies the nonthreatening features of the memory or situation and the capacity of the patient to master these reminders [50]. The convergent finding that other CBT components do not markedly enhance exposure suggests that exposure is a critical ingredient in facilitating recovery from PTSD [51]. As exposure typically includes a form of cognitive reframing in which the therapist discusses the mastery of the exposure to trauma reminders, it seems that the change mechanisms underpinning exposure and cognitive restructuring may be overlapping. Although there is some evidence that imaginal and in vivo exposure are equally efficacious [52], more work is needed on this issue. In summary, the largest body of evidence supports the use of exposure-based CBT, which will typically employ exposure to trauma memories and feared situations, as well as reframing the fears that patients have about confronting these experiences. It is important to note that CBT has been shown to be efficacious across many different trauma-exposed populations, including survivors of traumatic injury and assault [49, 52, 53], sexual assault [14, 48], combat [54], terrorist attacks [55] and child sexual abuse [56].

Several variants of CBT have been introduced in recent years, which have modified specific components. CPT is predominantly a cognitive therapy that was developed to address the needs of rape victims [15]. It uses cognitive restructuring techniques to address maladaptive beliefs about safety, trust, control, esteem and intimacy; it also engages trauma memories by requiring the patient to write detailed accounts of the trauma and relate these accounts to the therapist. Three randomised controlled trials on CPT have reported strong effects relative to wait-list [47, 59, 60]. A recent trial that compared (i) full CPT, (ii) the writing component and (iii) the cognitive component found that the writing component did not provide any additive gain over the cognitive element [61].

Recently there has been concern over the extent to which CBT effectively treats more complex cases of PTSD. Complex PTSD refers to cases of PTSD in which the patient has marked difficulties with emotion regulation, which may manifest in strong mood swings, difficulty stabilising emotional reactions, self-harm behaviour, impulsive behaviours and difficulties with interpersonal relationships [62]. In recognition of this pattern, recent adaptations of CBT have prepared patients with complex PTSD presentations with emotion-regulation training prior to commencing CBT. This approach teaches patients skills in distress tolerance, labelling emotions and emotion management. Two randomised trials have now demonstrated that this modified form of CBT is efficacious in treating complex PTSD, and there is evidence that it is more effective than standard CBT for patients with complex PTSD [63, 64]. Considering that many people suffer enduring or severe traumatic exposures that result in emotion-regulation difficulties, it appears that this approach may enhance the treatment gains of standard CBT. For example, it can be beneficial to people suffering the effects of childhood abuse, torture or refugee experience, or prolonged military or emergency-responder service.

CBT for children

Relative to CBT for adults, there has been much less study of the efficacy of this treatment for children. Overall, children appear to experience PTSD as often as adults, although there have been proposals that symptom manifestation may be different in children [65]. Accordingly, treatment programmes for children often modify standard CBT by integrating strategies that teach regulation of affect or behaviour, including parents in treatment, adapting treatment delivery to the developmental stage of the child and placing strong emphasis on rapport factors between therapist and patient [66]. Table 5.2 presents a summary of the few meta-analyses that have been published on psychological interventions for childhood-related PTSD; these have focused on CBT and EMDR. Consistent with the adult literature, these trials indicate that both trauma-focused CBT and EMDR are efficacious, and the treatment of choice in treating childhood PTSD.

Table 5.2 Summary of systematic reviews of cognitive behaviour therapy for children.

Study	Number of studies	Major finding	Conclusion
NICE [67]	5	CBT vs supportive therapy: SMD = −0.55	Limited evidence favouring CBT for children over seven years
McDonald *et al.* [68]	10	CBT vs wait-list/supportive therapy: SMD = −0.43	CBT efficacious in reducing PTSD
Rodenburg *et al.* [44]	–	EMDR vs wait-list: effect size = 0.66	EMDR efficacious in reducing PTSD
	–	EMDR vs other therapy: effect size = 0.25	EMDR has a small benefit compared to other therapies

SMD, standard mean difference.

Prophylactic approaches

Early intervention for all trauma-exposed individuals

Over the past three decades, psychological debriefing has arguably been the popular approach to managing stress reactions after disasters. The most widely disseminated form of debriefing was originally Critical Incident Stress Debriefing (CISD) [69]. Although this approach was initially developed for emergency service personnel, it has been proposed to be effective for a wide variety of victims of trauma [70]. A CISD session typically occurs within 48 hours of the event, and involves education about trauma reactions, requires participants to describe what occurred and their cognitive and emotional responses to the event, enquires about psychological or physical symptoms, and provides suggestions for stress reduction.

Despite its widespread use, systematic reviews of studies indicate that people who receive CISD do not enjoy better outcomes than those who do not receive CISD (see Table 5.3). In short, these reviews have concluded that single-session interventions provided to all trauma survivors in the immediate aftermath of trauma exposure do not result in prevention of subsequent PTSD. Apart from meta-analyses, this conclusion has also been ratified by recent systematic reviews and treatment guidelines [71, 72]. These developments have resulted in original conceptualisations of CISD being expanded to Critical Incident Stress Management, which is conceptualised as a multimodal and staged process that recognises that a single-session intervention may be only an initial strategy, which can be supplemented by more targeted interventions for those who require them [73].

Table 5.3 Summary of systematic reviews of early intervention for all trauma-exposed individuals.

Study	Number of studies	Major finding	Conclusion
NICE [67]	7	Debriefing vs wait-list: SMD = 0.11	No evidence that debriefing reduces subsequent PTSD severity
Rose *et al.* [74]	15	Debriefing vs wait-list: SMD = 0.11	No evidence that debriefing reduces subsequent PTSD severity
van Emmerik *et al.* [75]	5	CISD vs wait-list: effect size = 0.13	No evidence that debriefing reduces subsequent PTSD severity
Cuijpers *et al.* [76]	4	Debriefing vs wait-list: RR = 1.33	No evidence that debriefing reduces subsequent PTSD severity

SMD, standard mean difference; RR, relative risk.

One of the concerns about single-session interventions is that they may impede natural recovery processes that typically occur following trauma exposure. There is some evidence that people who receive single-session debriefing, especially those who are highly distressed, have higher PTSD levels at follow-up than those who do not receive debriefing [77]. It is possible that requiring people to ventilate their emotions within days of trauma exposure may hasten arousal and strengthen their trauma memories, which may impede natural recovery. In the context of prevailing models that noradrenergic activation at the time of trauma facilitates fear conditioning and consolidation of trauma memories [18], it is possible that emotional expression of the trauma memory in the context acute debriefing may be detrimental. This possibility is consistent with accumulating evidence that acute markers of PTSD include elevated heart and respiratory rates [78]. It also accords with evidence that agents that reduce noradrenergic activation in the initial 48 hours after exposure, such as propranolol [79] and morphine [80], are associated with reduced PTSD or conditioned responses to trauma reminders. In response to these concerns, agencies are tending towards interventions that provide support, assistance and referral rather than encouraging trauma survivors to engage trauma memories within the acute period after trauma [81].

In the wake of increasing evidence that immediate debriefing does not prevent PTSD, there has been a shift in recent years to policies that provide less intrusive interventions. Although these approaches are not yet evidence-based, they attempt to be informed by available evidence regarding adaptive responses to trauma. A recent commentary outlined five key principles that are important to facilitating adaptation after disasters and traumas [82]. The first principle is promoting a sense of safety: threat to perception of safety after trauma is one of the strongest predictors of post-traumatic problems [83], while enhancing safety is associated with reductions in adverse mental health outcomes [84]. The second principle is to promote 'calming', which aims to reduce the hyperarousal that is frequent after disaster. This principle emerges from evidence that hyperarousal in the acute aftermath of trauma is strongly predictive of subsequent PTSD [85]. Strategies that help to calm an individual include relaxation training, breathing control, problem-solving and adaptive self-talk. The third principle involves promoting a sense of self-efficacy, which entails the belief that one's actions will lead to positive outcomes. This perception is important as it encourages individuals and communities to regain a sense of control over their environment. Problem-solving is a core strategy in this goal, because it allows the individual to develop skills and successfully overcome their immediate problems. The fourth principle is promoting social connectedness, because of strong evidence that accessing social support is one of the strongest buffers against problems after trauma exposure [86]. The fifth principle is instilling hope, because optimism can be an important predictor of successful outcomes after trauma [87]. This is often achieved by cognitive reframing of one's expectations so they are not overly negative. These principles have led to the development of 'Psychological First Aid' (PFA) as an alternative to psychological debriefing [88]. This approach has three major goals: to facilitate adaptive coping and problem-solving; to reduce acute stress reactions; and to guide the survivor to additional resources that enhance coping. Importantly, PFA does not directly encourage ventilation of the trauma experience. It should be noted that there is currently no evidence regarding the outcomes of PFA.

Early intervention for post-traumatic stress disorder/acute stress disorder

As an altenrative to providing interventions to all trauma survivors after exposure, there has been a focus on providing interventions to survivors who are deemed high-risk for developing PTSD. One of the challenges in implementing secondary prevention for PTSD in the acute phase after trauma is identifying the individuals who are at high risk for PTSD development. This step is important because of the logistic and ethical problems in providing early intervention to all trauma survivors. There is considerable evidence that while many people experience elevated levels of PTSD symptoms in the initial weeks after trauma exposure, many of these symptoms remit in the following three to six months [89]. For example, whereas 94% of rape victims displayed sufficient PTSD symptoms two weeks post-trauma to meet criteria (excluding the one-month time requirement), this rate dropped to 47% 11 weeks later [90]. This pattern has also been observed in survivors of nonsexual assault [91], motor-vehicle accidents [92], terrorist attacks [93] and natural disasters [94].

In 1994 DSM-IV [95] introduced ASD as a new diagnosis to (i) describe stress reactions in the initial month after a trauma and (ii) discriminate between people who are having a transient stress reaction and those having a reaction that will develop into PTSD. [96] The major differences between ASD and PTSD are the timeframe and the former's emphasis on dissociative reactions to the trauma. ASD refers to symptoms manifested during the period from two days to four weeks post-trauma, whereas PTSD can only be diagnosed from four weeks. The diagnosis of ASD requires that the individual has at least three of the following: (i) a subjective sense of numbing or detachment; (ii) reduced awareness of their surroundings; (iii) derealistion; (iv) depersonalisation; or (v) dissociative amnesia.

One of the advantages of the new ASD diagnosis was that it stimulated considerable research into early intervention for PTSD, because it proposed that survivors who met criteria for ASD were at high risk for developing chronic PTSD. In fact, a series of early studies highlighted that the majority of people who satisfied ASD criteria did suffer chronic PTSD [97, 98]. Modifications to CBT were made insofar as it was abridged to be a briefer form of therapy, typically comprising five to six sessions that were offered within a month of trauma exposure. The common factor across interventions for ASD/acute PTSD is that they have used a trauma-focused exposure approach that has involved imaginal or in vivo exposure. Table 5.4 presents a summary of recent meta-analyses of early CBT for ASD/acute PTSD. The convergent finding is that CBT (primarily involving exposure and/or cognitive restructuring) is effective in reducing subsequent PTSD, and further evidence that CBT prevents subsequent PTSD more than supportive counselling. Overall, the evidence indicates the use of exposure-based therapies for early intervention in people with ASD/acute PTSD.

A challenge exists for clinicians to identify those trauma survivors who are at high risk for PTSD, because although the ASD diagnosis has been successful insofar as the majority of people who meet the criteria for the diagnosis subsequently develop PTSD, a review of 22 studies that longitudinally assessed people with ASD found that the majority of people who eventually developed PTSD did not initially meet criteria for ASD [100]. That is, identification of recently exposed people who are at high risk for PTSD probably requires indexing of severe PTSD reactions that persist after several weeks rather than focusing narrowly on those who meet the stringent criteria for PTSD. In this context, it is worth noting that the proposal for DSM-5 is that ASD no longer be conceptualised as a predictor of PTSD, and that the requirement for dissociative symptoms to be present be removed [101].

Eye-movement desensitisation reprocessing

Table 5.5 presents a summary of major systematic reviews that conducted meta-analyses of controlled trials of EMDR. It is apparent that across controlled trials,

Table 5.4 Summary of systematic reviews of cognitive behaviour therapy for acute provision of CBT.

Study	Number of studies	Major finding	Conclusion
NICE [67]	9	CBT vs wait-list: SMD = −1.7	CBT more effective than wait-list
Roberts *et al.* [43]	7	CBT vs wait-list: RR = 0.72	CBT more effective secondary prevention than no treatment
Kornør *et al.* [99]	7	CBT vs supportive counselling: RR = 0.56	CBT more effective secondary prevention than supportive counselling

SMD, standard mean difference; RR, relative risk.

EMDR is an effective treatment for PTSD relative to wait-list. Further, there is a convergent finding that EMDR and CBT perform comparably in reducing PTSD symptoms. Accordingly, EMDR is recommended, along with trauma-focused CBT, as a frontline treatment in a number of recent treatment guidelines [57, 67, 102]. There are several caveats, however, that should be noted regarding EMDR. Several reviews concluded that eye movements were not pivotal in the treatment effects of EMDR [42, 57]. This conclusion is based on findings from several studies that manipulated eye movement with other strategies and found that the eye movements themselves were not important in relieving the symptoms relative to the other components of EMDR [103–105]. Further, the Australian NHMRC guidelines concluded that EMDR was as efficacious as CBT only when EMDR also included in vivo exposure [57].

CLINICAL GUIDELINES

Timing of treatment

There is consensus that it is unnecessary, and potentially harmful, to provide mental health interventions too soon after trauma exposure. As noted above, the majority of trauma survivors will experience natural reemission of symptoms in the months following exposure [89]. Although the early provision of CBT for people with ASD has been shown to limit subsequent development of PTSD, there is consensus that CBT should not commence until immediately after trauma exposure. This conclusion is based on two findings. First, the sooner one attempts to identify a person as being at high risk for PTSD development, the more likely

Table 5.5 Summary of systematic reviews of studies of EMDR for PTSD.

Study	Number of studies	Major finding	Conclusion
Bradley *et al.* [40]	4	EMDR vs wait-list: effect size = 1.25	EMDR reduces symptoms
Davidson *et al.* [42]	34	Post-treatment EMDR pre-post: effect size = 0.63	EMDR reduces symptoms but movements not beneficial
		EMDR vs EMDR – eye movements: effect size = 0.10	
NICE [67]	5	EMDR vs wait-list: SMD = −1.54	EMDR reduces symptoms
		EMDR vs stress management: SMD = −0.40	No evidence of differential effects of EMDR and stress management
	5	CBT vs EMDR: SMD = −0.06	No evidence of differential effects of EMDR and CBT
Seidler *et al.* [45]	7	EMDR vs CBT: effect size = 0.13	EMDR and CBT equally efficacious

SMD, standard mean difference; RR, relative risk.

that a false positive identification will be made. For example, the predictive power of ASD is markedly stronger when it is diagnosed four weeks after exposure than when it is diagnosed 10 days after exposure [106]. Second, patients may not be able to cope with the demands of trauma-focused therapy. Accordingly, controlled trials of CBT have typically commenced treatment at least two weeks after trauma exposure. There have been concerns that providing treatment too soon after trauma may overload the patient when they have excessive demands upon them [107].

In deciding when to provide treatment, one should not simply consider the time that has elapsed since the traumatic event, but also the context in which survivors find themselves. Many traumatic events may be described as discrete incidents that occur in a relatively stable environment; in these cases, one may expect recovery to occur within several months. In cases when a trauma persists because of social upheaval or community destruction, the ongoing stressors may indicate that trauma-focused therapy will be overly demanding on the patient. For example, following Hurricane Katrina, many people's lives were massively disrupted for lengthy periods because of relocation, lack of housing and loss of basic infrastructures. In such cases, it may be more appropriate to provide supportive counselling, problem-solving techniques and possibly medication than trauma-focused therapy. In short, the decision to provide treatment should be influenced by (i) the extent to which a threat still exists for the patient and (ii) the extent to which the patient has sufficient resources to manage the demands of therapy.

Psychological versus psychopharmacological treatments

Very few studies have examined the relative effects of psychological and pharmacological interventions for PTSD. One study that compared paroxetine and CBT reported a slight improvement in PTSD symptoms in CBT relative to paroxetine [108]. In terms of combining psychological and pharmacological interventions, a study that compared 10 weeks of sertraline alone with 10 weeks of sertraline followed by exposure therapy found a trend for greater PTSD in the combined condition [109]. Another study found that combining sertraline with CBT led to greater symptom reduction than sertraline alone in women with PTSD who had previously been resistant to pharmacological treatment [110]. Despite the limited evidence, it appears that CBT is a preferred option to pharmacotherapy, and that greater treatment gains will be achieved by augmenting pharmacotherapy with CBT.

Treatment format

CBT and its variants (including EMDR, CPT and virtual-reality exposure therapy) are provided on an individual basis, primarily because of the specific needs of addressing an individual's trauma memories. There is some evidence that providing CBT in a group format can be efficacious. The NICE guidelines identify three studies that investigated group-administered CBT, and conclude that whereas there is some evidence that this is efficacious relative to wait-list (relative risk = 0.56), there is no evidence that it is more effective than group therapy that does not involve CBT (relative risk = 0.98) [67]. Therapy typically lasts for 90 minutes, incorporating a review of the previous week and of homework, at least 40 minutes of exposure tasks, a period of cognitive restructuring, and preparation for the following week. Across most treatment studies, outcomes are based on treatments that involve between 8 and 12 sessions.

Predictors of treatment outcome

Although trauma-focused therapies are the treatment of choice for PTSD, meta-analyses indicate that a significant minority of patients do not significantly benefit from treatment [40]. Across most studies, it appears that demographic factors, such as economic status, education, age and intelligence, are not associated with treatment outcome. A range of factors have been shown to predict treatment outcome, however. Poorer response has been shown in patients with comorbid depression [111], generalised anxiety disorder (GAD) [112], borderline personality disorder [113], anger [114], substance-use disorder [115], social alienation [116] and emotion-regulation difficulties [63]. There is recent evidence suggesting that the same neural networks implicated in extinction learning are also involved in successful CBT. Specifically, positive response to CBT is predicted by a larger rostral anterior cingulate [117]. Also consistent with extinction models, poor response to CBT has been predicted by stronger amygdala activation during fear processing prior to treatment [118]. There is also preliminary genetic influence on response to CBT. A recent study reported that PTSD patients with the 5-HTTLPR low-expression genotype responded more poorly to CBT than other patients, suggesting that serotonergic availability may influence response to CBT [119]. Taken together, these data suggest that patients with a tendency towards greater amygdala activity and fear conditioning may respond more poorly to CBT.

COMORBIDITY

There is overwhelming evidence that PTSD often occurs in the context of comorbid conditions, including depression, other anxiety disorders, substance use and complicated grief [86, 120, 121]. Accordingly, treating PTSD often requires addressing conditions that may be causing as much impairment as the PTSD symptoms themselves.

Depression

Depression can develop secondarily to PTSD, and as PTSD resolves the depression will reduce. There is indirect support for this proposition insofar as effective treatments of PTSD often find associated decreases in depression [57, 67]. Despite this pattern, depression may not necessarily resolve with PTSD reduction. Although little research has been conducted on the nature of post-traumatic depression, it appears that established depression-management approaches apply to these cases: antidepressant medication, cognitive restructuring, mood monitoring and pleasant event and activity scheduling [122]. These strategies should be applied if depressive symptoms do not adequately resolve with standard trauma-focused programmes. Patients with severe depression should be considered for antidepressant medication for two reasons: first, CBT may be impaired by the impaired attentional focus, mental slowing and listlessness that can be experienced in severe depression; and second, patients who are severely suicidal should not be treated with trauma-focused therapy that involves exposure to trauma reminders unless adequate protections are put in place to manage exacerbation of suicidal intent.

Generalised anxiety disorder

Many trauma survivors develop GAD, as they worry about a range of potential future harmful events [121]. This possibility is particularly significant in post-trauma settings where threat exists, such as in contexts of terrorist attack, war zones or areas that are at high risk for natural disasters. Although concern about realistic threat can be adaptive, many studies have shown that people with PTSD are likely to exaggerate concerns, and this can generalise to a wide range of events in their lives [31, 123].

Managing concerns about potential threat after trauma may require a different approach than one typically uses with GAD. Whereas GAD involves clearly irrational fears about potentially adverse events, fears of terrorism or disaster may be reasonably justified. Largely as a result of recent concerns about managing the effects of ongoing terrorist threats, specific attention has been given to developing principles to address risk appraisals with trauma survivors who continue to face some degree of realistic threat [124]. The first step is to clarify the person's belief. It is essential to determine whether the belief is rational or excessive in light of available evidence. Second, one should challenge the validity of the belief by discerning between what is 'likely risk' versus 'acceptable risk'. This approach recognises that all people live with acceptable levels of risk (e.g. driving in traffic), because the risk results in significant benefit. This phase focuses on the common tendency of trauma survivors to unrealistically seek zero levels of risk. The third step involves highlighting the benefits and losses associated with the belief that threat is imminent. Marshall *et al*. [124] cite the example of a New Yorker who avoided Manhattan after 9/11; although this strategy could provide short-term relief of anxiety, it could also lead to loss of job, career advancement and social interaction. The fourth step requires the patient to engage in behavioural experiments that demonstrate that excessive fears are not justified.

Complicated grief

It is very common in the context of PTSD for people to suffer traumatic loss in the case of a traumatic death of someone close to them. The last decade has seen much data emerge to indicate that complicated grief is a distinct construct [125]. Complicated grief is characterised by yearning for the deceased, bitterness about the loss, inability to proceed with life, preoccupation with the loss, hopelessness about the future and preoccupation with sorrow that persists for at least six months after the death. Many studies have demonstrated that complicated grief symptoms form a distinct syndrome that is separate from depression or anxiety [126, 127] and is predictive of substantial morbidity (e.g. depression, suicidal ideation), adverse health behaviours (e.g. increased smoking, alcohol consumption, insomnia) and quality-of-life impairment [128]. The available research suggests that complicated grief persists in approximately 10% of bereaved people [129].

Several meta-analyses have indicated that global counselling immediately after loss is not effective in alleviating subsequent disorder [130]. In contrast, there are now several randomised controlled trials that have demonstrated the efficacy of CBT for this condition [131, 132]. The available evidence suggests that treatment can include the following components: (i) emotional reliving/exposure, (ii) cognitive restructuring and (iii) goal setting and increasing activity schedules. There is clearly much overlap between treatment of PTSD and complicated grief, insofar as it facilitates emotional processing of the death and loss. The additional component of treating complicated grief focuses on forward-planning issues, such as enhancing social interactions, fostering positive memories of the deceased and planning activities. In the context of complicated grief, therapy can also use a technique to facilitate cognitive restructuring that involves 'communicating' with the deceased via 'empty chair' techniques that encourage the individual to express any outstanding issues that need to be resolved. An important caveat in treating complicated grief is that one needs to be sensitive that people require different periods of time to grieve; whereas PTSD may be treated shortly after a traumatic event, complicated grief may require intervention after at least 6 or 12 months have transpired since the death.

Post-traumatic agoraphobia and panic disorder

Agoraphobia and panic disorder are commonly reported following trauma [121]. Panic attacks play an important role in psychopathological responses to trauma; they are common during traumatic experiences [133]. Building on fear-conditioning models, it has been proposed that panic reactions that occur at the time of trauma may strengthen fear conditioning, and accordingly subsequent reminders may trigger cued panic attacks. Treatment of panic disorder typically occurs with interoceptive exposure, in which the patient is exposed to aversive somatic sensations in order to learn that they do not result in catastrophic outcomes [134]. One model posits that comorbid PTSD/panic disorder should be treated by initially treating panic attacks with interoceptive exposure, and subsequently progressing to trauma-related exposure activities [135]. It is questionable whether trauma-related panic requires this approach, particularly when the attacks experienced by trauma survivors are linked to trauma memories. Often, treating trauma memories with prolonged exposure results in successful reduction of panic attacks, presumably because of generalisation of extinction to trauma reminders (including somatic cues). Interoceptive exposure may be warranted, however, if the patient has marked panic disorder that persists after CBT for trauma-related memories and reminders.

Substance-use disorder

There is strong evidence that PTSD is associated with substance-abuse disorders [136]. The most common model of post-traumatic substance-use disorders is that people self-medicate to minimise the distress associated with post-traumatic responses. It is proposed that this response can be highly maladaptive because substance use has both anxiety-producing and stress-response-dampening effects. Substance use may be maintained by the immediate reinforcement of anxiety reduction, but it contributes to an overall worsening of anxiety which in turn promotes further substance use. There is evidence that it is more difficult to treat substance-use disorder that is comorbid with PTSD than substance-use disorder alone [137]. Accordingly, it is important to manage both conditions, because untreated PTSD can impede successful treatment of the substance abuse. Importantly, PTSD treatment is related to better substance-use outcomes, with remission of substance-use problems lasting through five-year follow-up assessments [138].

At this point in time, there is a dearth of well-conducted trials to shape practice for comorbid PTSD and substance-use disorder. Several uncontrolled treatment studies have adopted collaborative-care approaches that integrate motivational interviewing, case management and trauma-focused CBT [139]. One study combined a 12-step self-help programme with PTSD treatment and found that after controlling for substance-use therapy, PTSD patients were 3.7 times more likely to be in remission five years later than those who did not receive PTSD therapy [140]. At this point it appears that comorbid PTSD and substance-use disorder should be addressed by treating both conditions simultaneously, ensuring that substance abuse is addressed via motivational interviewing, stimulus-control strategies, coping skills and case management [141].

Mild traumatic brain injury

Although not a psychiatric disorder, another frequent complicating feature for many trauma survivors involves mild traumatic brain injury (MTBI). MTBI commonly occurs following motor-vehicle accidents, assaults, combat and industrial accidents. Enormous attention has been paid in recent years to the interplay between MTBI and post-traumatic psychiatric disorders, and there is a long-standing debate over the extent to which PTSD can develop after MTBI [142]. Earlier commentators argued that people who sustain an MTBI are unlikely to develop PTSD because they have suffered impaired consciousness secondary to the brain injury and do not encode the necessary mental representations of the traumatic experience to cause fear reactions [143]. In more recent years, it has been shown that PTSD can occur after MTBI, usually because patients with MTBI can still have 'islands' of memory for the traumatic experience;

trauma can also occur following resolution of post-traumatic amnesia and some fear conditioning can occur despite impaired consciousness [142]. There is even some evidence that MTBI may be associated with an increased risk for PTSD, recently documented in both combat troops returning from Iraq and Afghanistan [144, 145] and survivors of civilian trauma [121]. The prevailing model of PTSD proposes that the disorder develops as a result of impaired functioning of the medial prefrontal cortex, which limits regulation of the amygdala [146]. It has been suggested that damage to the prefrontal networks during the course of the MTBI may compromise their functioning and contribute to PTSD [147].

There is a very limited evidence base for treating PTSD following MTBI. One small controlled trial compared CBT and supportive counselling for ASD after MTBI and found considerably superior effects for CBT relative to the counselling condition [148]. CBT for patients with MTBI may require minor adjustments to standard CBT. First, as MTBI often results in islands of amnesia, imaginal exposure needs to focus on those aspects of the memory that can be recalled; alternatively, more focus may be placed on in vivo exposure to activate fear networks, with less reliance on retrieving memories. Second, in recognition of possible cognitive impairment (which is reasonably rare in MTBI), cognitive restructuring may need to be simplified so that successful therapy does not require sustained attention or cognitive flexibility.

Sequencing the treatment of comorbid conditions

When a patient presents with comorbid conditions, several principles can be applied. First, it is imperative that the patient's safety be addressed. Suicidal intent, substance dependence and self-harm tendencies should be managed with appropriate strategies to ensure that the patient is safe and stabilised. Second, if a comorbid condition is likely to interfere with CBT, it may be wise to address that condition prior to CBT. For example, if a patient is attending sessions intoxicated and cannot fully engage in exposure, it is imperative to manage the alcohol use prior to CBT. Third, it is useful to address aspects of the clinical presentation that will lead to generalised benefit. For example, if a patient presents with PTSD and insomnia, it is very likely that sleeping difficulties will be reduced once nightmares and associated PTSD issues are reduced. Accordingly, one should treat the PTSD, and only address the insomnia if it persists beyond PTSD remission. Finally, it is important to focus treatment on those core strategies that will achieve maximum therapy gain. Although many patients may prefer to focus on anxiety-management skills (e.g. breathing retraining, relaxation skills) rather than exposure, it is important to focus as quickly as possible on exposure and cognitive restructuring because these approaches will most effectively achieve change.

TRAUMA-FOCUSED THERAPY CONTRAINDICATIONS

Although trauma-focused therapies are the treatment of choice for PTSD, they are not necessarily suitable for all patients. This section addresses some of the contraindications for implementing trauma-focused therapy, and particularly exposure-based therapies, as well as other clinical presentations that warrant specific care in implementing trauma-focused therapy.

Excessive avoidance

Although strong avoidance tendencies will be present in nearly all cases of PTSD, in a proportion of individuals their avoidance impedes any form of exposure-based therapy. These patients may express such extreme avoidant tendencies that they are not willing or able to think or speak about the trauma. In these cases, the therapist should carefully explore the concerns that the patient may hold. In most cases these concerns are irrational and exposure should proceed. In some cases, however, the patient may fear that they will not be able to manage their reactions based on prior experiences. For example, patients who have experienced marked suicidal ideation, self-harming behaviour or even psychotic episodes as a result of being exposed to extreme distress may reasonably decide to avoid this form of therapy.

Anger

Anger is a very common response following a traumatic experience [149]. Anger may serve to inhibit anxiety following a trauma, especially when effortful avoidance is unsuccessful [150]. There is evidence that patients who display anger during narration of their trauma experience tend not to respond positively to exposure therapy [114]. In contrast, there is evidence that patients suffering post-traumatic anger can benefit from treatment that integrates anger-management strategies incorporating anxiety management and cognitive-therapy restructuring [151].

Catastrophic thinking

Although not a contraindication, one needs to be cautious in treating patients with entrenched and ruminative maladaptive thinking about their trauma. One study found that exposure was not successful if the patient's narrative of the trauma was characterised by mental defeat or lack of mastery over the situation [116]. These individuals often require careful cognitive restructuring, and only when their tendency to ruminate is modified should exposure be considered.

Techniques that emphasise 'mindfulness' strategies teaching the patient not to focus on the content of their thoughts may also be beneficial [152].

Severe depression/suicide risk

Individuals who are considered a marked suicide risk require containment and possibly antidepressant medication or hospitalisation. The risk of providing suicidal individuals with exposure-based therapy is that it may enhance their attention towards the negative aspects of their experience and heightened distress at a time when they are not able to tolerate it. These possibilities indicate that seriously suicidal people should have their depression and suicide managed, and post-traumatic stress reactions should be addressed after these more urgent problems are dealt with. Additionally, patients with severe depressive presentations, including psychomotor retardation, may not be able to sustain attention or motivation sufficiently to engage in trauma-focused therapy. Antidepressant medication or other therapies may be warranted, and trauma-focused therapy can be provided once the depression has alleviated to a point at which adequate cognitive resources can be allocated to therapy.

Ongoing stressors

Many trauma survivors experience marked stressors after trauma exposure, which can compound the PTSD response [153]. Severe pain, surgery, financial loss, criminal investigations, property loss, interpersonal breakdown and community fragmentation are some of the stresses that may impact on PTSD patients. Other patients may experience ongoing threats, such as domestic violence or the aftershocks of earthquakes. It is important to determine the extent to which the patient's stressors are not exceeding their capacity to undertake therapy. The demanding nature of trauma-focused therapy, and the homework and exercises that are commonly assigned between therapy sessions, may not be suitable for patients who are managing significant stressors. Clinicians need to determine the optimal time to provide therapy, and should be cautious about overloading patients who are stressed by ongoing stressors or threats.

CONCLUSION

Trauma-focused therapies have been the focus of many well-controlled studies in the past two decades. The convergent finding across many of these studies is that CBT, and the lesser-studied EMDR, have proven efficacy in reducing PTSD symptoms and increasing functioning and/or quality of life. There is agreement internationally that trauma-focused therapies are the treatment of choice for

PTSD. Despite their success, we need to recognise some important limitations in our current knowledge. Many patients do not respond adequately to these therapies, and there is a need to explore means to augment or modify trauma-focused therapies to increase the number of patients who do respond. There is also a dearth of effectiveness studies that implement trauma-focused therapies in community settings. This is a critical issue because of evidence that (i) many people do not seek mental health services following trauma [154] and (ii) a proportion of clinicians are reluctant to employ exposure-based therapies [155]. One of the major challenges for the field is to extend beyond current efficacy evidence and evaluate more rigorously the benefits and obstacles to trialing trauma-focused therapies in various community settings.

REFERENCES

1. Excellence NIoC (2005) *The Management of PTSD in Adults and Children in Primary and Secondary Care*, Wiltshire.
2. Defense DoVADo (2004) *Clinical Practice Guideline for the Management of Posttraumatic Stress, Version 1.0*, Washington, DC.
3. Health ACfPM (2007) *Australian Guidelines for the Treatment of Adults with Acute Stress Disorder and Posttraumamtic Stress Disorder*, Melbourne.
4. Frank, E., Anderson, B., Stewart, B.D. *et al*. (1988) Efficacy of cognitive behavior therapy and systematic desensitization in the treatment of rape trauma. *Behavior Therapy*, **19**, 403–420.
5. Meichenbaum, D. (1985) *Stress Inoculation Training*, Pergamon Press, New York.
6. Foa, E.B. and Goldstein, A. (1978) Continuous exposure and complete response prevention in the treatment of obsessive-compulsive neurosis. *Behavior Therapy*, **9**, 821–829.
7. Emery, J.R. and Krumbolz, J.D. (1967) Standard versus individualized hierarchies in desensitization to reduce test anxiety. *Journal of Counseling Psychology*, **14**, 204–209.
8. Mathews, A.M., Johnston, D.W., Lancashire, M. *et al*. (1976) Imaginal flooding and exposure to real phobic situations: treatment outcome with agoraphobic patients. *British Journal of Psychiatry*, **129**, 362–371.
9. Beck, A.T. (1976) *Cognitive Therapy and the Emotional Disorders*, International Universities Press, New York.
10. American Psychiatric Association (1980) *Diagnostic and Statistical Manual of Mental Disorders*, 3rd edn, American Psychiatric Association, Washington, DC.
11. Becker, J.V. and Abel, G.G. (1981) Behavioral treatment of victims of sexual assault, in *Handbook of Clinical Behavior Therapy* (eds S.M. Turner, K.S. Calhoun and H.E. Adams), John Wiley & Sons, Inc., New York, pp. 347–379.
12. Cooper, N.A. and Clum, G.A. (1989) Imaginal flooding as a supplementary treatment for PTSD in combat veterans: a controlled study. *Behavior Therapy*, **20** (3), 381–391.

13. Keane, T.M., Fairbank, J.A., Caddell, J.M. and Zimering, R.T. (1989) Implosive (flooding) therapy reduces symptoms of PTSD in Vietnam combat veterans. *Behavior Therapy*, **20** (2), 245–260.
14. Foa, E.B., Rothbaum, B.O., Riggs, D.S. and Murdock, T.B. (1991) Treatment of posttraumatic stress disorder in rape victims: a comparison between cognitive-behavioral procedures and counseling. *Journal of Consulting and Clinical Psychology*, **59** (5), 715–723.
15. Resick, P.A. and Schnicke, M.K. (1993) *Cognitive Processing Therapy for Sexual Assault Victims: A Treatment Manual*, Sage Publications, Newbury Park, CA.
16. Rothbaum, B.O., Hodges, L.F., Ready, D. *et al*. (2001) Virtual reality exposure therapy for Vietnam veterans with posttraumatic stress disorder. *Journal of Clinical Psychiatry*, **62** (8), 617–622.
17. Marks, I., Lovell, K., Noshirvani, H. *et al*. (1998) Treatment of posttraumatic stress disorder by exposure and/or cognitive restructuring: a controlled study. *Archives of General Psychiatry*, **55** (4), 317–325.
18. Charney, D.S., Deutch, A.Y., Krystal, J.H. *et al*. (1993) Psychobiologic mechanisms of posttraumatic stress disorder. *Archives of General Psychiatry*, **50**, 294–305.
19. Orr, S.P., Pitman, R.K., Lasko, N.B. and Herz, L.R. (1993) Psychophysiological assessment of posttraumatic stress disorder imagery in World War II and Korean combat veterans. *Journal of Abnormal Psychology*, **102** (1), 152–159.
20. Orr, S.P., Lasko, N.B., Metzger, L.J. *et al*. (1998) Psychophysiologic assessment of women with posttraumatic stress disorder resulting from childhood sexual abuse. *Journal of Consulting and Clinical Psychology*, **66** (6), 906–913.
21. Pitman, R.K., Orr, S.P., Forgue, D.F. *et al*. (1987) Psychophysiologic assessment of posttraumatic stress disorder imagery in Vietnam combat veterans. *Archives of General Psychiatry*, **44** (11), 970–975.
22. Davis, M. and Myers, K.M. (2002) The role of glutamate and gamma-aminobutyric acid in fear extinction: clinical implications for exposure therapy. *Biological Psychiatry*, **52** (10), 998–1007.
23. Guthrie, R.M. and Bryant, R.A. (2006) Extinction learning before trauma and subsequent posttraumatic stress. *Psychosomatic Medicine*, **68** (2), 307–311.
24. Rothbaum, B.O. and Davis, M. (2003) Applying learning principles to the treatment of post-trauma reactions. *Annals of the New York Academy of Sciences*, **1008**, 112–121.
25. Ehlers, A. and Clark, D.M. (2000) A cognitive model of posttraumatic stress disorder. *Behaviour Research and Therapy*, **38** (4), 319–345.
26. Foa, E.B., Steketee, G. and Rothbaum, B.O. (1989) Behavioral/cognitive conceptualizations of post-traumatic stress disorder. *Behavior Therapy*, **20** (2), 155–176.
27. Brewin, C.R., Gregory, J.D., Lipton, M. and Burgess, N. (2010) Intrusive images in psychological disorders: characteristics, neural mechanisms, and treatment implications. *Psychological Review*, **117** (1), 210–232.
28. Ehlers, A., Mayou, R.A. and Bryant, B. (1998) Psychological predictors of chronic posttraumatic stress disorder after motor vehicle accidents. *Journal of Abnormal Psychology*, **107** (3), 508–519.

29. Engelhard, I.M., van den Hout, M.A., Arntz, A. and McNally, R.J. (2002) A longitudinal study of 'intrusion-based reasoning' and posttraumatic stress disorder after exposure to a train disaster. *Behaviour Research and Therapy*, **40** (12), 1415–1424.
30. Andrews, B., Brewin, C.R., Rose, S. and Kirk, M. (2000) Predicting PTSD symptoms in victims of violent crime: the role of shame, anger, and childhood abuse. *Journal of Abnormal Psychology*, **109** (1), 69–73.
31. Smith, K. and Bryant, R.A. (2000) The generality of cognitive bias in acute stress disorder. *Behaviour Research and Therapy*, **38** (7), 709–715.
32. Warda, G. and Bryant, R.A. (1998) Cognitive bias in acute stress disorder. *Behaviour Research and Therapy*, **36** (12), 1177–1183.
33. Rothbaum, B.O. and Mellman, T.A. (2001) Dreams and exposure therapy in PTSD. *Journal of Traumatic Stress*, **14** (3), 481–490.
34. Rothbaum, B.O. and Schwartz, A.C. (2002) Exposure therapy for posttraumatic stress disorder. *American Journal of Psychotherapy*, **56** (1), 59–75.
35. Shapiro, F. (1995) *Eye Movement Desensitization and Reprocessing: Basic Principles, Protocols, and Procedures*, Guilford Press, New York, p. 398.
36. Shapiro, F. and Maxfield, L. (2002) Eye Movement Desensitization and Reprocessing (EMDR): information processing in the treatment of trauma. *Journal of Clinical Psychology*, **58** (8), 933–946.
37. (IOM) Institute of Medicine (2008) *Treatment of Posttraumatic Stress Disorder: An Assessment of the Evidence*, The National Academies Press, Washington, DC.
38. Australian Centre for Posttraumatic Mental Health (2007) *Australian Guidelines for the Treatment of Adults with Acute Stress Disorder and Posttraumatic Stress Disorder*, ACPMH, Melbourne.
39. Foa, E.B., Keane, T.M., Friedman, M.J. and Cohen, J.A. (eds) (2009) *Effective Treatments for PTSD: Practice Guidelines from the International Society of Traumatic Stress Studies*, 2nd edn, Guilford Press, New York.
40. Bradley, R., Greene, J., Russ, E. *et al*. (2005) A multidimensional meta-analysis of psychotherapy for PTSD. *American Journal of Psychiatry*, **162** (2), 214–227.
41. Munoz-Solomando, A., Kendall, T. and Whittington, C.J. (2008) Cognitive behavioural therapy for children and adolescents. *Current Opinion in Psychiatry*, **21** (4), 332–337.
42. Davidson, P.R. and Parker, K.C. (2001) Eye movement desensitization and reprocessing (EMDR): a meta-analysis. *Journal of Consulting and Clinical Psychology*, **69** (2), 305–316.
43. Roberts, N.P., Kitchiner, N.J., Kenardy, J. and Bisson, J.I. (2009) Systematic review and meta-analysis of multiple-session early interventions following traumatic events. *American Journal of Psychiatry*, **166** (3), 293–301.
44. Rodenburg, R., Benjamin, A., de Roos, C. *et al*. (2009) Efficacy of EMDR in children: a meta-analysis. *Clinical Psychology Review*, **29** (7), 599–606.
45. Seidler, G.H. and Wagner, F.E. (2006) Comparing the efficacy of EMDR and trauma-focused cognitive-behavioral therapy in the treatment of PTSD: a meta-analytic study. *Psychological Medicine*, **36** (11), 1515–1522.

46. Tarrier, N., Pilgrim, H., Sommerfield, C. *et al*. (1999) A randomized trial of cognitive therapy and imaginal exposure in the treatment of chronic posttraumatic stress disorder. *Journal of Consulting and Clinical Psychology*, **67** (1), 13–18.
47. Resick, P.A., Nishith, P., Weaver, T.L. *et al*. (2002) A comparison of cognitive-processing therapy with prolonged exposure and a waiting condition for the treatment of chronic posttraumatic stress disorder in female rape victims. *Journal of Consulting and Clinical Psychology*, **70** (4), 867–879.
48. Foa, E.B., Hembree, E.A., Cahill, S.P. *et al*. (2005) Randomized trial of prolonged exposure for posttraumatic stress disorder with and without cognitive restructuring: outcome at academic and community clinics. *Journal of Consulting and Clinical Psychology*, **73** (5), 953–964.
49. Bryant, R.A., Moulds, M.L., Guthrie, R.M. *et al*. (2003) Imaginal exposure alone and imaginal exposure with cognitive restructuring in treatment of post-traumatic stress disorder. *Journal of Consulting and Clinical Psychology*, **71** (4), 706–712.
50. Foa, E.B. (2000) Psychosocial treatment of posttraumatic stress disorder. *Journal of Clinical Psychiatry*, **61** (Suppl. 5), 43–51.
51. Cahill, S.P., Rothbaum, B.O., Resick, P.A. and Follette, V.M. (2009) Cognitive-behavioral therapy for adults, in *Effective Treatments for PTSD: Practice Guidelines from the International Society of Traumatic Stress Studies* (eds E.B. Foa, T.M. Keane, M.J. Freidman and J.A. Cohen), Guilford Press, New York, pp. 139–222.
52. Bryant, R.A., Moulds, M.L., Guthrie, R.M. *et al*. (2008) A randomized controlled trial of exposure therapy and cognitive restructuring for posttraumatic stress disorder. *Journal of Consulting and Clinical Psychology*, **76** (4), 695–703.
53. Blanchard, E.B., Hickling, E.J., Devineni, T. *et al*. (2003) A controlled evaluation of cognitive behavioural therapy for posttraumatic stress in motor vehicle accident survivors. *Behaviour Research and Therapy*, **41** (1), 79–96.
54. Schnurr, P.P., Friedman, M.J., Foy, D.W. *et al*. (2003) Randomized trial of trauma-focused group therapy for posttraumatic stress disorder: Results from a Department of Veterans Affairs cooperative study. *Archives of General Psychiatry*, **60** (5), 481–489.
55. Duffy, M., Gillespie, K. and Clark, D.M. (2007) Post-traumatic stress disorder in the context of terrorism and other civil conflict in Northern Ireland: randomised controlled trial. *British Medical Journal*, **334** (7604), 1147.
56. McDonagh, A., Friedman, M., McHugo, G. *et al*. (2005) Randomized trial of cognitive-behavioral therapy for chronic posttraumatic stress disorder in adult female survivors of childhood sexual abuse. *Journal of Consulting and Clinical Psychology*, **73** (3), 515–524.
57. Australian Centre for Posttraumatic Mental Health (2007) *Australian Guidelines for the Treatment of Adults with Acute Stress Disorder and Posttraumatic Stress Disorder: Practitioner Guide*, ACPMH, Melbourne.
58. Mendes, D.D., Mello, M.F., Ventura, P. *et al*. (2008) A systematic review on the effectiveness of cognitive behavioral therapy for posttraumatic stress disorder. *International Journal of Psychiatry In Medicine*, **38** (3), 241–259.

59. Monson, C.M., Schnurr, P.P., Resick, P.A. *et al*. (2006) Cognitive processing therapy for veterans with military-related posttraumatic stress disorder. *Journal of Consulting and Clinical Psychology*, **74** (5), 898–907.
60. Chard, K.M. (2005) An evaluation of cognitive processing therapy for the treatment of posttraumatic stress disorder related to childhood sexual abuse. *Journal of Consulting and Clinical Psychology*, **73** (5), 965–971.
61. Resick, P.A., Galovski, T.E., O'Brien Uhlmansiek, M. *et al*. (2008) A randomized clinical trial to dismantle components of cognitive processing therapy for posttraumatic stress disorder in female victims of interpersonal violence. *Journal of Consulting and Clinical Psychology*, **76** (2), 243–258.
62. Cloitre, M., Miranda, R., Stovall-McClough, K.C. and Han, H. (2005) Beyond PTSD: emotion regulation and interpersonal problems as predictors of functional impairment in survivors of childhood abuse. *Behavior Therapy*, **36** (2), 119–124.
63. Cloitre, M., Koenen, K.C., Cohen, L.R. and Han, H. (2002) Skills training in affective and interpersonal regulation followed by exposure: a phase-based treatment for PTSD related to childhood abuse. *Journal of Consulting and Clinical Psychology*, **70** (5), 1067–1074.
64. Cloitre, M., Chase Stovall-McClough, K., Nooner, K. *et al*. (2010) Treatment for PTSD related to childhood abuse: a randomized controlled trial. *American Journal of Psychiatry*, **167**, 915–924.
65. Salmon, K. and Bryant, R.A. (2002) Posttraumatic stress disorder in children – the influence of developmental factors. *Clinical Psychology Review*, **22** (2), 163–188.
66. Cohen, J.A., Mannarino, A.P., Deblinger, E. and Berliner, L. (2009) Cognitive-behavioral therapy for children and adolscents, in *Effective Treatments for PTSD: Practice Guidelines from the International Society of Traumatic Stress Studies* (eds E.B. Foa, T.M. Keane, M.J. Friedman and J.A. Cohen), Guilford Press, New York, pp. 223–244.
67. Excellence NNIfC (2005) *The Management of PTSD in Adults and Children in Primary and Secondary Care*, Wilshire.
68. Macdonald, G.M., Higgins, J.P. and Ramchandani, P. (2006) Cognitive-behavioural interventions for children who have been sexually abused. *Cochrane Database of Systematic Reviews*, (4) (Art. No.: CD001930). doi: 10.1002/14651858
69. Mitchell, J.T. (1983) When disaster strikes: the critical incident stress debriefing process. *Journal of Emergency Medical Services*, **8**, 36–39.
70. Everly, G.S. Jr and Mitchell, J.T. (1999) *Critical Incident Stress Management (CISM): A New Era and Standard of Care in Crisis Intervention*, 2nd edn, Chevron, Ellicott City, MD.
71. McNally, R.J., Bryant, R.A. and Ehlers, A. (2003) Does early psychological intervention promote recovery from posttraumatic stress? *Psychological Science*, **4**, 45–79.
72. Bisson, J.I., McFarlane, A.C., Rose, S. *et al*. (2009) Psychological debriefing for adults, in *Effective Treatments for PTSD: Practice Guidelines from the International Society for Traumatic Stress Studies* (eds E.B. Foa, T.M. Keane, M.J. Freidman and J.A. Cohen), 2nd edn, Guilford Press, New York, pp. 83–105.

73. Mitchell, J.T. and Everly, G.S. Jr (2000) Critical incident stress management and critical incident stress debriefings: evolutions, effects and outcomes, in *Psychological Debriefing: Theory, Practice and Evidence* (eds B. Raphael and J.P. Wilson), Cambridge University Press, New York, pp. 71–90.
74. Rose, S., Bisson, J. and Wessely, S. (2003) A systematic review of single-session psychological interventions ('debriefing') following trauma. *Psychotherapy and Psychosomatics*, **72** (4), 176–184.
75. van Emmerik, A.A.P., Kamphuis, J.H., Hulsbosch, A.M. and Emmelkamp, P.M.G. (2002) Single session debriefing after psychological trauma: a meta-analysis. *Lancet*, **360** (9335), 766–771.
76. Cuijpers, P., Van Straten, A. and Smit, F. (2005) Preventing the incidence of new cases of mental disorders: a meta-analytic review. *Journal of Nervous and Mental Disease*, **193** (2), 119–125.
77. Hobbs, M., Mayou, R., Harrison, B. and Worlock, P. (1996) A randomised controlled trial of psychological debriefing for victims of road traffic accidents. *British Medical Journal*, **313** (7070), 1438–1439.
78. Bryant, R.A., Creamer, M., O'Donnell, M. *et al*. (2008) A multisite study of initial respiration rate and heart rate as predictors of posttraumatic stress disorder. *Journal of Clinical Psychiatry*, **69** (11), 1694–1701.
79. Pitman, R.K., Sanders, K.M., Zusman, R.M. *et al*. (2002) Pilot study of secondary prevention of posttraumatic stress disorder with propranolol. *Biological Psychiatry*, **51** (2), 189–192.
80. Bryant, R.A., Creamer, M., O'Donnell, M. *et al*. (2009) A study of the protective function of acute morphine administration on subsequent posttraumatic stress disorder. *Biological Psychiatry*, **65** (5), 438–440.
81. Watson, P.J. and Shalev, A.Y. (2005) Assessment and treatment of adult acute responses to traumatic stress following mass traumatic events. *CNS Spectrums*, **10**, 123–131.
82. Hobfoll, S.E., Watson, P., Bell, C.C. *et al*. (2007) Five essential elements of immediate and mid-term mass trauma intervention: empirical evidence. *Psychiatry*, **70** (4), 283–315; discussion 316–269.
83. Mikulincer, M. and Solomon, Z. (1988) Attributional style and combat-related posttraumatic stress disorder. *Journal of Abnormal Psychology*, **97** (3), 308–313.
84. Ozer, E.J., Best, S.R., Lipsey, T.L. and Weiss, D.S. (2003) Predictors of posttraumatic stress disorder and symptoms in adults: a meta-analysis. *Psychological Bulletin*, **129** (1), 52–73.
85. Bryant, R.A. (2006) Longitudinal psychophysiological studies of heart rate: mediating effects and implications for treatment. *Annals of the New York Academy of Sciences*, **1071**, 19–26.
86. Norris, F.H., Friedman, M.J. and Watson, P.J. (2002) 60,000 disaster victims speak: Part I. An emirical review of the empirical literature, 1981–2001. *Psychiatry*, **65**, 207–239.
87. Antonovsky, A. (1979) *Health, Stress, and Coping*, Jossey-Bass, San Francisco, CA.

88. Young, B.H. (2006) The immediate response to disaster: guidelines for adult psychological first aid, in *Interventions Following Mass Violence and Disasters: Strategies for Mental Health Practice* (eds E.C. Ritchie, P.J. Watson and M.J. Friedman), Guilford Press, New York, pp. 134–154.
89. Bryant, R.A. (2003) Early predictors of posttraumatic stress disorder. *Biological Psychiatry*, **53** (9), 789–795.
90. Rothbaum, B.O., Foa, E.B., Riggs, D.S. *et al.* (1992) A prospective examination of post-traumatic stress disorder in rape victims. *Journal of Traumatic Stress*, **5** (3), 455–475.
91. Riggs, D.S., Rothbaum, B.O. and Foa, E.B. (1995) A prospective examination of symptoms of posttraumatic stress disorder in victims of nonsexual assault. *Journal of Interpersonal Violence*, **10** (2), 201–214.
92. Blanchard, E.B., Hickling, E.J., Barton, K.A. and Taylor, A.E. (1996) One-year prospective follow-up of motor vehicle accident victims. *Behaviour Research and Therapy*, **34** (10), 775–786.
93. Galea, S., Vlahov, D., Resnick, H. *et al.* (2003) Trends of probable post-traumatic stress disorder in New York City after the September 11 terrorist attacks. *American Journal of Epidemiology*, **158** (6), 514–524.
94. van Griensven, F., Chakkraband, M.L.S., Thienkrua, W. *et al.* (2006) Mental health problems among adults in tsunami-affected areas in southern Thailand. *JAMA-Journal of the American Medical Association*, **296** (5), 537–548.
95. American Psychiatric Association (1994) *Diagnostic and Statistical Manual of Mental Disorders*, 4th edn, American Psychiatric Association, Washingtonm, DC.
96. Harvey, A.G. and Bryant, R.A. (2002) Acute stress disorder: a synthesis and critique. *Psychological Bulletin*, **128** (6), 886–902.
97. Harvey, A.G. and Bryant, R.A. (2000) Two-year prospective evaluation of the relationship between acute stress disorder and posttraumatic stress disorder following mild traumatic brain injury. *American Journal of Psychiatry*, **157** (4), 626–628.
98. Bryant, R.A. and Harvey, A.G. (1998) Relationship between acute stress disorder and posttraumatic stress disorder following mild traumatic brain injury. *American Journal of Psychiatry*, **155** (5), 625–629.
99. Kornor, H., Winje, D., Ekeberg, O. *et al.* (2008) Early trauma-focused cognitive-behavioural therapy to prevent chronic post-traumatic stress disorder and related symptoms: a systematic review and meta-analysis. *BMC Psychiatry*, **8**, 81.
100. Bryant, R.A. (2011) Acute stress disorder as a predictor of posttraumatic stress disorder: a systematic review. *Journal of Clinical Psychiatry*, **72**, 233–239.
101. Bryant, R.A., Friedman, M.J., Spiegel, D. *et al.* A review of acute stress disorder in DSM-V. *Depression and Anxiety*, in press.
102. Spates, C.R., Koch, E., Cusack, K. *et al.* (2009) Eye movement desensitization and reprocessing, in *Effective Treatments for PTSD: Practice Guidelines from the International Society for Traumatic Stress Studies* (eds E.B. Foa, T.M. Keane, M.J. Freidman and J.A. Cohen), Guilford Press, New York, pp. 279–305.

103. Renfrey, G. and Spates, C.R. (1994) Eye movement desensitization: a partial dismantling study. *Journal of Behavior Therapy and Experimental Psychiatry*, **25** (3), 231–239.

104. Foley, T. and Spates, C.R. (1995) Eye movement desensitization of public-speaking anxiety: a partial dismantling. *Journal of Behavior Therapy and Experimental Psychiatry*, **26** (4), 321–329.

105. Sanderson, A. and Carpenter, R. (1992) Eye movement desensitization versus image confrontation: a single-session crossover study of 58 phobic subjects. *Journal of Behavior Therapy and Experimental Psychiatry*, **23** (4), 269–275.

106. Murray, J., Ehlers, A. and Mayou, R.A. (2002) Dissociation and post-traumatic stress disorder: two prospective studies of road traffic accident survivors. *British Journal of Psychiatry*, **180**, 363–368.

107. Bryant, R.A. and Harvey, A.G. (2000) *Acute Stress Disorder: A Handbook of Theory, Assessment, and Treatment*, American Psychological Association, Washington, DC.

108. Frommberger, U., Stieglitz, R.D., Nyberg, E. *et al*. (2004) Comparison between paroxetine and behaviour therapy in patients with posttraumatic stress disorder (PTSD): a pilot study. *International Journal of Psychiatry in Clinical Practice*, **8** (1), 19–23.

109. Rothbaum, B.O., Cahill, S.P., Foa, E.B. *et al*. (2006) Augmentation of sertraline with prolonged exposure in the treatment of posttraumatic stress disorder. *Journal of Traumatic Stress*, **19** (5), 625–638.

110. Otto, M.W., Hinton, D., Korbly, N.B. *et al*. (2003) Treatment of pharmacotherapy-refractory posttraumatic stress disorder among Cambodian refugees: a pilot study of combination treatment with cognitive-behavior therapy vs sertraline alone. *Behaviour Research and Therapy*, **41** (11), 1271–1276.

111. van Minnen, A., Arntz, A. and Keijsers, G.P.J. (2002) Prolonged exposure in patients with chronic PTSD: predictors of treatment outcome and dropout. *Behaviour Research and Therapy*, **40** (4), 439–457.

112. Tarrier, N., Sommerfield, C., Pilgrim, H. and Faragher, B. (2000) Factors associated with outcome of cognitive-behavioural treatment of chronic post-traumatic stress disorder. *Behaviour Research and Therapy*, **38** (2), 191–202.

113. Feeny, N.C., Zoellner, L.A. and Foa, E.B. (2002) Treatment outcome for chronic PTSD among female assault victims with borderline personality characteristics: a preliminary examination. *Journal of Personality Disorders*, **16** (1), 30–40.

114. Foa, E.B., Riggs, D.S., Massie, E.D. and Yarczower, M. (1995) The impact of fear activation and anger on the efficacy of exposure treatment for posttraumatic stress disorder. *Behavior Therapy*, **26** (3), 487–499.

115. Steindl, S.R., Young, R.M., Creamer, M. and Crompton, D. (2003) Hazardous alcohol use and treatment outcome in male combat veterans with posttraumatic stress disorder. *Journal of Traumatic Stress*, **16** (1), 27–34.

116. Ehlers, A., Clark, D.M., Dunmore, E. *et al*. (1998) Predicting response to exposure treatment in PTSD: the role of mental defeat and alienation. *Journal of Traumatic Stress*, **11** (3), 457–471.

117. Bryant, R.A., Felmingham, K., Whitford, T.J. *et al*. (2008) Rostral anterior cingulate volume predicts treatment response to cognitive-behavioural therapy for posttraumatic stress disorder. *Journal of Psychiatry and Neuroscience*, **33** (2), 142–146.
118. Bryant, R.A., Felmingham, K., Kemp, A. *et al*. (2008) Amygdala and ventral anterior cingulate activation predicts treatment response to cognitive behaviour therapy for post-traumatic stress disorder. *Psychological Medicine*, **38** (4), 555–561.
119. Bryant, R.A., Felmingham, K.L., Falconer, E.M. *et al*. (2010) Preliminary evidence of the short allele of the serotonin transporter gene predicting poor response to coognitive behavior therapy in posttraumatic stress disorder. *Biological Psychiatry*, **67**, 1217–1219.
120. North, C.S., Tivis, L., McMillen, J.C. *et al*. (2002) Psychiatric disorders in rescue workers after the Oklahoma City bombing. *American Journal of Psychiatry*, **159** (5), 857–859.
121. Bryant, R.A., Creamer, M., O'Donnell, M. *et al*. (2010) The psychiatric sequelae of traumatic injury. *American Journal of Psychiatry*, **167**, 312–320.
122. Hollon, S.D., Stewart, M.O. and Strunk, D. (2006) Enduring effects for cognitive behavior therapy in the treatment of depression and anxiety. *Annual Review of Psychology*, **57**, 285–315.
123. Dunmore, E., Clark, D.M. and Ehlers, A. (2001) A prospective investigation of the role of cognitive factors in persistent Posttraumatic Stress Disorder (PTSD) after physical or sexual assault. *Behaviour Research and Therapy*, **39** (9), 1063–1084.
124. Marshall, R.D., Bryant, R.A., Amsel, L. *et al*. (2007) The psychology of ongoing threat: relative risk appraisal, the September 11 attacks, and terrorism-related fears. *American Psychologist*, **62** (4), 304–316.
125. Prigerson, H.G., Horowitz, M.J., Jacobs, S.C. *et al*. (2009) Prolonged grief disorder: psychometric validation of criteria proposed for DSM-V and ICD-11. *PLoS Medicine*, **6** (8), e1000121.
126. Lannen, P.K., Wolfe, J., Prigerson, H.G. *et al*. (2008) Unresolved grief in a national sample of bereaved parents: impaired mental and physical health 4 to 9 years later. *Journal of Clinical Oncology*, **26** (36), 5870–5876.
127. Zhang, B., El-Jawahri, A. and Prigerson, H.G. (2006) Update on bereavement research: evidence-based guidelines for the diagnosis and treatment of complicated bereavement. *Journal of Palliative Medicine*, **9** (5), 1188–1203.
128. Prigerson, H.G., Shear, M.K., Jacobs, S.C. *et al*. (1999) Consensus criteria for traumatic grief. A preliminary empirical test. *British Journal of Psychiatry*, **174**, 67–73.
129. Bonanno, G.A. and Kaltman, S. (2001) The varieties of grief experience. *Clinical Psychology Review*, **21** (5), 705–734.
130. Currier, J.M., Neimeyer, R.A. and Berman, J.S. (2008) The effectiveness of psychotherapeutic interventions for bereaved persons: a comprehensive quantitative review. *Psychological Bulletin*, **134** (5), 648–661.
131. Shear, K., Frank, E., Houck, P.R. and Reynolds, C.F. III (2005) Treatment of complicated grief: a randomized controlled trial. *The Journal of the American Medical Association*, **293** (21), 2601–2608.

132. Boelen, P.A., de Keijser, J., van den Hout, M.A. and van den Bout, J. (2007) Treatment of complicated grief: a comparison between cognitive-behavioral therapy and supportive counseling. *Journal of Consulting and Clinical Psychology*, **75** (2), 277–284.
133. Nixon, R.D. and Bryant, R.A. (2003) Peritraumatic and persistent panic attacks in acute stress disorder. *Behaviour Research and Therapy*, **41** (10), 1237–1242.
134. Otto, M.W., Pollack, M.H. and Maki, K.M. (2000) Empirically supported treatments for panic disorder: costs, benefits, and stepped care. *Journal of Consulting and Clinical Psychology*, **68** (4), 556–563.
135. Falsetti, S.A., Resnick, H.S. and Davis, J.L. (2008) Multiple channel exposure therapy for women with PTSD and comorbid panic attacks. *Cognitive Behaviour Therapy*, **37** (2), 117–130.
136. Chilcoat, H.D. and Breslau, N. (1998) Posttraumatic stress disorder and drug disorders: testing causal pathways. *Archives of General Psychiatry*, **55** (10), 913–917.
137. Najavits, L.M., Harned, M.S., Gallop, R.J. *et al*. (2007) Six-month treatment outcomes of cocaine-dependent patients with and without PTSD in a multisite national trial. *Journal of Studies on Alcohol and Drugs*, **68** (3), 353–361.
138. Read, J.P., Brown, P.J. and Kahler, C.W. (2004) Substance use and posttraumatic stress disorders: symptom interplay and effects on outcome. *Addictive Behaviors*, **29** (8), 1665–1672.
139. Najavits, L.M., Ryngala, D. and Back, S.E. (2009) Treatment of PTSD and comorbid disorders, in *Effective Treatments for PTSD*, 2nd edn (eds E.B. Foa, T.M. Keane, M.J. Friedman and J.A. Cohen), Guilford, New York, pp. 508–535.
140. Ouimette, P., Humphreys, K., Moos, R.H. *et al*. (2001) Self-help group participation among substance use disorder patients with posttraumatic stress disorder. *Journal of Substance Abuse Treatment*, **20** (1), 25–32.
141. Miller, W.R. and Rollnick, S. (2002) *Motivational Interviewing: Preparing People for Change*, Guilford Press, New York.
142. Bryant, R.A. (2001) Posttraumatic stress disorder and traumatic brain injury: can they co-exist? *Clinical Psychology Review*, **21** (6), 931–948.
143. Sbordone, R.J. and Liter, J.C. (1995) Mild traumatic brain injury does not produce post-traumatic stress disorder. *Brain Injury*, **9** (4), 405–412.
144. Hoge, C.W., McGurk, D., Thomas, J.L. *et al*. (2008) Mild traumatic brain injury in US Soldiers returning from Iraq. *New England Journal of Medicine*, **358** (5), 453–463.
145. Schneiderman, A.I., Braver, E.R. and Kang, H.K. (2008) Understanding sequelae of injury mechanisms and mild traumatic brain injury incurred during the conflicts in Iraq and Afghanistan: persistent postconcussive symptoms and posttraumatic stress disorder. *American Journal of Epidemiology*, **167** (12), 1446–1452.
146. Rauch, S.L., Shin, L.M. and Phelps, E.A. (2006) Neurocircuitry models of posttraumatic stress disorder and extinction: human neuroimaging research-past, present, and future. *Biological Psychiatry*, **60** (4), 376–382.
147. Bryant, R.A. (2008) Disentangling mild traumatic brain injury and stress reactions. *New England Journal of Medicine*, **358** (5), 525–527.

148. Bryant, R.A., Moulds, M., Guthrie, R. and Nixon, R.D. (2003) Treating acute stress disorder following mild traumatic brain injury. *American Journal of Psychiatry*, **160** (3), 585–587.
149. Chemtob, C.M., Novaco, R.W., Hamada, R.S. *et al*. (1997) Anger regulation deficits in combat-related posttraumatic stress disorder. *Journal of Traumatic Stress*, **10** (1), 17–36.
150. Foa, E.B., Riggs, D.S. and Gershuny, B.S. (1995) Arousal, numbing, and intrusion: symptom structure of PTSD following assault. *American Journal of Psychiatry*, **152** (1), 116–120.
151. Chemtob, C.M., Novaco, R.W., Hamada, R.S. and Gross, D.M. (1997) Cognitive-behavioral treatment for severe anger in posttraumatic stress disorder. *Journal of Consulting and Clinical Psychology*, **65** (1), 184–189.
152. Kuyken, W., Byford, S., Taylor, R.S. *et al*. (2008) Mindfulness-based cognitive therapy to prevent relapse in recurrent depression. *Journal of Consulting and Clinical Psychology*, **76** (6), 966–978.
153. Solomon, Z., Mikulincer, M. and Flum, H. (1988) Negative life events, coping responses, and combat-related psychopathology: a prospective study. *Journal of Abnormal Psychology*, **97** (3), 302–307.
154. Kessler, R.C., Sonnega, A., Hughes, M. and Nelson, C.B. (1995) Posttraumatic stress disorder in the national comorbidity survey. *Archives of General Psychiatry*, **52**, 1048–1060.
155. Becker, C.B., Zayfert, C. and Anderson, E. (2004) A survey of psychologists' attitudes towards and utilization of exposure therapy for PTSD. *Behaviour Research and Therapy*, **42** (3), 277–292.

COMMENTARY

5.1 Psychological Interventions for PTSD in Children

Lucy Berliner

Harborview Center for Sexual Assault & Traumatic Stress, School of Social Work, University of Washington, Seattle, WA, USA

Our comments focus on psychotherapy for post-traumatic stress disorder (PTSD) in children. Trauma-focused cognitive behaviour therapies (CBTs) have the strongest empirical support for reducing PTSD in children, as is true for adults (see Commentry of Chapter 3). Although the current PTSD symptom algorithm may need adjustment for children, especially younger children, child and adult conceptualisations of trauma impact and the typical content of CBT interventions are comparable. Treatment models target emotional memories, avoidance and maladaptive cognitions, and contain the same basic components: psychoeducation, relaxation and coping skills, exposure via some level of direct discussion of the trauma and cognitive processing to address inaccurate or unhelpful cognitions [1].

Developmentally appropriate adjustments are common but do not stray from basic CBT principles and strategies. For example, the delivery methods for the treatments include using play and non-verbal strategies for younger children to accomplish the treatment components [2]. Most models incorporate parents/caregivers to some extent. Inclusion of parents is intended to lower parental distress or avoidance that may interfere with support for the children and to engage parents in reinforcing skill practice between sessions. Scheeringa *et al*. [3] document that with active parental participation CBT can be accomplished even with preschool children.

Systematic reviews find that trauma-focused CBT is effective for childhood PTSD and clinically significant post-traumatic stress (e.g. [4–6]). Randomised trials have compared trauma-focused CBTs to wait-list, treatment as usual and supportive treatment. They are shown to be effective for many types of trauma

Post-traumatic Stress Disorder, First Edition. Edited by Dan Stein, Matthew Friedman, and Carlos Blanco.

(e.g. physical and sexual abuse, exposure to community and domestic violence, war), for boys and girls, for children from a broad range of ethnicities and backgrounds, and for children with multiple trauma history and comorbidities.

Several versions of trauma-focused CBT for children have been empirically tested. Cohen *et al.* [2] have conducted a series of studies of their 12-week structured approach that involves children and caregivers receiving approximately equivalent amounts of active treatment. Several other investigators have demonstrated the effectiveness of their versions of trauma-focused CBT [7–9]. School-based group versions have also been found to be effective (e.g. [10, 11]). As in the adult studies, eye-movement desensitisation reprocessing (EMDR) has empirical support, although study sample sizes are small and the function of the eye movements and other attentional activities has not yet been established [12].

Many of the issues raised by Bryant regarding adult interventions have parallels in the child literature. A key issue is how much exposure is necessary. A recent multisite dismantling study [13] directly investigated this question. Children were randomly assigned to one of four conditions: 8 or 16 weeks' CBT with explicit exposure or 8 or 16 weeks' CBT without explicit exposure. The 8-week exposure-based condition had the best results for PTS, with only minimal additional benefit for the 16-week condition; the 16-week CBT without explicit exposure produced the best results for behaviour problems. The authors hypothesised that exposure is necessary but may have diminishing returns at some point, whereas longer CBT may be better for behaviour problems because of the increased opportunity for parents to learn and practise skills.

Comparable to the standards for adults, the National Child Traumatic Stress Network (http://www.nctsnet.org) recommends psychological first aid for the acute response to children and families [14]. Few randomised trials have been carried out for early brief CBT interventions with children. Berkowitz *et al.* [15] report promising results for a four-session psychoeducation and coping skills intervention compared to a supportive condition.

A key question, as with adults, is whether brief structured CBTs for children can be successfully applied to 'complex trauma'. While it is likely that children with severe psychological problems beyond PTSD and comorbid depression and anxiety will require treatments that are somewhat longer and multicomponent, the evidence suggests that CBT-based interventions are the best candidates. For example, Runyon *et al.* [16] found that a multicomponent parent–child group CBT improved PTS and parenting skills for families where the parent had physically abused the child. Adaptations of dialectical behaviour therapy, a CBT, seem logical as an approach when the clinical presentation involves extreme emotion dysregulation and suicidality.

In accord with Bryant's review of psychotherapy for adults, trauma-focused CBT is the first-line treatment for children affected by trauma, although there is much yet to be learned, especially for the more complex presentations. Of critical importance are more studies addressing implementation in real-world settings (see e.g. [17]).

COMMENTARY

5.2 Challenges in the Dissemination and Implementation of Exposure-Based CBT for the Treatment of Hispanics with PTSD

Rafael Kichic,[1] **Mildred Vera,**[2] **and María L. Reyes-Rabanillo**[3]

[1] *Anxiety Clinic, Institute of Cognitive Neurology (INECO) and Institute of Neurosciences, Favaloro University, Buenos Aires, Argentina*

[2] *Department of Health Services Administration, Medical Sciences Campus, University of Puerto Rico, San Juan, Puerto Rico*

[3] *Psychiatry Service, Veterans Affairs Caribbean Healthcare System, San Juan, Puerto Rico*

Dr Bryant's chapter makes a thorough revision of the literature on the efficacy of trauma-focused treatments for PTSD across the lifespan, with special emphasis on CBT for PTSD. He concludes that trauma-focused therapies have been the focus of many well-controlled studies that evidence the efficacy of exposure-based CBT for PTSD. However, he acknowledges that important limitations in our current knowledge still remain, highlighting the dearth of effectiveness studies that examine benefits and obstacles when implementing trauma-focused therapies in community settings.

Speaking to this issue, in sharp contrast to the large body of evidence supporting the efficacy, and, to a lesser extent, the effectiveness of CBT for PTSD in English-speaking samples, there is a lack of outcome studies for Hispanics in spite of data that suggest high risk for PTSD among this group. Findings from a

Post-traumatic Stress Disorder, First Edition. Edited by Dan Stein, Matthew Friedman, and Carlos Blanco.

national sample of Vietnam veterans revealed that Hispanic veterans, particularly Puerto Ricans, had higher rates of PTSD and experienced more severe symptoms than non-Hispanic white veterans [18]. Although available research suggests that ethnic-group affiliation can have a direct impact on PTSD, there is limited information on the acceptability, efficacy and effectiveness of PTSD treatment in ethnic minorities. To address this limitation the Institute of Medicine Committee on Treatment of PTSD recommended designing intervention studies tailored to these populations [19].

With the goal of making advances in the treatment of PTSD available for the Hispanic community, our initial efforts have focused on establishing the groundwork to examine the efficacy of exposure-based CBT with Puerto Rican veterans. We first translated the prolonged exposure manual from English to Spanish [20]. Prolonged-exposure therapy, developed by Foa *et al.* [21–23], incorporates repeated imaginal exposure (i.e. revisiting, recounting and processing of the traumatic memories) and in vivo exposure (i.e. approaching trauma-related distressing situations). Next, we evaluated the sociocultural compatibility of the translated intervention, which involved the assessment of the sociocultural compatibility of the intervention per se and the identification of factors within the sociocultural environment of Puerto Ricans that either facilitated or served as barriers to receiving PTSD treatment. Prior to initiating these activities, clinicians received training from intervention developers with the goal of having a clear understanding of the core components of prolonged exposure relevant for adapting the manual and maintaining treatment fidelity.

The cultural adaptation of the prolonged-exposure treatment manual included key informant interviews, expert review by mental health clinicians and focus groups with Spanish-speaking veterans. The prolonged exposure manual was examined to evaluate whether the vocabulary was clear and understandable. Results allowed the manual to be revised so it reflected situations, vocabulary and issues relevant to the Hispanic population. The importance of family members, particularly veterans' spouses, was highlighted when discussing their attitudes and views about the proposed intervention. Patients strongly preferred that spouses receive information about the treatment so they would have a better understanding of the therapeutic process the patient would be undergoing. To strengthen this dimension within the manual we developed an optional introductory session targeted at participants' spouses or other family members, explaining the principles, goals and methods of prolonged exposure, as well as its relevance for veterans' recovery. The provision of prolonged exposure by Hispanic therapists facilitated important aspects of the treatment such as the appropriate use of culturally sound idiomatic expressions and examples.

The next step involved pilot testing the culturally-adapted prolonged-exposure intervention with a small sample of veterans with PTSD. A major barrier identified in the implementation of prolonged exposure is clinicians' concern that the intervention may lead to increases in anxiety symptoms and negatively impact the patient [24]. In response, clinical researchers identified three essential prerequisites for the use of exposure interventions [25]: that clinicians have trust in the intervention, feel comfortable administering it and are confident in their ability to address clients' reactions during exposures. They suggested that these prerequisites can be achieved through a combination of instruction, supervised practice while administering exposure treatment, and peer consultation.

Therefore, a big challenge was to obtain adequate training and supervision in prolonged exposure for PTSD. For that reason it was necessary to request collaboration with experts, including those able to understand Spanish. Many Hispanic countries lack this clinical expertise, limiting the advancement and dissemination of prolonged exposure for Hispanics. Based on the trainers' model [24], the Spanish-speaking supervisor, who had prior training in using prolonged exposure, was trained as a consultant by Dr Foa and Dr Hembree and received supervision from the latter on an as-needed basis. The supervision involved an additional on-site three-day training session in Spanish right before the recruitment started, weekly group supervisions via teleconferencing technology and written feedback for each videotaped session, also in Spanish. Five therapists from varied backgrounds (psychiatry, psychology) with no prior expertise in using exposure-based interventions for trauma treated six cases.

Adequate training in the underlying principles of prolonged exposure helped the research team to become familiarised with the model, to redesign exposures when obstacles were encountered (e.g. how to help clients drop their safety behaviours) and to deal with misconceptions regarding the treatment. The group-supervision format was found to be particularly helpful in overcoming therapists' concerns about using the imaginal exposure. Therapists learned from each others' cases how to handle different clinical difficulties before treating their own case. As a result, their confidence in implementing the imaginal exposure increased throughout the study.

In summary, our experience suggests that Hispanic therapists share the same specific concerns as therapists from other countries, mainly pertaining to the use of the imaginal exposure [24]. However, language is an important obstacle for implementing prolonged exposure, not only for Spanish-speaking therapists who need to obtain expertise in prolonged exposure, but also for therapist–patient communication. In this study, we were able to combine human and financial resources to overcome typical problems encountered in Spanish-speaking countries (e.g. lack of research funding, expertise or organisational support) and more importantly, to develop the foundation to support larger outcome studies for Spanish-speaking veterans with PTSD.

COMMENTARY

5.3 What Else Do We Need to Know about Evidence-Based Psychological Interventions for PTSD?

Karina Lovell
The School of Nursing, Midwifery and Social Work, The University of Manchester, Manchester, UK

This excellent chapter by Bryant examines and synthesises the evidence base for psychological interventions for PTSD. In essence the key message emerging from the literature is that trauma-focused psychological interventions are effective for PTSD. The psychological treatments with the strongest evidence base include CBT and EMDR. In terms of replicable intervention, 'CBT' is somewhat meaningless as it encompasses a wide range of interventions which aim to alter behavioural, cognitive or physiological aspects. Systematic reviews demonstrate that of the CBT interventions, exposure-based interventions are considered the treatment of choice for PTSD.

However, what is most striking about this chapter is the dearth of literature focusing on the essential components of the evidence-based interventions for PTSD. Thus, despite the increasing evidence base, there remains ambiguity concerning the 'active ingredients' of CBT and EMDR interventions for PTSD, including the specific content of the intervention, the delivery style, where the intervention should take place and the skills and expertise required to deliver it.

For example, Bryant states that CBT for chronic PTSD is typically between 8 and 12 sessions but 'typical' is derived from the overall mean number of sessions from randomised controlled trials rather than from carefully conducted session-by-session analysis. Thus the minimum number of sessions required to achieve a sufficient health benefit is unclear. Session length is based on tradition rather than

Post-traumatic Stress Disorder, First Edition. Edited by Dan Stein, Matthew Friedman, and Carlos Blanco.

a theoretical rationale; it is notable that the average duration of session length is between 60 and 90 minutes regardless of the psychological intervention being delivered. Although it is likely that exposure is a critical ingredient, other key ingredients remain unidentified. Even for exposure there are many other factors which require further investigation. For example, Bryant highlights that there is some but insufficient evidence that imaginal and in vivo exposure are equally efficacious. Further, there is literature suggesting that exposure may lead to a worsening or exacerbation of symptoms [26], noncompliance, lack of engagement and high attrition [27–29]. Such findings are important and warrant further exploration.

Recent literature has focused on the development and evaluation of complex interventions [30, 31]. Complex interventions are used in health- and social-care research and can be defined as interventions which have several separate but interacting components. It is imperative that we define the critical ingredients of both CBT and EMDR to exactly specify how and why these interventions are effective. In addition, understanding and correctly estimating duration and timing of sessions is critical in our quest to provide treatments in the most cost-effective way possible. We need to go beyond the 'does it work?' question and incorporate significantly more process evaluation [32] in future studies.

It is perplexing that as researchers and clinicians we insist on the importance of evidence-based interventions to improve outcomes for patients but mostly neglect to evaluate the way we deliver these interventions. In short, we have an evidence-based treatment but its delivery is based on tradition. Such lack of knowledge impacts on the implementation of interventions into the real clinical world.

It is disturbing that the majority of PTSD studies have failed to examine perhaps the most important element of any intervention: are these interventions acceptable to the patients receiving them? It could be argued that the single most important issue in first developing evidence-based intervention and hence ensuring that the intervention will be implemented into clinical practice is whether it is acceptable to both patients and the therapists delivering it.

Although there is promising evidence of the efficacy of both CBT and EMDR there is only limited literature on their acceptability. Successfully implementing research into clinical practice requires that new interventions are accepted and welcomed by those receiving them. The acceptability of an intervention involves making a normative judgement based on the extent to which it can be tolerated and considered reasonable. Judgements of acceptability of new treatments are likely to be made with reference to what has been used within everyday normal practice and to judgements about existing forms of treatment and practice related to the management of PTSD. Qualitative methods are the most appropriate method to explore views and also offer the opportunity to examine facilitators and barriers of change. However, there is a near absence of studies that examine the acceptability of CBT or EMDR for PTSD from the patient's perspective.

This is surprising given that both exposure therapy and EMDR focus on painful memories and by their very nature are distressing treatments for the individual.

Similarly, there are limited studies that adequately explore the acceptability of delivering either CBT or EMDR from the therapist's perspective. Research findings will not be implemented into clinical practice if those delivering the intervention are either unable to deliver the intervention (due to lack of training) or do not find it acceptable for delivery. So despite the evidence base and international guidelines for the use of PTSD therapies, studies of therapists working in the clinical area demonstrate only a minority of clinicians utilise exposure-based treatments for PTSD [33].

In summary, it could be argued that we have two evidence-based interventions but that they are not being implemented into the clinical arena by therapists for a variety of reasons, we don't know whether they are acceptable to patients and there is a lack of literature concerning the critical ingredients. Future research must focus on addressing these deficiencies and some carefully conducted preparatory studies should be carried out to delineate the critical ingredients. In addition, there is a very great need to examine the acceptability to both those receiving these interventions and those delivering them – only by doing so will such interventions be successfully implemented into clinical practice and thereby be able to improve the lives of those individuals experiencing PTSD.

COMMENTARY

5.4 Another Perspective on Exposure Therapy for PTSD

Barbara Olasov Rothbaum
Department of Psychiatry, Trauma and Anxiety Recovery Program, Emory University School of Medicine, Atlanta, GA, USA

In 'Psychological Interventions for Trauma Exposure and PTSD', Richard Bryant covers the topic in a most impressive manner. It is completely comprehensive, yet succinct and very well-written. He begins with a historical overview of cognitive behaviour interventions for PTSD, reviews the major interventions for chronic PTSD and early interventions and prophylactic approaches and the evidence for their use for both adults and children, presents evidence-based clinical guidelines, and even discusses the implications of the major comorbid or complicating factors often associated with PTSD. He includes five tables summarising the systematic reviews of CBT for PTSD, of CBT for children, of early interventions, of CBT provided acutely and of EMDR. Overall, this chapter provides a wealth of information in a succinct package. He is to be congratulated.

Dr Bryant covers the material in a scientifically objective manner, so generally there is not a great deal of controversy in his presentation. This author agrees with his assertion that there is more similar than different in the outcomes and mechanisms of action between cognitive processing therapy (CPT) [34] and prolonged exposure [35], for example. The emphasis is different in the two treatments: in prolonged exposure, exposure to the memory and reminders of the traumatic experience are prominent and more time is spent on exposure (imaginal in-session and imaginal and in vivo between sessions) than any other technique or intervention, whereas in CPT exposure to the trauma memory is conducted in writing and only a few times, and more for the purpose of identifying stuck points. CPT highlights the cognitive-therapy aspects of treatment within sessions and for homework, whereas in prolonged exposure this is reserved for the 'processing' that occurs in-session following the imaginal exposure. However, in prolonged exposure, we know that processing occurs, possibly less formally,

Post-traumatic Stress Disorder, First Edition. Edited by Dan Stein, Matthew Friedman, and Carlos Blanco.

when *therapeutic* exposure [36] to the memory and reminders takes place. A very recent article [37] reported that negative cognitions reduced just with exposure therapy and no formal cognitive therapy, and that this reduction was preceded by reductions in distress. The processing in prolonged exposure after imaginal exposure helps the patient to identify the patterns of distress with exposure and whether they change with unhelpful cognitions, and assists in evaluating them. However, oftentimes patients come back after listening to the tape of their imaginal exposure for homework and report changes in cognitions without any more formal techniques. We often have them keep these 'revised' thoughts in mind as they engage in exposure. I suspect that the optimal endpoint is the same for most PTSD therapies: survivors can be reminded of the traumatic experience without inordinate distress or interference and can think about it realistically in ways that don't impede their current functioning.

However, I do take issue with Dr Bryant's distinction of generalised anxiety disorder (GAD) and agoraphobia/panic disorder as separate, comorbid disorders. We have taken the approach, as instructed in the DSM, that if one disorder is 'better accounted for' by another disorder, that diagnosis should be assigned, rather than both. Many PTSD patients will worry excessively, can't sleep, are tense and so on; that is, they would meet criteria for GAD if these symptoms were taken at face value. Similarly with agoraphobia and panic disorder: we often recruit best for PTSD studies when we also have a panic-disorder study, as patients resonate with the experience of panic attacks, but in the context of PTSD these are all feared situations. We believe that agoraphobia works along the same lines – patients with PTSD by definition are avoidant, but if all of their avoided situations are trauma-related, then it is best accounted for by PTSD. Although Dr Bryant doesn't mention social anxiety disorder (SAD), we find that the same holds true for SAD. Many of our PTSD patients, particularly those who served in the military, are very avoidant of social situations. They don't go to movies or sporting events and avoid going out on the town with their buddies. However, this avoidance is not motivated by factors that influence social anxiety, namely fear of negative evaluation, but rather by PTSD-related fears. It is certainly possible to have PTSD and a truly comorbid anxiety disorder, but in our experience the new onset of symptoms following the traumatic event most usually occurs within the context of PTSD. Conversely, when the PTSD is successfully treated, these other symptoms decrease as well.

Dr Bryant discusses the combination of psychotherapy and pharmacotherapy for the treatment of PTSD. He reviews one of our studies in which all patients received 10 weeks of open-label sertraline then were randomly assigned to just continue the sertraline for five more weeks or to continue sertraline in addition to a full course of twice-weekly prolonged exposure. The most prominent finding of that study was in a *post hoc* analysis that found that prolonged exposure added to the medication benefits but only for patients who were weaker medication responders. For the strong medication responders, the addition of prolonged exposure didn't offer much advantage. I think this mirrors what we see in clinical practice. Patients who respond well to medication alone are (hopefully) maintained on that medication and don't require further therapy. However, for the significant number of patients who receive only a partial or no benefit from the medication alone, the addition of therapy can almost get them to the same point as the strong medication responders.

It is true that combining 'traditional' pharmacotherapy (typically selective serotonin reuptake inhibitors, SSRIs) and CBT for patients with anxiety disorders seems to offer no advantage over CBT alone, although this has not been tested in a well-controlled design for PTSD [38]. However, Dr Bryant doesn't mention the excitement surrounding the addition of a novel medication to CBT, probably because the data for this in PTSD have not yet been published. In this model, pharmacotherapy is aimed at improving the learning that takes place during CBT (specifically exposure-based therapy) and not at treating the symptoms of anxiety. D-cycloserine (DCS), an NMDA partial agonist, has been shown in animal studies to facilitate the extinction of learned fear. In studies with patients with various anxiety disorders, DCS combined with exposure therapy has also been found to facilitate extinction [39]. Studies combining DCS with exposure therapy in PTSD patients are currently ongoing.

REFERENCES

1. Cohen, J.A., Bukstein, O., Walter, H. *et al*. (2010) Practice parameter for the assessment and treatment of children and adolescents with posttraumatic stress disorder. *Journal of the American Academy of Child and Adolescent Psychiatry*, **49**, 414–430.
2. Cohen, J., Mannarino, A. and Deblinger, E. (2006) *Treating Trauma and Traumatic Grief in Children and Adolescents*, Guilford, New York.
3. Scheeringa, M.S., Weems, C.F., Cohen, J.A. *et al*. (2010) Trauma-focused cognitive-behavioral therapy for posttraumatic stress disorder in three through six year-old children: a randomized clinical trial. *Journal of Child Psychology and Psychiatry*. doi: 10.1111/j.1469-7610.2010.02354.x
4. Harvey, S.T. and Taylor, J.E. (2010) A meta-analysis of the effects of psychotherapy with sexually abused children and adolescents. *Clinical Psychology Review*, **30**, 517–535.
5. McDonald, G.M., Higgins, J.P.T. and Ramchandi, P. (2006) Cognitive-behavioral interventions for children who have been sexually abused. *Cochrane Database of Systematic Reviews*, 4 (Art. No.: CD001930). doi: 10.1002/14651858
6. Silverman, W.K., Ortiz, C.D., Viswesvaran, C. *et al*. (2008) Evidence-based psychosocial treatments for children and adolescents exposed to traumatic events. *Journal of Clinical Child and Adolescent Psychology*, **37**, 156–183.
7. Smith, P., Yule, W., Perrin, S. *et al*. (2007) Cognitive-behavioral therapy for PTSD in children and adolescents: a preliminary randomized control trial. *Journal of the American Academy of Child and Adolescent Psychiatry*, **46**, 1051–1061.

8. Gilboa-Schechtman, E., Foa, E., Shafran, N. *et al*. (2010) Prolonged exposure versus dynamic therapy for adolescent PTSD: a pilot randomized controlled trial. *Journal of the American Academy of Child and Adolescent Psychiatry*, **49**, 1034–1042.
9. Ruf, M., Schauer, M., Neuner, F. *et al*. (2010) Narrative exposure therapy for 7- to 16-year-olds: a randomized controlled trial with traumatized refugee children. *Journal of Traumatic Stress*, **23**, 437–445.
10. Berger, R., Pat-Horenczyk, R. and Gelkopf, M. (2007) School-based intervention for prevention and treatment of elementary-students' terror-related distress in Israel: a quasi-randomized controlled trial. *Journal of Traumatic Stress*, **20**, 541–551.
11. Stein, B.D., Jaycox, L.H., Kataoka, S.H. *et al*. (2003) A mental health intervention for schoolchildren exposed to violence: a randomized controlled trial. *Journal of the American Medical Association*, **290**, 603–611.
12. Rodenburg, R., Benjamin, A., De Roos, C. *et al*. (2009) Efficacy of EMDR in children: a meta-analysis. *Clinical Psychology Review*, **29**, 599–606.
13. Deblinger, E., Mannarino, A.P., Cohen, J.A. *et al*. (2010) Trauma-focused cognitive behavioral therapy for children: impact of the trauma narrative and treatment length. *Depression and Anxiety*. doi: 10.1002/da.20744
14. NCTSN (2006) *Psychological First Aid: Field Operations Guide for Community Religious Professionals*, PFA, Los Angeles, CA.
15. Berkowitz, S.J., Stover, C.S. and Marans, S.R. (2010) The child and family traumatic stress intervention: secondary prevention for youth at risk of developing PTSD. *Journal of Child Psychology and Psychiatry*. doi: 10.1111/j.1469-7610.2010.02321.x
16. Runyon, M., Deblinger, E. and Steer, R. (2010) Group CBT for parents and children at risk for physical abuse. *Journal of Child and Family Behavior Therapy*, **32**, 196–218.
17. Jaycox, L.H., Cohen, J.A., Mannarino, A.P. *et al*. (2010) Children's mental health care following Hurricane Katrina: a field trial of trauma-focused psychotherapies. *Journal of Traumatic Stress*, **23**, 223–231.
18. Ortega, A.N. and Rosenheck, R. (2000) Posttraumatic stress disorder among Hispanic Vietnam veterans. *American Journal of Psychiatry*, **157**, 615–619.
19. Institute of Medicine (2008) *Treatment of Posttraumatic Stress Disorder: An Assessment of the Evidence*, National Academic Press, Washington, DC.
20. Foa, E.B., Hembree, E.A. and Dancu, C.V. (2002) Prolonged exposure manual – Revised version. Unpublished manuscript.
21. Foa, E.B., Dancu, C.V., Hembree, E.A. *et al*. (1999) A comparison of exposure therapy, stress inoculation training, and their combination for reducing posttraumatic stress disorder in female assault victims. *Journal of Consulting and Clinical Psychology*, **67**, 194–200.
22. Foa, E.B., Hembree, E.A., Cahill, S.P. *et al*. (2005) Randomized trial of prolonged exposure for posttraumatic stress disorder with and without cognitive restructuring: outcome at academic and community clinics. *Journal of Consulting and Clinical Psychology*, **73**, 953–964.
23. Foa, E.B., Hembree, E.A. and Rothbaum, B.O. (2007) *Prolonged Exposure Therapy for PTSD: Emotional Processing of Traumatic Experiences. Therapist Guide*, Oxford University Press, New York.

24. Cahill, S.P., Foa, E.B., Hembree, E.A. *et al.* (2006) Dissemination of exposure therapy in the treatment of posttraumatic stress disorder. *Journal of Traumatic Stress*, **19**, 597–610.
25. Gunther, R.W. and Whittal, M.L. (2010) Dissemination of cognitive-behavioral treatments for anxiety disorders: overcoming barriers and improving patient access. *Clinical Psychology Review*, **30**, 194–202.
26. Foa, E.B., Zoellner, L.A., Feeny, N.C. *et al.* (2002) Does imaginal exposure exacerbate PTSD symptoms? *Journal of Consulting and Clinical Psychology*, **70**, 1022–1028.
27. Scott, M.J. and Stradling, S.G. (1997) Client compliance with exposure treatments for posttraumatic stress disorder. *Journal of Traumatic Stress*, **10**, 523–526.
28. Chemtob, C.M., Novaco, R.W., Hamada, R.S. *et al.* (1997) Anger regulation deficits in combat-related posttraumatic stress disorder. *Journal of Traumatic Stress*, **10**, 17–35.
29. Hemree, E.A., Foa, E.B., Dorfan, N.M. *et al.* (2003) Do patients drop out prematurely from exposure therapy for PTSD? *Journal of Traumatic Stress*, **16**, 555–562.
30. Craig, P., Dieppe, P., Macintyre, S. *et al.* (2008) Developing and evaluating complex interventions: the new Medical Research Council guidance. *British Medical Journal*, **337**, 1655.
31. Campbell, N.C., Murray, E., Darbyshire, J. *et al.* (2007) Designing and evaluating complex interventions to improve health care. *British Medical Journal*, **334**, 455.
32. Oakley, A., Strange, V., Bonnell, C. *et al.* (2006) Process evaluation in randomised controlled trials of complex interventions. *British Medical Journal*, **332**, 413.
33. Black Becker, C., Zayfert, C. and Anderson, E. (2004) A survey of psychologists' attitudes towards and utilization of exposure therapy for PTSD. *Behaviour Research and Therapy*, **42**, 277.
34. Resick, P.A. and Schnicke, M.K. (1993) *Cognitive Processing Therapy for Sexual Assault Victims: A Treatment Manual*, Sage Publications, Newbury Park, CA.
35. Foa, E.B., Hembree, E. and Rothbaum, B.O. (2007) *Prolonged Exposure Therapy for PTSD: Emotional Processing of Traumatic Experiences, Therapist Guide*, Oxford University Press, New York.
36. Davis, M., Ressler, K., Rothbaum, B.O. and Richardson, R. (2006) Effects of D-cycloserine on extinction: translation from preclinical to clinical work. *Biological Psychiatry*, **60**, 369–375.
37. Hagenaars, M.A., van Minnen, A. and de Rooij, M. (2010) Cognitions in prolonged exposure therapy for posttraumatic stress disorder. *International Journal of Clinical and Health Psychology*, **10**, 421–434.
38. Rothbaum, B.O. (2008) Critical parameters for D-cycloserine enhancement of cognitive behavioral therapy for obsessive compulsive disorder. *American Journal of Psychiatry*, **165**, 293–296.
39. Ressler, K.J., Rothbaum, B.O., Tannenbaum, L. *et al.* (2004) Facilitation of psychotherapy with D-cycloserine, a putative cognitive enhancer. *Archives of General Psychiatry*, **61**, 1136–1144.

CHAPTER 6

(Disaster) Public Mental Health

Joop de Jong
Department of Psychiatry, VU University Amsterdam, The Netherlands; Boston University, USA; Rhodes University, South Africa

INTRODUCTION

Therapist, context and technique: how important is the context in healing?

In an overview of the evidence of the effectiveness of psychotherapy, Asay and Lambert [1] ascribed 30% of the variance in psychotherapy to universal therapist variables, 40% to contextual variables, 15% to placebo and 15% to technique. In the course of our professional lives, we spend large amounts of time on learning therapeutic techniques and relatively little on handling contextual variables. While we try to keep up with new developments in therapy, controlled studies suggest these new psychotherapies, despite their 'evidence-based' status, are no more effective than older ones such as psychodynamic therapies [2]. The best evidence suggests that the 'specific ingredient' in any given therapy – that which theoretically makes it work – adds little to the nonspecific effects of psychotherapy. Moreover, clinical success is more a function of differences among therapists than among therapies [3], and the success of therapists is primarily related to the quality of their alliance with patients [4]. Similarly, we go to great lengths to keep up with new developments in psychopharmacology, but in general various types of antidepressants (tricyclic, selective serotonin reuptake inhibitors (SSRIs), serotonin noradrenaline reuptake inhibitors (SNRIs), etc.) have identical efficacy despite their action on different neurotransmitters. In addition, they have proven effective in multiple psychiatric conditions (such as generalised anxiety disorder, phobic disorders, panic disorder, post-traumatic stress disorder (PTSD), eating disorders) [5, 6]. Trauma experts agree there is limited evidence for pharmacological agents in the treatment of PTSD in the early response phases. There is some evidence for a small positive effect of

Post-traumatic Stress Disorder, First Edition. Edited by Dan Stein, Matthew Friedman, and Carlos Blanco.

medication on chronic PTSD, and more for other post-traumatic disorders such as depression, but further evidence is still needed [7].

In the next decades, the mental health of populations will continue to depend less on developments in neurosciences or psychopharmacology and more on broader political and sociocultural trends influencing people's lives. For example, the increase in alcoholism-related mortality after the collapse of the Soviet Union [8] was not due to a genetic mutation or a decline in mental health services, but to the elimination of Soviet-era restrictions on alcohol consumption in the context of social and economic dislocation [9]. Similarly, many studies argue that, despite a paucity of psychiatric services, outcomes in schizophrenia are better in rural, low-income countries than in industrialised high-income societies [10, 11]. A country like Burundi provides comprehensive mental health services to 8 million people with 1.6 psychiatric hospital beds per 100 000 people, compared to 130 beds/100 000 in Germany and the Netherlands[1] and 62 beds/100 000 in the UK (H. Ndayisaba 2010, personal communication) [13]. These huge differences in service delivery between high- and low-income countries cannot be explained by variations in psychopathology. They can be explained in terms of political, sociocultural and contextual variables, and to some extent they can be addressed with a public mental health approach, as outlined in this chapter. This chapter does not intend to play down the importance of new clinical developments, but it primarily attempts to illustrate the importance of a complementary public mental health approach.

Political violence, war and disaster

How do these considerations play out in situations of armed conflict, complex humanitarian emergencies and natural disasters?

The World Health Organization (WHO) [14] distinguishes three broad categories of violence: self-directed violence, interpersonal violence and collective violence. Political violence belongs to the third category of collective violence and includes war and violent conflicts, state violence, terrorist acts and mob violence. In 2000, an estimated 1.6 million people worldwide died as a result of violence. Nearly half of these deaths were suicides, one third were homicides and one fifth were war-related [14]. Estimates of disability-adjusted life years (DALYs) due to war injuries will increase between 2010 and 2019 [15]. Armed conflict is often associated with forced displacement of people and with increasing poverty, hunger and malnutrition [16, 17]. A local conflict can develop into a national conflict, which can sometimes spill over into neighbouring countries and thus may destabilise an entire region, as in the Great Lake area in Africa or in the Middle East [18, 19].

[1] Despite the fact that the Netherlands has a longstanding history of deinstitutionalisation, a decennia-old moratorium on new psychiatric beds, complex substitution programmes and the highest expenditure on mental health worldwide (22% of the health budget, indirect costs not included) [12].

The ratio of involvement in collective violence of low- and middle-income countries (LAMICs) versus high-income countries is 10 to 1 [14]. Political violence particularly affects LAMICs: 88% of the 34 armed conflicts recorded in 2007 took place in lower-income settings, the majority in Asia (41%) and Africa (35%) [20]. At the global level, the total number of armed conflicts rose steadily from the early 1950s through 1994 and then declined sharply until 2004. The decline after the Cold War was largely due to the resolution of old conflicts rather than the prevention of new conflict, and many dormant societal conflicts reemerged after 2004 [21].

In modern warfare, 10% of the people who are killed are soldiers and 90% civilians – one half of which are children. Despite this, few psychosocial and mental health intervention models have been reported for children, especially in situations of political violence [22, 23].

Regarding natural disasters: cyclones and hurricanes occur three times more often in rich than in poor countries, but 81% of the casualties take place in the latter. Floods typically have a disproportionate impact on poor people, who may live in relatively dangerous places, a problem that will increase with global warming.

Poor countries also carry the brunt of the migration problem often caused by disasters or oppression. Of the almost 1 billion refugees who sought a better life in 2009, about 75% did so within the boundaries of their own country; 200 million went to another poor developing country (such as Sudan, Colombia, Iraq, Somalia or Pakistan) and 70 million, less than 8%, went to a rich country (cf. Index of Global Reports 2009–2010).

Treatment needs and treatment gap

The burden of disease in LAMICs caused by mental disorders (11%) is larger than the combined contribution of tuberculosis, HIV/AIDS and malaria. Nevertheless, there are generally few mental health resources in terms of infrastructure, human resources and policies in these countries, resulting in a large gap between needs and availability of care [24]. Even in normal times, there is a huge discrepancy between prevalence rates and service provision. The WHO World Mental Health Survey Consortium [25] showed that 35.5–50.3% of serious adult cases in developed countries and 76.3–85.4% in less-developed countries received no treatment in the 12 months before the interview. There is also a vast gap between child and adolescent mental health needs and mental health resources in LAMIC [26]. Similarly, there is very little evidence-based consensus with regard to effective interventions in complex emergencies [27]. These figures are not representative for any current post-disaster area, where the treatment gap impresses as invariably larger [28]. The post-9/11 efforts to provide services were a vivid example of the discrepancy between needs and the availability of adequate intervention models and services, especially for immigrants, even in the city of New York, with the highest density of mental health professionals worldwide [29].

The treatment gap in conflict and disaster areas in LAMICs

LAMICs struggle with additional complexities, and the psychosocial and mental health consequences of conflict and disaster cannot easily be handled with psychological and psychiatric approaches common to high-income countries for the following reasons [30, p. 24]:

First, approaches from the West require highly trained professionals. However, as noted above, within Africa, Asia and parts of Latin America, there are only small numbers of any one type of mental health professional [24]. For example, African conflict-affected countries such as Angola, Eritrea, Rwanda, Burundi and Mozambique have one psychiatrist each and a few psychologists. Even if a country does have mental health professionals, violence may cause an exodus of intellectuals (cf. Algeria, Iraq and Afghanistan) or they may have been killed in the genocide (cf. Cambodia, Rwanda).

Second, knowledge from high-income settings has limited applicability in LAMIC settings due to differences in sociocultural context. For example, many survivors of emergencies in non-Western societies are not aware of mental disorders and services. They may show variations in the expression of psychopathology, including PTSD [31–33]. They often experience suffering in spiritual, religious, family or community terms. They may experience intense stress if they are unable to engage in normal religious, spiritual or cultural practices, as is often the case in post-disaster situations.

Third, local health professionals and teachers may lack understanding of mental health problems or explain them solely in magic-religious terms. In general, health professionals have not been trained in models that are appropriate to dealing with mass traumatic stress. Their working models are often determined by social or colonial history and need thorough transformation to be effective in post-war circumstances (e.g. the former Yugoslavia, the Caucasian republics, Cambodia and Vietnam were heavily influenced by the Soviet approach, with its emphasis on medical and psychiatric authority and hospital-based care). Moreover, psychologists may have little training and experience in psychotherapy, let alone trauma-focused therapy, when leaving academia (cf. China and Algeria).

Fourth, refugees, internally displaced persons (IDPs) and survivors of disasters may belong to different ethnic groups and reside in peripheral or rural areas, which are not the preferred sites for urban intellectuals to work.

Fifth, the state mental health care sector is often weak, offering little opportunity for professional employment. In order to survive, the few existing professionals may have to work a substantial amount of their time in private practice in cities, at the expense of the public sector and the rural areas.

Sixth, many middle-class urban professionals have difficulties relating to refugee populations or disaster victims who express their plight in a specific discourse, show different illness behaviour and use different explanatory models.

For all these reasons, the aforementioned treatment gap is much larger in LAMIC countries.

Summary

To summarise, despite remarkable achievements in psychotherapy and psychopharmacology, we need to give more attention to contextual variables in dealing with the burden of mental health. Low-income countries are disproportionally affected by disasters and conflicts, with increased internal and external migration flows, poverty and a large burden of mental health problems. Even though trained human resources are limited in LAMIC settings, there is a reservoir of talented people who have missed the opportunity to receive training and who have the capacity to use the universal nonspecific therapist variables that appear to be so important even among highly trained academic professionals. Finally, in the aftermath of emergencies there is a large treatment gap and a need to develop contextually relevant and culturally appropriate preventive and curative interventions: the main theme of this chapter.

SCOPE OF THE CHAPTER

This chapter is based on a number of principles and limitations, as summarised in Table 6.1.

1. The public mental health model presented focuses on LAMICs, although most interventions also apply to medium- and large-scale emergencies in high-income countries. Although the nature of violence or disaster may be different around the globe, the impact of violence or disaster can be similar in war areas in Asia or Africa, in townships in South Africa, in *favelas* in Brazil, in inner cities in the USA, in earthquake areas in China or Haiti, after flooding in New Orleans, Bangladesh or Pakistan, and after bombing in Bagdad, Kabul, Kampala or London.[2]
2. The chapter describes a generic and adaptable disaster public mental health (DPMH) model. The model can be used for both adults and children and is resilience-, ecology- and family-oriented (cf. [36, 37]). The DPMH model

[2] Sexual assault and combat are more likely to lead to PTSD than accidents or disasters [34, 35].

uses a spectrum approach towards mental health and psychosocial issues. It emphasises the complementarity between both domains and stipulates that both mental health and psychosocial issues should be incorporated into any disaster plan.

3. The model uses a transdisciplinary approach combining the fields of public health, psychology, psychiatry, anthropology and epidemiology. Risk and protective factors are addressed by combining primary, secondary and tertiary interventions with their implementation on the levels of the society-at-large, the community, the family and the individual. The interventions are multi- or intersectoral, multiagency, multimodal, multilevel, ecological and systems-oriented, involving the sectors of public health, mental health and psychosocial care, education, human rights and rural development.
4. The model uses a time perspective and provides minimum responses that ought to be implemented in the emergency preparation phase, the emergency phase[3] and subsequently in the more comprehensive efforts during the stabilisation and reconstruction phases. The model acknowledges that the distinction in phases may be important for agencies, scholars and professionals, but is generally irrelevant to the subjective experience of people coming to terms with a disaster.
5. The model shows the complementarity of and strengthens collaboration between humanitarian actors and mental health professionals, ranging from community-based organisations to nongovernmental organisations (NGOs), government authorities, United Nations (UN) organisations and donors operating in emergency settings at local, national and international levels.
6. Emergencies and major incidents erode protective supports and tend to amplify preexisting problems of social injustice, poverty and inequality, demographic pressures, ethnic tensions, discrimination, marginalisation and political oppression [38, 39]. During and after an emergency, social support is a prophylactic to protect and promote well-being. Social approaches are fundamental, consistent with findings that the presence of PTSD is associated with perceived lack of social support [40, 41]. Social approaches are also fundamental for the five intervention principles proposed by Hobfoll *et al.* [42]: promotion of sense of safety, sense of self- and community-efficacy, connectedness, calming, and hope. Whereas the indigenous reconstruction of a protective shield of social support should be promoted, there is also a clear need for selective psychological and psychiatric interventions.
7. This DPMH model consists of a series of generic and universal phases and steps that can be applied in an eclectic and integrative way. It does not require that actors or agencies implement every intervention, though it does require adaptation of the generic principles to the specific context. Professionals may

[3] Sometimes subdivided into: initial response, first week; early response, first month; response between one and three months.

decide to start with a few core interventions covering a substantial population (e.g. 50,000–500,000 people) and gradually add more, or proceed the other way around: develop a comprehensive package in a small area for a few thousand people, and after monitoring the outcome disseminate the package towards a larger target population. Similarly, they may start with a grass-roots community-based psychosocial programme and gradually collaborate with mental health services; or, conversely, an academic centre of excellence may decide to work top-down towards mental health in primary care and extend its services to a community psychosocial approach. This chapter describes the generic steps that can often be applied universally around the globe. Specific and culturally relevant issues related to natural disasters, political violence, combat, interpersonal and family violence, culture and socioeconomic status will only be mentioned when necessary.

8. This chapter focuses on what mental health professionals can do in DPMH. Based on decades of experience around the globe, in my opinion the most difficult tasks for practitioners are (i) to learn to think in public (mental) health terms instead of focusing on the dyadic practitioner–patient interaction; (ii) to adapt academic knowledge to different and often complex health systems, to emergency settings and to culturally diverse groups; (iii) to question the cultural premises of their own native culture; and (iv) to reflect on and transform the culture of psychiatry, psychology, nursing and social work in which they are socialised.
9. DPMH is not totally different from our day-to-day care and therefore does not need to be perceived as a threat (which obviously would be a disaster per se, especially in emergencies with a scarcity of professionals). There is a continuum of care of social, physical and psychological support that stretches from normal circumstances to emergencies and catastrophes. Therefore, the model described in this chapter can be applied equally in times of conflict, disaster and peace.[4]
10. The model is compatible with other models such as the community-based rehabilitation approach (CBR),[5] the protective or child rights approach[6] and the conservation of resources (COR) model [45].

---

[4] And hence perhaps the word 'disaster' could be deleted from the model or from the title of the chapter.

[5] CBR is an intersectoral, comprehensive rehabilitation and social mobilisation program which falls mostly outside the health sector. It has been described in terms of a framework of goals (human rights, socioeconomic development and poverty alleviation), principles (participation, inclusion, sustainability and self-advocacy) and areas of activity (health, education, livelihoods, empowerment and social integration).

[6] Protective approaches concentrate on the legal and professional response to cases of maltreatment. Children's rights as laid out in the United Nations Convention on the Rights of the Child (UNCRC) provide a framework for understanding child maltreatment [43, 44] as part of a range of violence, harm and exploitation at the individual, institutional and societal levels. The greatest strength of an approach based on the UNCRC is that it provides a legal instrument for implementing policy, accountability and social justice, all of which enhance public health responses.

Table 6.1 Basic principles of the public mental health model arranged according to a set of continua.

From	To	Remark
Low-income	High-income country	The nature of disaster may be different, the impact similar.
Children	Adults	Resilience-, ecology- and family-oriented.
Psychosocial	Mental health	Both should be incorporated in any disaster plan.
Mono-	Multidisciplinary	Public health, psychology, psychiatry, anthropology and epidemiology.
Mono-	Multisectoral/ agency/modal/ level	Sectors of public health, mental and psychosocial care, education, human rights and rural development. Use a matrix combining prevention with societal levels.
Primary	Tertiary prevention	Address both risk and vulnerability factors.
Emergency	Reconstruction phase	Phases are less important for survivors.
Community organisations	United Nations	Emphasises complementarity and collaboration.
Social support	Neurobiology	Address predictors of political violence: social injustice, poverty, demography, ethnic tensions, discrimination, marginalisation and oppression
Eclectic, integrative and small population	Generic, universal and large target population	Few core interventions in a substantial population, or a comprehensive package in a small area. Bottom-up or top-down. No fundamental difference between natural disaster and political violence.
Common mental health expertise	Disaster-specific expertise	Required additional expertise: Public Mental Health (PMH), complex systems, diversity and reflection on (professional) culture. Care continuum (social, physical and psychological) from normal circumstances to catastrophes.
Public mental health	Other models	e.g. community-based rehabilitation (CBR), child rights, conservation of resources (COR).

CORE CONCEPTS AND DEFINITIONS

A health system *consists of all organisations, people and actions whose primary intent is to promote, restore or maintain health*. Its six building blocks are quality service delivery, health workforce, health information system, access to essential products and technologies, a financing system, and leadership and governance [46].

Complex interventions contain interacting components, and have other characteristics that one should take into account (such as number and difficulty of behaviours, number of organisational levels, variability of outcomes and the tailoring of interventions [47].

Public mental health is defined as the discipline, the practice and the systematic social actions that protect, promote and restore mental health of a population [30, p. 24]. Since public mental health is part of public health, most public mental health concepts are derived from or overlap with public health views and policies.

'Psychosocial' is defined as the close relation between psychological factors (emotion, behaviour and cognition) and the sociocultural context. The terms mental health and psychosocial support overlap. Aid agencies tend to speak of psychosocial well-being. Health agencies tend to speak of mental health, yet historically have used the terms 'psychosocial rehabilitation' and 'psychosocial treatment' to describe nonbiological interventions for people with mental disorders. In this chapter, the concept of *mental health and psychosocial support (MHPSS)* will be used to describe *any type of local or outside support that aims to protect or promote psychosocial well-being and/or prevent or treat mental disorder* [48].

Although mental health and psychosocial problems in emergencies are interconnected, problems of a predominantly *social* nature may be induced by: (i) the emergency itself (e.g. family separation, disruption of social networks, destruction of community structures, hope, trust and resources, increased gender-based and family violence); (ii) humanitarian aid (e.g. by reinforcing dependency behaviour in refugee or IDP camps, by undermining resilient coping styles, or by undermining community structures or traditional support mechanisms); or (iii) political parties (e.g. by countries that do not follow international rules regarding asylum, deny refugees the right to employ their capacities, or use combat veterans for political purposes).

Similarly, problems of a predominantly *psychological* nature are often aggravated by: (i) the emergency itself (e.g. severe mental disorder, alcohol/substance abuse, grief, nonpathological distress, depression and anxiety disorders including PTSD); (ii) humanitarian aid (e.g. anxiety due to splitting up of families, overcrowded reception centres or refugee camps, or a lack of information about food distribution); or (iii) political parties (e.g. anxiety caused by a protracted reaction of the international community to an imminent genocide, by exaggerating rumours about impending danger, or by denying veterans access to appropriate or anonymous care).

'Traumascape' refers to the systemic dynamics of local and international representations and actions around extreme stress [49, p. 247].

In our current world, the conceptualisation of distress and traumatic stress and the social and power relations related to the cultural construction of these concepts are in constant flux and prone to cybernetic looping. For example, a cascade of events – determined by the media, the role of the UN, NGOs, governments, local stakeholders and funders, humanitarian agencies, identification with a disaster, and discrimination – will often determine the focus, the size and the nature of assistance for a group of survivors of a natural or human-made disaster. In addition, media hype, pop musicians and movie stars, possibly in combination with geopolitical and voter-dependent considerations, may determine whether human rights, child rights, quality of governance, terrorism, gender-based violence, domestic violence, child soldiers or combat veterans are the main concern of the international community, and, subsequently, whether funds will go to a specific region or a specific type of disaster, often to the detriment of other catastrophes (e.g. the invasion in several areas of Asia by psychosocial programmes after the 2004 tsunami deflected funds from areas such as Darfur and other parts of Sudan, and raised the status of even daily hassles to a 'trauma'). Professionals have to bear in mind that epidemiological considerations are often dominated by the (inter)national dynamics of the traumascape. Mental health professionals have to accept that at times they are sweepers of the debris caused by faulty political and economic institutions. The rest of the chapter looks at the different phases of development of a DPMH programme.

PHASE 1. ASSESSMENT: PRE-PROGRAMME AND CYCLICAL

In doing a pre-programme assessment, it is important to maximise the participation of males, females and youth in the design, implementation, monitoring and evaluation of emergency, rehabilitative and reconstruction services. From the beginning onwards, it is important to conceptualise the programme in a sustainable way (see below).

Depending on the (post-)disaster stage of involvement, one has to decide how rapidly an assessment should be carried out. For an emergency programme, the assessment must be sufficiently rapid and short to be used effectively in the early planning of interventions. When an MHPSS team gets involved in a later stage, the assessment can be more rigorous and may even include an epidemiological survey. Assessments should be repetitive and should preferably be related to the management cycle of the programme. It is wise to repeat the assessment after one and two years to adapt the programme to changing community needs, to the dynamics of the recovery after disaster, and to policy resistance and the dynamic complexity of the system.[7] In general, it is advisable to have an assessment process consisting of two phases:

1. *Initial ('rapid') assessment of 10 – 14 days*, focusing mostly on understanding the basics of the care system, the stake holders, the experiences and the current situation of the affected population, together with community and organisational capacities, in line with phase 2:
2. *Detailed assessments of one to two months*, addressing the following issues from the macro to the micro level:
   2.1 What are the *core characteristics of the emergency situation* according to politicians and policy-makers, the UN, the NGOs and community-based organisations, the representatives of the district and the local community, as well as the heads of the family? It is important to get insight into:
      i. agency and interagency national policies and plans for MHPSS emergency response, as well as the plans of stakeholders and focal points in the health, social and educational systems with which collaboration and coordination is needed. Insight into the health system and other sectors is fundamental to developing interventions that can be anchored in the public sector to make them sustainable;
      ii. people's experiences of the emergency, how individuals, communities and organisations respond to the emergency and how this affects their mental health and psychosocial well-being;
      iii. threats to and capacities for mental health and psychosocial well-being, as well as an inventory of risk, protective and resilience factors.
   2.2 What are the *resources*, as well as the *needs*? It is important to:
      i. map existing human resource capacity and training resources in the government and NGO sectors of, for example, health, social welfare, women's and youth organisations, human rights and rural development;
      ii. identify current community action and social support mechanisms as well as the mechanisms that existed in the local communities before the disaster;
      iii. get insight into individual coping skills, both positive and negative, as well as life skills;
      iv. try to understand topics or behaviours surrounded with stigma, taboos and shame in relation to differential sensitivity to gender (regarding e.g. sexual issues, rape and domestic violence);
      v. involve community leaders and traditional healers in identifying communal and individual cultural, religious and spiritual supports and coping mechanisms as well as rituals and ceremonies;

[7] Policy resistance is the tendency for interventions to be defeated by the systems response to them; dynamic complexity is the often counterintuitive behaviour of complex systems that arises from the interactions of agents over time [47].

vi. ask these stakeholders about local interpretations of the (spiritual) causes and effects of the emergency, about proper mourning, reconciliation or cleansing rituals, the appropriate timing of the rituals, guidance on involving the ritual and healing complex, and on the prevention of spiritual harm caused by, for example, suicide, homicide or filth [39, 49]. For example, former child soldiers among the Acholi in northern Uganda were often haunted by spirits called Cen [50], southern Sudanese people by Jok Jok, Mozambicans by Gamba spirits (Igreja [51]), and Bissau Guineans by Kiyang-yang spirits [52, 53]. Adolescents in a Bhutanese refugee camp in Nepal were possessed and experienced 'spirit' attacks in the form of fainting and dizziness, due to the belief that the spirits of two lovers who had committed suicide were still on earth and were disturbed by the camp's filth, violation of cultural sanitary beliefs and thoughts of premarital sex [54].

2.3 *Communities*. Since communities are the main vehicles for a contextual approach it is important to strengthen a feeling of ownership and control over the emergency response, and to conduct participatory mapping and context analysis of the local communities and neighbourhoods (current situation, resources, services and practices). A risk analysis should be conducted, a community response plan, including an early warning system, should be considered, and the local capacity to implement such a plan should be strengthened.
Protection issues should be investigated, such as the cause of the violence, past and present perpetrators and family separation: the fate of separated or unaccompanied children, the elderly and disabled, and those living in institutions and hospitals. Current safety and security concerns should also be addressed (e.g. attacks by rebels and bandits on refugee camps, or the risk of sexual violence to women when getting water).
An attempt should be made to find out how groups in the community handle(d) protection threats in the past and present, and how previously active protection systems and coping mechanisms have been affected. It is important to establish whether presumed protective resources – such as police, soldiers, peacekeepers or schools – are in reality protection threats. Community-owned social support activities and community plans on protecting and supporting early childhood development should be set up. Reconciliation can be facilitated by providing space for victims and survivors to discuss issues of reparation and compensation.

2.4 *Monitoring, evaluation and the management cycle*. Monitoring and evaluation are related to repetitive cyclical assessments and to the management cycle. The management cycle moves from problem definition to problem clarification, policy development, decision taking, implementation and evaluation of the policy [55]. It enables the DPMH programme to adapt itself to changing conditions. The first step is problem definition (e.g. a lack of insight into the mental health status of the population, accessibility or affordability of services, or the absence of adequate mental health indicators). The second step aims at problem clarification (e.g. lack of information or awareness among the population). The third step, policy development, aims to define clear goals and objectives. During the decision phase, the DPMH programme makes decisions that will be implemented in the implementation phase. The final phase is the evaluation phase, which coincides with the aforementioned repetitive assessment after one, two or four years.

One of the crucial decisions of the management cycle is the determination of which quality aspects are to be evaluated at what level, and which indicators and criteria to use. Process, satisfaction and outcome indicators should be formulated that are consistent with predefined objectives.[8] They should span both the minimum response during the emergency phase and the long-term reconstruction phase. Indicators need to be measured before and after the intervention to see if there has been any change. A more rigorous design is required to determine whether the intervention caused the change. Moreover, the indicators should be SMART (Specific, Measurable, Achievable, Relevant and Timebound), be chosen on the principle of 'few but powerful', and be disaggregated by age, gender and location whenever possible (for a list of indicators, see [48]).

2.5 *Data collection techniques (phase 1).* The main techniques for collecting data during the assessment phase are operational, action-oriented and participatory; for example: (i) an inventory of government, UN and NGO documents and the (grey) literature; or (ii) qualitative techniques such as focus groups, key informant (KI) interviews with groups of individuals, community meetings, participant observation, in-depth interviews and thick descriptions at all the abovementioned system levels (for the techniques of focus groups, KI and in-depth interviews and rapid appraisals, see [30, 56, 57, p. 48–51; 58–60]).

[8] Process indicators describe activities and cover the quality, quantity coverage and utilisation of services and programmes (e.g. number of self-help meetings). Satisfaction indicators describe the satisfaction of the affected population with the activity (satisfaction indicators may be seen as a subtype of process indicators). Outcome indicators describe changes in the lives of the population according to predefined objectives. These indicators aim to describe the extent to which the intervention was a success or a failure. Although certain outcome indicators are likely to be meaningful in most contexts (e.g. level of daily functioning), deciding what is to be meant by 'success' in an MHPS programme should form part of the participatory discussions with the affected population. Although process and satisfaction indicators are useful tools for the management cycle, outcome indicators provide the strongest data for informed action.

PHASE 2. SELECTION CRITERIA DEFINING PRIORITIES FOR MENTAL HEALTH AND PSYCHOSOCIAL INTERVENTIONS

In order to achieve adequate coverage of the population with limited human and financial resources one has to carefully select interventions. This section lists 10 different selection criteria, explaining the rationale for each and suggesting methods to apply them in the field. The criteria are listed in rank order of importance, although policy considerations and professional background may influence the weight one attributes them. It is no surprise that these selection criteria also apply to the training of the staff that will implement the interventions.

The first criterion: community concern

Community concern is the perceived need of people, communities, families and individuals to cope with their lives. It is related to daily hassles, social structures, mental health beliefs, stigma and the meaning given to the events. For example, it may make quite a difference whether a culture attributes the plight of a community to the deeds of their ancestors in a previous life (e.g. Cambodians attributing the plight of the Khmer Rouge to bad karma) or to a heroic struggle for autonomy (as happens among Israelis and Palestinians, for example). Measurement of community concern belongs to the field of qualitative, operational and action research. In carrying out such measurement, one must try to understand social phenomena from the perspective of those being studied (i.e. an emic perspective).

Changes in population 'norms' due to the disaster

Community concern can be hard to assess in (post-)conflict or disaster circumstances. Victims may have been so seriously deprived of basic human needs such as shelter, water or food for a considerable amount of time that these issues form the gestalt of any interview. Or they may be so conditioned to ask for material help from agencies – the 'dependency syndrome' – that the idea of bringing forward any other issue does not occur to them. They may also be so accustomed to the effects of traumatic stress that a distortion has taken place in the population norm – an important yardstick in cross-cultural work for assessing normality, deviancy and pathology. For example, during focus group discussions in a war-ridden area in East Africa, the mothers stated they believed that their children were not affected by the war, while many of the children had night terrors or were wetting their bed up to the age of 12 in an area where being potty trained at the age of one year was not exceptional. Other examples: in some parts of countries such as Congo or South Africa, sexual violence has almost become as 'normal' as the massive conversion to Pentecostal or spiritistic churches, whereas in some other areas dissociative behaviour such as non-epilectic psychogenic seizures, trance and possession have increased.

The second criterion: prevalence and the role of epidemiology

The second criterion is the *prevalence* of the problem. Commentary of Chapter 1 explained how epidemiology helps to assess needs, to distinguish individuals who develop a disturbance versus those who are resilient, to explain the relative contribution of exposure, protective and vulnerability factors, and to plan services. Ideally, an epidemiological survey includes studying help-seeking behaviour that provides information about the distribution of distress and psychopathology in different health care sectors. When designing a study in an emergency setting, it is advisable to pursue 'directness' – how long it takes before knowledge results in concrete interventions; to pursue 'intersectorality' – the extent to which answering the research question will encourage collaboration of community and intersectoral domains in the implementation of interventions; and to study 'transferability' – the capacity of a research question to add to the transfer of research knowledge to a local context. In my opinion, there is no need for additional cross-sectional research on prevalence with instruments such as the General Health Questionnaire, the Self Reporting Questionnaire or the Hopkins Symptom Checklist (HSCL-25) without a multistep translation and validation process including appropriate cut-points in the local culture (for culture-informed epidemiology cf. [57]). In contrast, there is a large need to show the cost-effectiveness of both preventive and curative interventions.

In short, to develop preventive and curative interventions, we need information on the incidence, the prevalence and the distribution of distress, disorders, disability and quality of life. Studying help-seeking behaviour provides information on the indigenous, the allopathic and the lay services where people try to get support.

The two most important selection criteria – community concern and epidemiology – are complementary in several aspects, as shown in Table 6.2.

Another way of illustrating the complementarity between community concern and prevalence is to compare the figures from an epidemiological survey with the nature of the problems presented by people to mental health and psychosocial programmes. For example, our team found an average lifetime prevalence rate in Algeria, Ethiopia, Palestine and Cambodia of 27% for PTSD, 25% for anxiety disorder and 12% for depressive disorder ([31], cf. Commentry of Chapter 1). However, when we looked at the rank order of the problems people would bring to some of our major public mental health programmes, they mentioned the following community concerns: (i) health (sleep, headache, body pain, epilepsy and neck/back/epigastric pain); (ii) mood (sadness, anxiety, aggression and nervousness); (iii) family (domestic violence, child problems and disharmony);

Table 6.2 Complementarity of the first and second criteria: community concern and prevalence.

Community concern	Prevalence
Qualitative research: participative/social science	Quantitative research: epidemiology
Assesses perceived concerns, idioms of distress, folk illnesses and culture-related syndromes	Assesses disorder and its distribution: for example, depression, anxiety, alcohol, schizophrenia, PTSD and epilepsy PTSD
Related to suffering and psychological pain	Assesses morbidity, mortality, disability and quality of life
Related to well-being and community involvement	Related to health
Technique: multimethod (focus groups, KI interviews, in-depth interviews, etc.)	Technique: culture-informed psychiatric epidemiology
Ongoing and cyclical (once/one to two years)	Cross-sectional, rarely longitudinal
Assessment plus reporting takes two to eight weeks	Survey plus reporting takes one to three years
Emic	Etic/emic

(iv) mental illness (psychosis and falling); (v) abuse (alcohol and drugs); (vi) social (lack of food, conflicts at work, poverty and unemployment); (vii) cognitive (concentration and memory problems); (viii) trauma; and (ix) stress (stress, suicide and spirits). In other words, the epidemiological survey yielded 27% PTSD as the most important problem, but when we looked at what the local populations brought forward to our programmes, cognitive problems, trauma and stress came out as the least important priorities.

The third criterion: seriousness

In emergencies, acute distress and minor psychological disorders affect almost the whole population. After a certain amount of time, a majority of the people generally cope with their problem without professional support. When developing a programme, one has to carefully weigh the management of psychosocial problems with the seriousness of major neuropsychiatric disorders that are brought forward by the population. Most programmes struggle with a discrepancy between a need for services and the availability of funding. A balance must therefore be found between the seriousness of disorders with high levels of disability among a minority of the population and the large amount of distress among the majority, which often dissipates in time. Treatment of serious disorders and problems such as schizophrenia, bipolar disorder, epilepsy and suicidality is a priority in areas without accessible and affordable mental health services. A complicating factor is that after a disaster an increase in the incidence of major psychiatric disorders may occur, partly caused by the absence of services during the disaster or war period [61]. In addition, other disturbances such as anxiety disorder, depressive disorder and substance abuse will be found.

Several guidelines provide a balanced choice on the optimal moment for intervention when extreme stress prevails [7, 48].

A further source of confusion in considering seriousness or perceived need is that subgroups in a population may show a differential response when mental health services are offered. For example, refugees who return to their home countries may have received mental health services in the refugee camps abroad, while the population that stayed behind had no treatment possibilities [62]. Such a difference, which can also occur with regard to other services such as water supply or food distribution, can fuel animosities between groups.

The fourth criterion: treatability or feasibility of treatment

The criterion of treatability or susceptibility to treatment is important. One needs to know if there are sufficient resources in terms of personnel, expertise, time and funds to manage or treat specific problems. Prior to initiating interventions, the likelihood of effective assistance and availability of resources must be evaluated during the preparatory assessment phase described above.

Thinking about treatability may include considerations of when and how to collaborate with the sector of complementary and alternative medicine (CAM). In developing countries, people may go to healers due to the scarcity of professionals, while in other countries a substantial part of the population may regularly attend the CAM sector for a variety of reasons; in the USA this amounts to 42% of its inhabitants. CAM does not exclude using Western medicine, although one should be careful about pharmacological interactions. People who use CAM may use more Western medicine than those who do not use CAM (cf. [63, 64]).

An example is collaboration in the field of epilepsy and psychogenic seizures or dissociative phenomena. In some areas of Africa, the prevalence of epilepsy is as high as 3.7–4.9%, it is highly stigmatised, and it often presents to psychiatric and primary health care services [65, 66]. All over Africa people tend to go to healers who have no effective treatments for epilepsy. The motivation to visit healers is likely related to a decrease in seizure frequency because the healer reduces the stress component related to the neurobiological disorder or to psychosocial stress. In addition, especially in situations of massive stress, a substantial number of people show symptoms of dissociation varying from individual possession as an 'idiom of distress' to classical fugue states and epidemics of mass psychogenic illness with or without non-epileptic psychogenic seizures (what we used to call 'hysteria'). These psychogenic fits may mimic generalised seizures without the classical symptoms of symmetric contractions, tongue bite, incontinence or serious accidents such as falling in a cooking fire, a well or a wet rice field [52, 54].[9]

While setting up services, one has to consider which health care sector is best equipped to deal with what type of seizure, whether neurological or dissociative in origin. Offering treatment to those with generalised epileptic seizures is a highly feasible option. With a few hours of training and a single low dosage of phenobarbital, primary health care workers can reach a diagnostic sensitivity of 80–90% and the average seizure frequency may decrease from 10 or above to about 0.3 per month [66, 67]. Dealing with the equally highly prevalent dissociative states requires sophisticated psychotherapeutic skills, which are often not available in LAMICs or are too time-consuming to employ in high-income countries.[10] It is tempting to propose triage of the epileptic patients and refer those with dissociative states to the local healers, healing churches or possession cults. The latter are often very effective in dealing with dissociative states and psychogenic seizures, for which a few sessions may suffice. In reality, this proposal is premature because we still have limited insight into the similarities and differences between expressions of behaviour that phenomenologically are similar (e.g. dissociative identity disorder (DID), complex PTSD, trauma-related borderline personality disorder, dissociative disorder not otherwise specified (DDNOS)-type 1, possession trance (disorder)) but may hide different forms of psychopathology [69]. This is but one example of the complexity of treatability and of the potential collaboration between different health care sectors.

The fifth criterion: sustainability

Sustainability is the potential to develop good-quality interventions and integrate them in local communities and services. Sustainability has to be a priority from the very beginning of a programme. It depends on quality, volume and time. If the *quality* or effectiveness is not sufficient, the interventions will dissipate and hence not be sustainable. *Volume* is related to building sufficient human resource and institutional capacity to cover a population and to reach new cohorts in the same area or in other countries. *Time* determines whether the endeavour can be maintained and developed over longer periods, and includes an adequate exit strategy.

[9] In LAMICs, one often still sees 'classical' dissociative phenomena (as described by Janet, Charcot and Freud during their time in the Salpêtrière in Paris).

[10] Brand *et al*. [68] mention that the prevalence of dissociative disorders in the West ranges from 12 to 38% among outpatients. Although after 8.4 years of treatment most patients had significantly improved, these so-called stage-five patients remained at clinically significant levels.

Factors promoting sustainability are:

1. rational project design,
2. local ownership and partnership,
3. adequate management and cost-effectiveness,
4. a small dependency gap in terms of external funding,
5. cultural sensitivity and acculturation of services,
6. adequate monitoring despite the possible volatility of the situation,
7. attention to gender issues, age groups and local health care concerns,
8. integration in local services and collaboration with local institutions such as universities, the government and other sectors,
9. continued provision of psychotropic medicines, and
10. long-term commitment.

Obstacles to sustainability are:

1. externally driven or externally implemented programmes (e.g. donor 'drivenness' and donor hype, as described in the Core Concepts and Definitions, above),
2. dependence on nonprofit funding, instead of mixed nonprofit/commercial funding,
3. a long-term monodisciplinary or monointervention approach,
4. interventions that do not suit the local needs,
5. lack of flexibility or adaptability when violence flares up or the disaster situation gets worse,
6. too-short funding periods in relation to agreed-upon objectives and target populations (cf. [30, pp. 54–58]).

In my experience, setting up a sustainable DPMH programme requires 5–10 years.

The sixth criterion: knowledge, skills and availability of (mental) health care professionals

Before setting up a programme, the number and types of humanitarian workers, mental health care professionals, general health workers and other possible trainees from sectors such as education or social services should be assessed, for example with the help of a semi-structured interview. The assessment should answer questions regarding: (i) their strengths and weaknesses and their ability to tolerate high-stress situations; (ii) their ability to recognise and handle different types of psychosocial and mental health problem; (iii) their normal duties and responsibilities; (iv) the kinds of problem they come across in their work; (v) the kind of training and supervision they need; (vi) the extent to which trainees themselves have been affected by the war or disaster; (vii) their formal qualifications; and (viii) a possible history of child abuse, or their voluntary involvement as a perpetrator.

The training should address their own traumatic experiences in order to allow them to support other people. After the training, a second assessment should be carried out to find out whether the trainees are able to deal with the experiences of others. Treating mental health problems in primary care need not increase the work burden of the primary care worker, as a study in Europe showed [70].

Group and individual debriefing, supervision and job rotation are all useful measures to prevent burn-out expressing itself in emotional exhaustion, a tendency to develop cynical and negative attitudes towards others or negative self-evaluation, especially regarding work (cf. [48, 71]).

The seventh criterion: political acceptability

It is relevant to seek to understand the sometimes hidden agenda of policy makers. For example, in epidemiological research it is common to assess exposure to stressors and life events before, during and after the disaster. The results play a central role in designing locally appropriate interventions. However, the results can also be used for other purposes, such as human rights work or advocacy against repressive governments or rebel groups, either at home or in a guest country. This may help democracy, respect for human rights and good governance. On the other hand, such research may raise the suspicion of local authorities, which may then try to hinder the DPMH programme. Governments are often reluctant towards mental health activities for a variety of reasons. Health ministries may not have a specific department, focal point or legislation for mental health, making it hard for mental health to compete with other health sectors, for example when it comes to sectoral funding. In addition, health ministries may not know the public health impact of mental health problems or the availability of interventions and therefore not regard mental health as a priority.

The eighth criterion: ethical acceptability

A DPMH programme must consider the possible harm that might be inflicted on others by research that lacks cultural sensitivity or that does not result in provision or improvement of services. All too often scholars are eager to collect data for publication without questioning whether the work will help in formulating preventive or curative interventions.

Interviews, both during the assessment of a programme and as part of an epidemiological survey, are an intervention in themselves. Survivors tend to create a ‘conspiracy of silence’ because they do not want to embarrass others with their traumatic past, because everyone is preoccupied with surviving, or because their culture may not facilitate disclosure of traumatic events. On the other hand, interviewees often perceive an interview as a unique event enabling them to share their problems and feel recognised in their suffering. It also gives them the possibility of giving testimony. The urge to be heard may create a dilemma for the interviewer. Knowledge that neutral cues and a moderate amount of empathy create less distress for the interviewee may run counter to the need of the latter to disclose the past. Methodologically, this dilemma poses a similar problem. An interview format often imposes time limitations, and allowing time for specific events may create memory bias. Handling these ethical and methodological dilemmas requires careful navigation and preparation on the part of the interviewers.

Another possible ethical problem is that informed consent with signatures on an elaborate consent form is expected in the West, but as Bromet [72] argued after the Chernobyl accident, such forms may be perceived with distrust and suspicion in other parts of the world. The procedure may evoke fear, as our team found in countries such as Cambodia, Ethiopia or Sudan. One way of solving this problem is to acquire verbal informed consent, preferably in the presence of a family member or friend (cf. [73]).

A final consideration relates to the abovementioned sustainability of the project, which might only be achieved after a decade. It may take years before a local training of trainers group has been trained, acquired field experience, received booster training, and subsequently trained and supervised sufficient secondary- and tertiary-level staff to ensure continuity of the work. Without long-term commitment, it is not ethical to start a programme.

The ninth criterion: cultural sensitivity

Culture defines reality for its members and serves two roles. It is integrative, that is it represents the beliefs and values that provide individuals with a sense of identity, and it is functional, that is it furnishes the rules for behaviour that enable the group to survive and provide for its welfare, while supporting an individual's sense of self-worth and belonging. These two functions are analogous to the warp and woof of a tapestry [74].

Culture has a collective and an individual dimension. The collective dimension of culture represents schemes that determine views of the ego and the self, with autonomy and individualisation as core values in the West, whereas interdependency, collectivism and dividuality are more common in LAMICs. The collective dimension influences the social origins of conflict and violence, and guides the meaning of suffering, healing and reconciliation, and stigma.

The individual dimension of culture represents influences on traumatic stressors and their appraisal, their modification by protective and vulnerability factors, and their expression in suffering, distress, psychopathology and post-traumatic growth, and its concomitants of disability, functioning, quality of life, well-being and resilience. Culture and history are intertwined. Both collective and individual history can challenge a culture to the extent that it has to adapt its collective and individual survival strategies and coping styles [49].

Each aspect of a DPMH programme has to be tested for its cultural assumptions in order to develop culturally appropriate interventions that reduce impact and help rebuild the care system, contributing to an equitable society. Local mental health care professionals – especially if they were trained abroad – should adapt their academic insights to their countrymen if they have different cultural backgrounds. In my opinion, academic mental health care professionals without proper training in cultural psychiatry and public mental health, and without expertise in working with immigrants or refugees, have to be cautious in offering their culture-bound expertise elsewhere.

An example of the influence of culture can be seen in suicide, a taboo in many places. Within a range of African cultures, when a person commits suicide their soul may not be able to join the ancestors and reincarnate in future generations. The soul may turn into a revengeful and capricious spirit attacking the living, and causing misfortune, illness (such as madness) or death. Apart from having a preventive effect, this taboo may lead to underreporting of suicidal ideation and suicide attempts in clinical work and research.

The same may happen with the soul of a person who is killed by homicide or as the consequence of political or criminal violence. The anxiety-provoking whims of the wandering spirit may decrease if a proper burial ritual has taken place. But in an armed conflict, it is often impossible to find the body, or part of it, which is required both in African local 'animist' cultures and in Islam to conduct a proper burial ceremony. Sometimes people find a solution for this problem: for example, in Mozambique the healers' associations decided that when due to the war corpses were not available for ceremonies, a piece of cloth or another material possession of the dead would be acceptable for a proper burial and permit the soul of the deceased to take its place among the ancestors.

The tenth criterion: cost-effectiveness

There are several cost-effective treatments for mental disorders in LAMICs [75]. Cost-effectiveness is an important criterion for developing a programme because:

1. It would be unethical to carrying out non-cost-effective interventions in view of the scarcity of funding available for any public health priority in LAMICs. Without such considerations, governments and donors are likely to move their focus to other issues.
2. We need information on effectiveness because it is theoretically possible that the current programmes are doing harm. For example, by focusing on the vulnerability of individuals, programmes may undermine resilience, cause

unnecessary distress or helplessness, create sick roles and thus increase health care expenditure.

3. We need more information on the outcome of different treatment modalities employed in LAMICs. For example, how is the effect of the treatment related to therapist/mental health worker/psychosocial counsellor/nurse/local healer variables, or to such variables as preliminary training, duration of training and supervision of treatment? How is the effect related to the duration and the content of the specific interventions? Will the outcomes of the interventions improve in the course of time? Are they related to improved and advanced training and supervision? How can we provide the best cost-effective services? All these issues are related to the costs and the quality of the intervention.

PHASE 3. INTERVENTIONS: A MULTIMODAL, MULTISECTORAL AND MULTILEVEL MODEL

The remaining part of this chapter focuses on prevention and practice.

Table 6.3 shows a matrix of the relation between primary, secondary and tertiary prevention, with three intervention levels. The first or macrolevel is the society-at-large, including (inter)national agencies and government. The second or mesolevel is the community and the neighbourhood, and the third or microlevel is the family and the individual (cf. [39, 76]).

The matrix offers a generic framework addressing the complementary relationship between important players such as the various UN agencies, governments and (international) nongovernmental organisations ((I)NGOs). Realising the complementarity between key agents may help to reduce unnecessary competition that hinders coordination and collaboration.

The first of the three intervention levels is the macrolevel, or the society-at-large level, which includes (inter)national agencies and governments. Interventions at this level are meant for all countries and belong to the realm of the UN and its Security Council, the United Nations Office for the Coordination of Humanitarian Affairs (UNOCHA), governments, politicians, policy-makers and several (I)NGOs. Interventions on the second level, or the community level, are directed at the total population in a disaster or conflict zone, including refugees and IDPs. Such interventions are often provided by more specialised international agencies such as the United Nations Refugee Agency (UNHCR), the World Food Program, the Food & Agricultural Organization, the United Nations Development Program, the World Bank, local governments, (I)NGOs and advocacy groups. On the third level are families and individuals. Interventions at this level are mostly covered by specialised UN agencies such as the United Nations Children's Fund (UNICEF), the WHO, the UN Women, the United Nations Entity for Gender Equality and the Empowerment of Women, governments, local NGOs, community and faith-based organisations and academic and private organisations. Depending on political will

Table 6.3 The scaffolding of the DPMH model 'mansion'. Matrix showing the relation between universal, selective and indicated preventive interventions, and primary, secondary and tertiary prevention.[a]

	Society-at-large/(inter)national	Community	Family and individual
Primary prevention: eliminating a disease or disorder state before it can occur	*Economy, governance and early warning* *Free media and press* *Resolving underlying root causes of violence* *(Inter)national laws* *Defining and condemning human rights violations* *Research into events and their consequences* *Setting standards for intervention and training* *Expanding security institutions* *The military's role of last resort* *Reinforcing peace initiatives and conflict resolution* *Arms and landmine control* *Preventing the reemergence of violence* **Transnational collaborative projects** *Humanitarian operations* *War tribunals and the persecution of perpetrators* *Peace-keeping forces* *Indicated preventive interventions* *Human rights advocacy*	**Rural development and food production** **Community empowerment** **Decreasing dependency and learned helplessness** **Public health and education** **Peace education and conflict resolution in schools and the community** **Public (psycho)education, community sensitisation and awareness raising** **Security measures**	**Including women and children in the distribution of economic growth** **Family reunion/family tracing** **Family/network building** **Improvement of physical aspects** **Resilience groups for children**

Secondary prevention: shortening the course of an illness or problem	**Humanitarian relief operations: shelter, food, water and sanitation** **(Cooccurring) natural disasters: quality standards** **Voluntary repatriation** **Reparation and compensation**	**Conflict prevention and resolution** **Crisis intervention** **Vocational skills training**	**Preventing recruitment of child soldiers** **Reparation and compensation for afflicted families** **Public health and disease control** **Mental health and psychosocial support (MHPSS)** **Crisis intervention**
Tertiary prevention: reducing chronicity through the prevention of complications and through active rehabilitation	*Peace-keeping and peace-enforcing troops* *Peace agreements*	**Reconciliation and mediation skills between groups**[b]	**Involving the family in rehabilitation and reconstruction**

[a]Some of the cells are compressed by taking universal, selective and indicated interventions together, in order to facilitate reading. Moreover, some interventions apply both to primary, secondary and tertiary intervention, and on a national and community level, such as reinforcing peace initiatives. Interventions in italics are published elsewhere, interventions in bold are described in this chapter.
[b]cf. sub-primary prevention, mentioned in the text: ‘Peace education and conflict resolution in schools and the community’.

and socioeconomic resources, most of the interventions at the community, family and individual level can be realised within a decade, whereas interventions at the level of society-at-large will likely take substantially more time.

The goal of primary prevention is to eliminate a disease or disorder state before it can occur.[11] Universal, selective and indicated preventive interventions are included within primary prevention. Universal preventive interventions are targeted at the general public or a whole population group that has not been identified on the basis of individual risk. Selective preventive interventions are targeted at subgroups or individuals whose risk of developing a problem (e.g. a psychosocial problem or a mental disorder) is significantly higher than average. The risk may be imminent, or it may be a lifetime risk: a distinction that is important when we think of the accumulation of risk factors during humanitarian emergencies.[12] Indicated preventive interventions are targeted at high-risk individuals who are identified as having minimal but detectable signs or symptoms foreshadowing a problem or a disorder. In the classical literature, secondary prevention aimed to shorten the course of an illness. The US Committee [82] relabelled secondary prevention as 'treatment', subdivided into 'case identification' and 'standard treatment' of known disorders. Similarly, the original tertiary prevention, which aimed to reduce chronicity through the prevention of complications and through active rehabilitation, has been relabelled as 'maintenance', subdivided into 'compliance with long-term treatment' (with the goal of reduction of relapse and recurrence) and 'aftercare' (including rehabilitation).

Primary prevention in the society-at-large

Primary prevention of armed conflict and disasters is paramount and depends on changes in the economic, governance, diplomatic, military, human rights, criminal justice, health and rural development sectors. Interventions related to prevention in these societal sectors are described elsewhere and fall outside the scope of this chapter [38, 39]. They are listed in the second column in Table 6.3 and are printed in italics.

[11] And when it comes to political economy, the military and diplomacy, the goal of primary prevention is to eliminate a conflict or disaster before it can occur. Universal preventive interventions are targeted at the community of nations, the general public or a whole population group. Selective preventive interventions are targeted at nations or states whose risk of developing collective violence is higher than average based on the presence of risk factors. Indicated preventive interventions are targeted at high-risk countries or (sub)regions that show signs of collective violence foreshadowing a serious armed or ethnic conflict ([77]; cf. [38]).

[12] Think, for example, of the gene × environment interaction (e.g. the serotonin transporter gene [78, 79]). Birth itself can also be a risk factor, especially in war or disaster circumstances, where often poor prenatal and perinatal care are compounded by the collapse of the public health care sector. Famine, starvation, nutritional deficiency, environmental health hazards, cerebral malaria, parasites, diarrhoeal diseases and respiratory infections may further negatively influence cognitive and bodily development both in utero and later in life [80, 81]. Family disruption, parental illness and death, possibly aggravated by the AIDS pandemic, can affect attachment, bonding, separation and socialisation and contribute to anxiety, depression, PTSD, attachment disorders of childhood and antisocial, borderline or traumatic personality development (cf. [49], p. 350).

Secondary prevention in the society-at-large

Humanitarian relief operations: shelter, food, water and sanitation

The provision of adequate shelter in emergencies saves lives and reduces morbidity, overcrowding and lack of privacy. The participation of people, especially women, affected by an emergency in decisions regarding shelter and site planning reduces the helplessness seen in many camps. A range of camp options should be explored in crises regarding location and layout, including self-settled camps. Although camps or collective centres are often the only option, displaced people, in certain situations, may be hosted with local families who provide shelter and social support. This is a useful option provided that services to the hosting families are strengthened.

Ignoring the interactions between psychosocial well-being and food and nutritional security may cause harm, resulting, for example, in programmes that require people to queue up for long hours to receive food, treat recipients as dehumanised passive consumers, or create conditions for violence in and around food deliveries. Sociocultural aspects of diet and nutrition are relevant (what food is eaten and how it is prepared and served; cultural taboos). Hunger and food insecurity can impact cognitive abilities, especially in young children (e.g. due to deficits of (micro)nutrients and nutraceuticals), result in harmful coping strategies (e.g. selling food, exchanging sex for food, taking children out of school, using food to brew alcohol). They may result in loss of hope or perspective on the future (e.g. in situations of protracted conflict or slow reconstruction after a disaster), in feelings of helplessness (e.g. after loss of livelihood) and in aggressive behaviour (e.g. in situations of perceived unfairness of food entitlement or distribution) [83].

In a similar way, water and sanitation supports can either improve or harm well-being. In some emergencies, poorly lit, unlocked latrines have become sites of gender-based violence, whereas in others, conflict at water sources, for example after the influx of new groups of survivors, has caused distress. Inattention to cultural norms can lead to the construction of latrines or water points that are never used. Members of the affected population should be involved in decisions on the siting and design of latrines and, if possible, of water points and bathing shelters. Consider incentives for water committees and user fees, remembering that both have potential advantages and disadvantages and need careful evaluation in the local context [48, 83].

(Cooccurring) natural disasters: quality standards

Natural disasters may cooccur with or be superimposed on the effects of political violence. (Inter)national initiatives and disaster-preparedness training of the disaster-prone segments of the population can have a preventive effect, such as setting quality standards for buildings in earthquake- or landslide-prone areas or river beds, setting higher quality standards for the construction of nuclear power stations, providing better access to land in areas with landslides, creating better alarm systems for floods, cyclones or hurricanes, and providing sheltered areas and evacuation plans in regions that are hit by volcano eruptions or typhoons.

Voluntary repatriation

Another universal preventive activity is to work towards political solutions that allow for voluntary migration or repatriation to the place of origin.

Reparation and compensation

Every state has the responsibility to redress human rights violations and to enable victims to exercise their right to reparation (economic, judicial and symbolic) and to compensation. Ensuring social justice, a criminal justice system, an international or local criminal court and a truth and reconciliation process will have a preventive and curative effect.

Primary prevention at the community level

Rural development and food production

In settings of extreme poverty, integration and inter- or multisectoral synergy are paramount. Livelihood or infrastructural programmes complement psychosocial support and vice versa [36]. Rural development initiatives help local populations, refugees and IDPs to enhance their economic capacities and increase their food security, resilience and quality of life. Rural development improves the rural infrastructure, living conditions and livelihood of the population. This can be achieved through increasing food production, improving its distribution, and by setting up small-scale income-generating projects. If focused on areas with instability or increasing grievances, these policies can play a role in reducing the risk of armed conflict, including riots triggered by high food prices [84]. These projects may compensate for a lack of land and prevent competition between local populations and IDPs or refugees. Rural development is one aspect of empowering a community.

Community empowerment

Community empowerment aims to revitalise helpful skills that are not utilised by the local people due to demoralisation, collective apathy or a lack of appropriate knowledge. Empowerment activities allow community members to help themselves, their families and their neighbours. They include the development of networks of families that cope with similar problems (see below). These interventions lead to a sense of self and community efficacy; to connectedness, providing social support activities such as problem-solving, sharing of experience and emotional understanding, and mutual instruction about coping; and to hope or the expectation that a positive future outcome is possible: elements that according to an expert panel are empirically supported intervention principles after a disaster [42]. Rural development and empowerment also diminish dependency.

Decreasing dependency and learned helplessness

Decreasing dependency and learned helplessness, which often tend to develop in the aftermath of disasters, is important in stimulating resilience and agency. Reduction of dependency and the promotion of autonomy can be stimulated by involving local people in community interventions, health and (public) educational activities, and management and administrative issues. Religious leaders and healers should be stimulated to continue their rituals and ceremonies. Musicians,[13] dancers and storytellers should be allowed to organise leisure activities in closed communities like refugee and IDP camps.

Public health and education

Armed conflict, military or rebel action and disaster often undermine public health and disease-control programmes well beyond the period of active warfare, with reduced health sector spending and reduced surveillance, prevention, treatment and vector control [85, 86]. Access to health and education is often reduced due to: (i) reduced geographic and economic access (e.g. because of security concerns when travel to public services is dangerous); (ii) the service infrastructure, logistics and equipment being affected or deliberately destroyed; and (iii) a scarcity of human resources due to personnel fleeing the area, leaving the country or being targeted by armed forces. As mentioned before, it is useful to facilitate linkages between health care and education ministries and NGOs to expand capacity building.

Health and education and other sectors can further conciliate and collaborate by: (i) setting a policy to strengthen equitable health and educational services; (ii) reconstructing the former infrastructure; (iii) developing human resources via a cascade of training levels; (iv) supplying educational materials, food and nutrition, medicines and vaccines; and (v) creating a monitoring and surveillance system [38, 39].

There are several good examples of 'peace through health' programmes at http://www.humanities.mcmaster.ca/peace-health.

[13] As stimulated by Musicians Without Borders, for example.

Peace education and conflict resolution in schools and in the community

Education is a force for reducing intergroup conflict by enlarging social identifications, creating a basis for identification across cultures and trying to provide a correct version of the historical events that led to the conflict. Pivotal educational institutions such as the family, schools, community-based organisations and the media can shape attitudes and skills towards decent human relations or towards hatred and violence. Much of what schools can accomplish is similar to what parents can do, such as employing positive discipline practices, teaching the capacity for responsible decision-making, fostering cooperative learning procedures and guiding children in pro-social behaviour both in and outside of schools. They can convey an interest in other cultures, making respect a core attribute of children's outlook on the world. It is obvious that these peace-education and conflict-resolution skills can be expanded to adults and religious and community leaders (e.g. the Ushi or Bashigantahe counsels that are currently discussed as a post-conflict peace-promoting approach in Burundi).

Public (psycho)education, community sensitisation and awareness raising

Public education is a community intervention with the potential to provide large numbers of people with information about aid, legal rights and any number of issues that will help them cope with their particular situation. In humanitarian crises, public education can be used to quell rumours and help the community to reach a more realistic view of the situation (cf. [42]). Public education and community awareness-raising campaigns can involve educating citizens on how to prevent violence of all types towards children, spouses, the elderly and individuals with disabilities. In addition, young people can be trained in methods of conflict resolution and help those who are more vulnerable because they have lost a family member or their possessions.

In our DPMH model, community sensitisation aims at acceptance of our proposed services, explains the rationale of our approach (reducing stigma), increases understanding, awareness and identification of psychosocial issues, and helps to mobilise existing community resources. For example, in working with children, sensitisation is used to achieve community-level awareness to promote acceptance and school-level awareness to help in identification and implementation of programmes for children with problems [87].

Security measures

Survivors of wars and other types of disaster are often retraumatised by robbers or gangs of armed bandits. Shelling, ambushes, land mines and unexploded ordnances are an additional plight and need to be addressed in order to create a safe environment, especially in camps with a majority of women and children (e.g. when women look for wood to cook or when children fetch water).

Secondary prevention at the community level

Conflict prevention and resolution

Local organisations may: (i) monitor conflicts and provide early warning to the media and (inter)national organisations; (ii) convene adversarial parties; (iii) undertake mediation between the parties and/or the population groups involved; (iv) develop and train conflict resolution methods, using a hybridisation of traditional or academic models (e.g. the Gacaca in Rwanda); (v) strengthen institutions for conflict resolution involving local and religious leaders, healers and the ritual complex (e.g. the Sraddhanjali mass grieving ceremony in Sri Lanka); and (vi) foster development of the rule of law.

Crisis intervention

This involves the intervention of police forces or peace-keeping troops when tensions between local groups erupt or when there are armed activities by paramilitary forces, rebels or criminals.

Vocational skills training

Vocational skills training can help the local community to develop economic activities. Farmers may have lost their land, civil servants their jobs and demobilised soldiers and child soldiers their positions, such that all have to learn a new trade in order to set up income-generating activities or earn a living.

Primary prevention at the level of the family and the individual

Include women and children in the distribution of economic growth

In vulnerable societies, women are an important source of community stability and vitality. Even under adverse circumstances, women are often engaged in small-scale trade or horticulture around the house. Women-operated businesses, microcredit programmes, education for girls and the involvement of women in decision-making are all important.

Children of different ages and genders have different resources, coping skills and vulnerabilities. Older children may be better able to grasp the complications of a disaster and draw on more effective coping strategies and a broader set of social supports during recovery. For children, education is the main vehicle for stabilisation and healing. In addition, children should have access to basic health services and not be exploited economically.

Family reunion/family tracing

A network, preferably the family, supports healing. Separated children need to be traced and reunified e.g., by contacting the proper reunification organisation. Western-style orphanages or children villages are a last resort – in cases of massive loss of family members due to war or a disease such as HIV, – because these facilities may create additional problems and can easily become a breeding place for bandits or prostitution. Abandoned or orphaned children should be accommodated within their extended family or within foster families, and international and local organisations should assess whether one or both parents or other first- or second-generation family members are alive.

Family/network building

Family/network building promotes the family network or other types of network so that groups with similar problems can help each other, share certain rituals or get involved in human rights work (see also the Empowerment section above).

Improvement of physical aspects

It is important to their well-being that families are involved in the development of their life world, including the physical aspects of their habitat or refugee camp. This includes discussing acceptable amounts of water, decreasing overcrowding, allotting land to grow vegetables, varying diets, draining the terrain and providing space for children to play and for mothers to take care of their babies or infants. As we have seen, relief agencies are not always aware of the cultural taboos surrounding the disposal of waste or excrement.

Resilience groups for children

Within a care package developed for children [87], child resilience groups provide a set of preventive semistructured group activities for children without indication for focused MHPSS. The first aim of these group activities is to strengthen existing resilience by encouraging social support systems, engagement in recreational or traditional activities and normalisation through peer-group discussion and activities. The second aim is to reduce stigmatisation due to (non)enrolment in psychosocial interventions for both the indicated and nonindicated groups of children.[14] Finally, the third aim is to conduct case identification through structured and recurring nontherapeutic group activities, using a screener such as the seven-item Child Psychosocial Distress Screener (CPDS), which includes the child's appraised traumatic and current distress and their resilience [88]. Activities range from recreational and traditional activities to theme-based discussion groups (e.g. life-skills-focused discussions combined with songs and dances in Sri Lanka; drumming and dancing or football practices resulting in intercommunity competition or presentations in Burundi) and among Sudanese refugees in Uganda.

Secondary prevention at the level of the family and the individual

Preventing recruitment of child soldiers

Children are often recruited when there are no other means of subsistence and hence become easy targets for government armies and rebel forces. Vocational skills training for child soldiers has already been mentioned. Such training would need to address the transition from a 'combat mode' to a 'civil mode' and use reconciliation and cleansing rituals to reintegrate children into their communities. Girl child soldiers are more likely to experience sexual assault and communities may respond differently to returning male and female child soldiers. One has to prevent reprisal attacks during their rehabilitation process. Rehabilitation services for combat-related injuries, such as loss of hearing, sight and limbs, as well as for psychosocial problems and poor control of aggression, will be required [89, 90].

Reparation and compensation for afflicted families

Compensation is a form of reparation that is paid in cash or provided in kind. Compensation-in-kind might include provision of health and mental health care, employment, housing, education or land. Transitional justice mechanisms may be employed (economic, symbolic and judicial – either modern, as happened in South Africa, Guatemala and Cambodia, or traditional, as in Rwanda). When a truth and reconciliation commission or a war tribunal is installed, old wounds may be reopened and a need for psychosocial support may arise [91, 92]. Compensation is often seen as part of the truth and reconciliation process, for example in South Africa.

[14] A potential risk of focused mental health and psychosocial support is that the indicated group is stigmatised or that the nonindicated group is 'envious' of those receiving care. Two strategies to overcome such challenges are community sensitisation (see above) and ensuring that all children receive some intervention, matched for the level of need for psychosocial care (cf. [87]).

Public health and disease control

Attention is required for the major causes of death in conflict-affected societies, particularly acute respiratory infections, diarrhoea, malaria, measles, neonatal causes and malnutrition. In emergencies in sub-Saharan Africa, particularly southern Africa, HIV/AIDS is also an important cause of morbidity and mortality. As we have seen, military action often undermines public health and disease-control programmes that extend well beyond the period of active warfare, with reduced health-sector spending and reduced surveillance, prevention, treatment and vector control [85, 86]. A series of recent emergencies in Afghanistan, Somalia, the Balkans and Iraq underscores the increasing role of the military in humanitarian emergencies, requiring more coherence between political and humanitarian objectives [93].

Mental health and psychosocial support (MHPSS)

Psychosocial support

Self-help groups

Self-help groups help people with similar problems to help each other and thus eliminate the need of a trained helper. I have found examples in a variety of African and Asian countries of these groups being organised for ex-combatants, ex-child soldiers, widows, unaccompanied minors, survivors of rape and torture, mothers of vulnerable groups such as handicapped children, the elderly and alcoholics [36].

Counselling

In view of the scarcity of mental health professionals, paraprofessional counsellors are often recruited among the target population. Counselling is a relatively easy-access level of care that targets more severe forms of distress, both nonspecific and common mental disorders, forming a link between informal and formal specialised care structures. In the humanitarian field, the term 'counselling' is so widely used that it is depleted of meaning, and it is often referred to as 'trauma counselling'.

The core practice elements are structured problem solving, symptom management, psychoeducation and emotional support. These occur in a relationship that offers trust and hope through a set of nonspecific therapeutic skills, intercultural sensitivity and structured steps that aim to reduce stressor-induced symptoms and to solve problem situations [94, 95]. In LAMICs, one has to be aware of cultural processes that influence the counselling process, such as the embodiment of meaning in psychophysiological reactions, the development of interpersonal attachments, the molding of collective and individual identity, the expression of illness experiences and idioms of distress, and the use of explanatory models by patients, healers and allopathic practitioners.

Local psychosocial counsellors are trained with a cascade model of training and supervision, often referred to as 'training of trainers'. Counselling is offered either in the home of the client or in community-based counselling centres. It may be conducted in a family setting, a group setting or on an individual basis. One of the major problems with families and family counselling is the high prevalence of violence against women [96]. Some scholars are of the opinion that violence can be prevented by promoting social awareness to change norms that condone violence against women, by equipping young people with skills for healthy relationships or by expanding women's access to economic and social resources and support services [97]. Others mention that there are no known approaches for preventing emotional abuse or exposure to intimate-partner violence, even though a specific parent-training programme has shown benefits in preventing recurrence of physical abuse of children. Cognitive-behavioural therapy for sexually abused children with symptoms of post-traumatic stress shows the best evidence [98].

Children

Classroom-based intervention

Schools are often recommended as the setting of choice for psychosocial support interventions as they offer a familiar, nonstigmatising setting and provide the broadest access to children and their families [99, 100]. Usually, group work is preferred over individual work: group members can recognise that they are not alone with their problems and can learn new strategies and coping skills from each other, and the group can function as a place to try out new problem-solving skills.

Classroom-based intervention (CBI) is a 15-session intervention that includes group activities such as cooperative games, music, drawing and psychodrama which focus on stabilisation and safety, individual coping strategies, traumatic exposure narratives and future-oriented resources [87]. A cluster randomised trial has shown that CBI is moderately effective in reducing PTSD and maintaining hope in Indonesia [101], with an effect size that is similar to CBI for children in the West [102]. In Nepal, another trial showed that CBI reduced psychological difficulties and aggression among boys and increased pro-social behaviour among girls [87]. Apart from these two studies, there are only three other randomised controlled trials regarding children in (post-)conflict: one showing the efficacy of group interpersonal therapy in reducing depression symptoms among adolescent girls in Uganda [15] [103]; one demonstrating the effectiveness of a trauma- and

[15] It is noteworthy that creative workshops showed no effect compared to the control condition, yet hundreds of children NGOs around the world continue to pursue such activity.

grief-focused group intervention in reducing PTSD and depression symptoms among school children (aged 13–18 years) in Bosnia [104]; and one showing a small positive effect on mothers' mental health, children's weight gain and children's psychological functioning in Bosnia [105].

Parental support

Targeting families, and specifically parents, to improve the psychosocial well-being of children is recommended because parents, as the natural child-raisers, are influential mediators of children's reactions to (nonfamilial) violence. Wallen and Rubin [106] summarised the role of the family in mediating negative effects of violence as follows:

1. physical availability of the parents;
2. protection and physical safety through parental awareness of potential dangers and subsequent installation of rules, education and supervision;
3. support in working through traumatic events via communication and emotional sensitivity;
4. child rearing that fosters moral development to counterbalance the moral erosion as a result of conflict; and
5. models of positive coping regarding safety, emotion regulation and sense of control.

This role can be translated in the provision of family-oriented supportive counselling, mostly through home visits, focused on parental capacities: for example, psychoeducation sessions with parents to increase problem identification and awareness, and subsequent extension to child-rearing support (i.e. simple behaviour modification techniques); introduction of the family to existing services and social support systems; provision of family problem-solving support (based on existing parental coping strategies); and individual counselling for parents [87].

Individual and family therapy

Psychotherapy requires extensive training and supervision. Examples are trauma therapy, testimony work, group therapy for survivors of violence including children, and systemic family therapy.

In countries with a considerable number of psychologists, professionals will employ forms of psychotherapy that are commonly used in high-income countries (cf. [107, 108]). These include culturally appropriate versions of cognitive behaviour therapy (CBT), including exposure therapy, cognitive therapy, cognitive processing therapy, stress-inoculation training, systematic desensitisation, assertiveness training, relaxation training, narrative exposure therapy and eye-movement desensitisation and reprocessing (EMDR) (see Chapter 3).

Mental health

In fragile states, public health services generally do not cater for mental health, referring these services to NGOs and community-based organisations. Larger programmes are frequently limited in terms of coverage and sustainability. Afghanistan is an exception, including mental health and disability services as one of the five pillars of the Basic Package of Health Services (BPHS). When compared to other BPHS components, scaling up of these services is proceeding at a snail's pace due to a lack of qualified staff, of awareness of rehabilitation services among BPHS staff, and of donor support. Because this is exemplary of the situation in many LAMICs, it is useful to have a closer look at some elements of this programme.

For each service level of the BPHS, training modules and a supervision system were developed. For health posts, staffed by (non-paid) community health workers, a three-day training course was provided, which focused on identification of persons with possible mental health problems in the community and follow-up of patients with chronic mental illness. For staff of the basic health centres/community health center (BHCs/CHC), 10-day training courses were organised. The training for doctors focused on diagnosis and biopsychosocial management of the most important mental disorders, while the training for nurses and midwives focused on basic principles of nonpharmacological mental health care management, including empathic listening skills and provision of social support. At the district hospitals, outpatient and inpatient services were made accessible for patients with mental problems, and each hospital had a mental health focal point: a full-time medical doctor responsible for referral cases from the surrounding health facilities. Supervisors of the mental health programme were to visit these trained health staff at least once a month. The programme has now started to integrate mental health into higher tiers of the care system, opening some psychiatric beds in the provincial hospitals and upgrading the national referral centre of 60 beds in Kabul.

Crisis intervention

A crisis team can intervene when health emergencies, suicide, domestic violence or attacks by rebels, the army or paramilitary forces occur. A quick response calms and supports the family, assists in referral and activates community and family support for victims.

Tertiary prevention at the level of the family and the individual

Involving the family in rehabilitation and reconstruction

The goal of tertiary prevention is to reduce anomia, apathy and chronic disabling conditions through active rehabilitation and the development of skills for peaceful conflict resolution. Collective violence in low-income countries often takes place in collectivistic and interdependent cultures where – as long as family members are around – rejection by the family is exceptional. Hence, there are ample opportunities to involve the family in rehabilitation.

Norris and Kaniasty [109] rightly mention that after mass trauma, initial periods of a high degree of social support are followed by a quick deterioration of the support system. This problem is compounded when many adults die due to war or AIDS, or when families seek refuge in the houses of other family members, turning a large extended family into a vulnerability factor.

CONCLUSION

This chapter has outlined a public mental health model that accommodates a variety of preventive interventions related to political violence and natural disasters. The model indicates how multisector, multimodal and multilevel preventive principles can be applied in an integrative and eclectic way. This public mental health approach also shows how prevention can be molded to the requirements of the specific sociocultural contexts. Moreover, it may help to clarify the complementary relationship between the UN and (non)governmental actors. It further shows how the social sector and the sectors of health, education, human rights, gender and rural development can collaborate. The model may help to identify gaps in our knowledge and to guide the future elaboration of a preventive approach.

There are several limitations to this model. One may question whether the distinction between primary, secondary and tertiary preventive interventions fits with the real world, and whether certain interventions should be located elsewhere in the matrix. Much more evidence is needed to determine whether the interventions are effective. We also need more insight into appropriate ways to scale up the delivery of priority interventions and into the components of successful large-scale programmes. Further efforts are needed to continue expanding the spectrum of effective preventive interventions, to improve their effectiveness and cost-effectiveness in varied settings, and to continue strengthening the evidence base. This will require a process of repeated evaluation of preventive policies and their implementation, and a coordinated and long-term effort and commitment.

REFERENCES

1. Asay, T.R. and Lambert, M.J. (1999) The empirical case for the common factors in therapy: quantitative findings, in *The Heart and Soul of Change: What Works in Therapy* (eds M.A. Hubble, B.L. Duncan and S.D. Miller), American Psychological Association, Washington, pp. 23–55.
2. Driessen, E., Cuijpers, P., de Maat, S.C. *et al.* (2010) The efficacy of short-term psychodynamic psychotherapy for depression: a meta-analysis. *Clinical Psychology Review*, **30**, 25–36.
3. Wampold, B.E. (2001) *The Great Psychotherapy Debate: Models, Methods and Findings*, Lawrence Erlbaum Associates, Mahwah (NJ).
4. Baldwin, S.A., Wampold, B.E. and Imel, Z.E. (2007) Untangling the alliance-outcome correlation: exploring the relative importance of therapist and patient variability in the alliance. *Journal of consulting and clinical psychology*, **65**, 842–852.
5. Freemantle, N., Anderson, I.M. and Young, P. (2000) Predictive value of pharmacological activity for the relative efficacy of antidepressant drugs. *The British Journal of Psychiatry*, **177**, 292–302.
6. Horwitz, A. (2002) *Creating Mental Illness*, University of Chicago Press, Chicago.
7. Bisson, J.I., Tavakoly, B., Witteveen, A.B. *et al.* (2010) TENTS guidelines: development of post-disaster psychosocial care guidelines through a Delphi process. *The British Journal of Psychiatry*, **196**, 69–74. doi: 10.1192/bjp.bp.109.066266.
8. Zaridze, D., Brenna, P.,Boreham, J. *et al.* (2009) Alcohol and cause specific mortality in Russia: A retrospective case-control study of 48,557 adult deaths. *Lancet*, **373**, 2201–2214.
9. Luchins, D.J. (2010) The future of mental health care and the limits of the behavioral neurosciences. *The Journal of Nervous and Mental Disease*, **198** (6), 395–398.
10. Hopper, K, Harrison. G, Janca, A and Sartorius, N (eds) (2007) *Recovery From Schizophrenia: An International Perspective*, Oxford University Press, Oxford (NY).
11. De Jong, J.T.V.M. and Komproe, I.H. (2006) A 15-year open study on a cohort of West-African outpatients with a chronic psychosis. *Social Psychiatry and Psychiatric Epidemiology*, **41** (11), 897–903.
12. Slobbe, L.C.J., Kommer, G.J., Smit, J.M. *et al.* (2003) *Kosten van Ziekten in Nederland 2003*, RIVM, Bilthoven, www.kostenvanziekten.nl (accessed 2010).
13. Priebe, S., Badesconyi, A., Fioritti, A. *et al.* (2005) Reinstitutionalisation in mental health care: comparison of data on service provision from six European countries. *British Medical Journal*, **330** (15), 123–126.
14. WHO (2002) *World Report on Violence and Health*, World Health Organization, Geneva.
15. Murray, C.J.L. and Lopez, A.D. (1997) Alternative projections of mortality and disability by cause 1990–2020: Global Burden of Disease Study. *Lancet*, **349**, 1498–1504.

16. Farmer, P. (2003) *Pathologies of Power: Health, Human Rights, and the New War on the Poor*, University of California Press, California.
17. Kleinman, A., Eisenberg, L. and Good, B. (1978) Culture, illness and care: clinical lessons from anthropologic and cross-cultural research. *Annals Internal Medicine*, **88**, 251–258.
18. Murdock, J.C. and Sandler, T. (2002) Economic growth, civil wars, and spatial spillovers. *Journal of Conflict Resolution*, **46** (1), 91–110.
19. Pinstrup-Andersen, P. and Shimokawa, S. (2008) Do poverty and poor health and nutrition increase the risk of armed conflict onset? *Food Policy*, **33**, 513–520.
20. Harbom, L., Melander, E. and Wallensteen, P. (2008) Dyadic dimensions of armed conflict, 1946–2007. *Journal of Peace Research*, **45**, 697–710.
21. Hewitt, J. (2008) *Trends in global conflict, 1946–2005, in Peace and Conflict 2008* (eds J. Hewitt, J. Wilkenfeld and T. Gurr), Paradigm Publisher, Boulder.
22. Tol, W.A. (2009) Healing in the aftermath of war: conceptualization and evaluation of mental health and psychosocial support for populations exposed to political violence in low-income settings. PhD Thesis. VU University, Amsterdam.
23. Jordans, M.J.D., Tol, W.A., Komproe, I.H. *et al*. (2010) Development of a multi-layered psychosocial care system for children in areas of political violence. *International Journal of Mental Health Systems*, **4**, 15, http://www.ijmhs.com/content/4/1/15 (accessed 2010).
24. World Health Organization (2005) *Mental Health Atlas*, World Health Organization, Geneva.
25. The WHO World Mental Health Survey Consortium (2004) Prevalence, severity, and unmet need for treatment of mental disorders in the World Health OrganizationWorld Mental Health surveys. *JAMA*, **291** (21), 2581–2590.
26. Patel, V., Flisher, A.J., Nikapota, A. and Malhotra, S. (2008) Promoting child and adolescent mental health in low- and middle-income countries. *The Journal of Child Psychology and Psychiatry*, **49** (3), 313–334.
27. Morris, J., Van Ommeren, M., Belfer, M. *et al*. (2007) Children and the Sphere standard on mental and social aspects of health. *Disasters*, **31** (1), 71–90.
28. De Jong, J.T.V.M. and Komproe, I.H. (2002) Closing the gap between psychiatric epidemiology and mental health in (post-)conflict situations. *Lancet*, **359**, 1793–1794.
29. Herman, D.B. and Susser, E.S. (2003) The World Trade Center attack: mental health needs and treatment implications. *Bulletin of the Board of International Affairs of the Royal College of Psychiatrists*, **1**, 8–9.
30. De Jong, J.T.V.M. (2002) *Trauma, War and Violence: Public Mental Health in Socio-Cultural Context*, Plenum-Kluwer, New York.
31. De Jong, J.T.V.M., Komproe, I.H., Van Ommeren, M. *et al*. (2001) Lifetime events and post-traumatic stress disorder in 4 post-conflict settings. *Journal of American Medical Association*, **286** (5), 555–562.

32. De Jong, J.T.V.M., Komproe, I. and Van Ommeren, M. (2003) Common mental disorders in post-conflict settings. *Lancet*, **361** (6), 2128–2130.
33. De Jong, J.T.V.M., Komproe, I.H. and O'Connell, K.A. (2005) *Effectiveness and Cost-effectiveness of Mental Health Care in Low-income Developing Countries: Burundi, Gaza, Nepal and Uganda*, World Bank, Washington, DC, pp. 1–120.
34. Kessler, R.C., Sonnega, A., Bromet, E. *et al.* (1995) Posttraumatic stress disorder in the National Comorbidity Survey. *Archives of General Psychiatry*, **52**, 1048–1060.
35. Creamer, M., Burgess, P. and McFarlane, A.C. (2001) Post-traumatic stress disorder: findings from the Australian National Survey of Mental Health and Well-being. *Psychological Medicine*, **31**, 1237–1247.
36. De Jong, J.T.V.M. (2002) Public mental health, traumatic stress and human rights violations in low-income countries: a culturally appropriate model in times of conflict, disaster and peace, in *Trauma, War and Violence: Public Mental Health in Sociocultural Context* (ed. T.V.M. Jongde), Plenum-Kluwer, New York, pp. 1–91.
37. Saltzman, W.R., Layne, C.M., Syeinberg, A.M. *et al.* (2003) Developing a culturally and ecologically sound intervention program for youth exposed to war and terrorism. *Child and Adolescent Psychiatric Clinics North America*, **12**, 319–342.
38. De Jong, J.T.V.M. (2010) A public health framework to translate risk factors related to political violence and war into multilevel preventive interventions. *Social Science and Medicine*, **70**, 71–79.
39. De Jong, J.T. (2010) A public-health view on the prevention of war and its consequences, in *Trauma Rehabilitation after War and Conflict* (ed. E. Martz), Springer Science, pp. 73–97.
40. Brewin, C.R., Andrews, B. and Valentine, J.D. (2000) Meta-analysis of risk factors for posttraumatic stress disorder in trauma-exposed adults. *Journal of Consulting and Clinical Psychology*, **68**, 748–766.
41. Ozer, E.J., Best, S.R., Lipsey, T.L. and Weiss, D.S. (2003) Predictors of posttraumatic stress disorder and symptoms in adults: a meta-analysis. *Psychological Bulletin*, **129**: 52–73.
42. Hobfoll, S.E., Watson, P., Bell, C.C. *et al.* (2007) Five essential elements of immediate and mid-term mass trauma intervention: empirical evidence. *Psychiatry*, **70** (4), 283–315.
43. Harriet, L. MacMillan, C. Nadine Wathen, J. *et al.* (2008) Interventions to prevent child maltreatment and associated impairment. *Lancet*, doi: 10.1016/S0140-6736(08)61708-0
44. Reading, R., Bissell, S., Goldhagen, J. *et al.* (2008) Promotion of children's rights and prevention of child maltreatment. *Lancet*. doi: 10.1016/S0140-6736(08)61709-2 (Published Online 3 December 2008).
45. Hobfoll, S.E. (1998) *The Ecology of Stress*, Hemisphere, New York.

46. World Health Organization (2007) Strengthening Health Systems to Improve Health Outcomes, World Health Organization, Geneva.
47. Craig, P., Dieppe, P. and Macintyre, S. (2008) Developing and evaluating complex interventions: the New Medical Research Council guidance. *British Medical Journal*, **337**, 979–983.
48. Inter Agency Standing Committee (2007) Guidelines on Mental Health and Psychosocial Support in Emergency Settings, IASC, Geneva.
49. De Jong, J.T.V.M. (2007) Traumascape: an ecological-cultural-historical model for extreme Stress, in *Textbook of Cultural Psychiatry* (eds D. Bhugra and K. Bhui), Cambridge University Press, Cambridge, pp. 347–364.
50. Akello, G., Richters, A. and Reis, R. (2009) Coming to terms with accountability: why the reintegration of former child soldiers in Northern Uganda fails, in *Memory, Narrative, and Forgiveness: Perspectives on the Unfinished Journeys of the Past* (eds P. Gobodo-Madikizela and C. van der Merwe), Cambridge Scholars Publishing, Cambridge, pp. 188–212.
51. Igreja, V. (2008) Gamba spirits, gender relations, and healing in post-civil war Gorongosa, Mozambique. *Journal of the Royal Anthropological Institute (N.S.)*, **14**, 350–367.
52. De Jong, J.T.V.M. (1987) *A Descent into African Psychiatry*, Royal Tropical Institute, Amsterdam. ISBN 90 6832 018 1.
53. de Jong, J.T. and Reis, R. (2010) Kiyang-yang, a West-African post-war idiom of distress. *Culture, Medicine and Psychiatry*, **34** (2), 301–321.
54. Van Ommeren, M., Sharma, B. and Komproe, I.H. (2001) Trauma and loss as determinants of culture-bound epidemic illness in a Bhutanese refugee community. *Psychological Medicine*, **31** (7), 1259–1267.
55. Minas, H. (2007) Developing mental health services for multicultural societies, in *Textbook of Cultural Psychiatry* (eds D. Bhuga and K. Bhui), Cambridge University Press, Cambridge.
56. Krueger, R.A. (1988) *Focus Groups. A Practical Guide for Applied Research*, Sage, Newbury Park, CA.
57. De Jong, J.T.V.M. and Van Ommeren, M.H. (2002) Toward a culture-informed epidemiology: combining qualitative and quantitative research in transcultural contexts. *Transcultural Psychiatry*, **39**, 422–433.
58. Creswell, J.W. (2003) *Research Design: Qualitative, Quantitative, and Mixed Method Approaches*, 2nd edn, Sage, Thousand Oaks, CA.
59. Ritchie, J. and Lewis, J. (eds) (2003) *Qualitative Research Practice. A Guide for Social Science Students and Researchers*, Sage, London.
60. Corbin, J.M. and Strauss, A.L. (2007) *The Basics of Qualitative Research: Techniques and Procedures for Developing Grounded Theory*, 3rd edn, Sage, London.
61. Cohen, R.E. and Ahearn, F.L. (1991) *Handbook of Mental Health Care for Disaster Victims*, John Hopkins University Press, London.
62. Somasundaram, D., de Put Van W.A.M., Eisenbruch, M. and de Jong, J.T.V.M. (1999). Starting mental health services in Cambodia. *Social Science and Medicine*, **48** (8), 1029–1046.

63. Eisenberg, D.M., Davis, R.B. and Ettner, S.L. (1998) Trends in alternative medicine use in the United States, 1990–1997. *The journal of the American Medical Association*, **280**, 1569–1575.
64. Bodeker, G. and Kronenenberg, F. (2002) A public health agenda for traditional, complementary, and alternative medicine. *American Journal of Public Health*, **92**, 1582–1591.
65. Adamolekum, B. (1995) The aetiologies of epilepsy in tropical Africa. *Tropical and Geographical Medicine*, **47** (3), 115–117.
66. de Jong, J.T.V.M. (1996) A comprehensive public mental health programme in Guinea-Bissau: A useful model for African, Asian and Latin-American countries. *Psychological Medicine*, **26**, 97–108.
67. De Jong, J.T.V.M., Komproe, I.H. and O'Connell, K.A. (2005) *Effectiveness and Cost-Effectiveness of Mental Health Care in Low-Income Developing Countries: Burundi, Gaza, Nepal and Uganda*, World Bank, Washington, DC, pp 1–120.
68. Brand, B., Classen, C. and Lanins, R. (2009) A naturalistic study of dissociative identity disorder and dissociative disorder not otherwise specified patients treated by community clinicians. *Psychological Trauma: Theory, Research, Practice, and Policy*, **1** (2), 153–171.
69. Van Duijl, M., Cardeña, E., de Jong, J.T.V.M. *et al*. (2005) The validity of DSM-IV dissociative disorders categories in South-West Uganda. *Transcultural Psychiatry*, **6**, 219–241.
70. Zantinge, E.M., Verhaak, P.F. and de Bakker, D.H. (2006) Does the attention general practitioners pay to their patients' mental health problems add to their workload? A cross sectional national survey. *BMC Family Practice*, **7**, 71.
71. Antares (2005) www.antaresfoundation.org.
72. Bromet, E.J. (1995) Methodological issues in designing research on community-wide disasters with special reference to Chernobyl, in *Extreme Stress and Communities: Impact and Intervention* (eds S.E. Hobfoll and M. W. De Vries) Kluwer, Dordrecht, The Netherlands, pp. 267–283.
73. ICH/CPMP (1997) *ICH/CPMP Guideline for Good Clinical Practice Including the Declaration of Helsinki and the Belmont Report*, ICH, London (7 Westferry Circus, Canary Wharf, London E14 4HB).
74. Kagawa-Singer, M. and Chi-Yung Chung, R. (1994) A paradigm for culturally based care in ethnic minority populations. *Journal of Community Psychology*, **22**, 192–208.
75. Hyman, S., Chisholm, D., Kessler, R., Patel, V., Whiteford, H. (2006) Mental disorders, in *Disease Control Priorities in Developing Countries*, 2nd edn, (eds D.T Jamison *et al*.), World Bank/ Oxford University Press, Washington/Oxford, pp. 605–625.
76. Fairbank, J., de JongJ., Friedman, M., GreenB. (2003) Integrated intervention strategies for traumatic stress, in *Trauma Interventions in War and Peace: Prevention, Practice, and Policy* (eds B. Green, M. Friedman, J. de Jong, T. Keane, S. Solomon, J.A. Fairbank, B. Donelan, E. Frey-Wouters), Plenum-Kluwer, New York.

77. Mrazek, P.J. and Haggerty, R.J., US Committee on Prevention of Disorder (1994) *Reducing Risks for Mental Disorders: Frontiers for Preventive Intervention Research*, National Academy Press, Washington, DC.
78. Caspi, A., Sugden, K., Moffitt, T.E. *et al.* (2003) Influence of life stress on depression: moderation by a polymorphism in the 5-HTT gene. *Science*, **301**, 386–389.
79. Kendler, K.S. (2005) 'A gene for...': The nature of gene action in psychiatric disorders. *The American journal of psychiatry*, **162**, 1243–1252.
80. West, K.P., Caballero, B. and Black, R.E. (2001) Nutrition, in *International Public Health: Diseases, Programs, Systems and Policies* (ed. M.H. Merson, R.E. Black and A.J. Mills), Aspen Publishers, Maryland, pp. 207–270.
81. Bangirana, P., Idro, R., John, C.C. and Boivin, M.J. (2006) Rehabilitation for cognitive impairments after cerebral malaria in African children: strategies and limitations. *Tropical Medicine and International Health*, **11** (9), 1–9.
82. Mrazek, P.J. and Haggerty, R.J. (1994) *Reducing Risks for Mental Disorders: Frontiers for Preventive Intervention Research*, National Academy Press, Washington, DC.
83. Sphere Project (2004) Minimum standards in water, sanitation and hygiene promotion, *Humanitarian Charter and Minimum Standards in Disaster Response*, Sphere Project, Geneva, pp. 51–102. http://www.sphereproject.org/handbook/index.htm.
84. Hegre, H. and Sambanis, N. (2006) Sensitivity analysis of empirical results on civil war onset. *The Journal of Conflict Resolution*, **50** (4), 508–535.
85. Beyrer, C., Villar, J.C.,Suwanvanichkij, V. *et al.* (2007) Neglected diseases, civil conflicts, and the right to health. *Lancet*, **370**, 619–627.
86. Ghobaraha, H.A., Huthb, P. and Russettc, B. (2004) The post-war public health effects of civil conflict. *Social Science & Medicine*, **59**, 869–884.
87. Jordans, M.J.D., Komproe, I.H. and Tol, W.A. (2010) Evaluation of a school based psychosocial intervention in Nepal: a randomized controlled trial. *Journal of Child Psychology and Psychiatry*, **51**, 818–826.
88. Jordans, M.J.D., Komproe, I.H. and Ventevogel, P. (2008) Development and validation of the child psychosocial distress screener in Burundi. *The American Journal of Orthopsychiatry*, **78**, 290–299.
89. Machel, G. (1996) *The Impact of Armed Conflict on Children*, United Nations, New York. Report submitted to General Assembly resolution 48/175.
90. UNICEF and the Coalition to Stop the Use of Child Soldiers (2003) Guide to the Optional Protocol on Children in Armed Conflict. http://www.unicef.org/publications/files/option_protocol_conflict.pdf.
91. Gibson, J.L. (2006) Overcoming apartheid: can truth reconcile a divided nation? *The Annals of the American Academy of Political and Social Science*, **603**, 82–110.
92. Sonis, J., Gibson, J.L. and De Jong, J.T. (2009) Probable posttraumatic stress disorder and disability in Cambodia: associations with perceived justice, desire for

revenge, and attitudes toward the Khmer Rouge Trials. *Journal of the American Medical Association*, **302** (5), 527–536.

93. Salama, P., Spiegel, P., Talley, L. and Waldman, R. (2004) Lessons learned from complex emergencies over past decade. *Lancet*, **364**, 1801–1813.
94. Egan, G., (1998) *The Skilled Helper. A Problem-management Approach to Helping*, 6th edn, Brooks/Cole, California, CA.
95. Ivey, A.E. and Ivey, M. (1999) *Intentional Interviewing and Counseling: Facilitating Client Development in a Multicultural Society*, 4th edn, Brooks/Cole, California.
96. Garcia-Moreno, C., Heise, L., Jansen, H.A.F.M. *et al*. (2005) Violence Against Women. *Science*, **310**, 1282–1283.
97. Garcia-Moreno, C., Jansen, H.A.F.M., Ellsberg, M., (on behalf of the WHO Multi-country Study on Women's Health and Domestic Violence against Women Study Team) *et al*. (2005) Prevalence of intimate partner violence: findings from the WHO multi-country study on women's health and domestic Violence, pp. 1260–1269. http://www.thelancet.com.
98. McMillan, D., Hastings, R.P., Salter, D.C. and Skuse, D.H. (2008) Developmental risk factor research and sexual offending against children: A review of some methodological issues. *Archives of Sexual Behavior*, **37**, 877–890.
99. Macy, R.D., Johnson-Macy, D., Gross, S.I. and Brighton, P. (2003) Healing in familiar settings: support for children in the classroom and community. *New Directions for Youth Development*, **98**, 51–79.
100. Stein, B.D., Jaycox, L.H. and Kataoka, S.H. (2003) A mental health intervention for school children exposed to violence: a randomized controlled trial. *Journal of the American Medical Association*, **290**, 603–611.
101. Tol, W.A., Komproe, I.H., Susanty, D. *et al*. (2008) Children and communal violence in Indonesia: cluster randomized trial of a psychosocial school-based intervention. *Journal of the American Medical Association*, **300**, 655–662.
102. Silverman, W.K., Ortiz, C.D., Viswesvaran, C. *et al*. (2008) Evidence-based psychosocial treatment for children and adolescents exposed to traumatic events. *Journal of Clinical Child and Adolescent Psychology*, **37**, 156–183.
103. Bolton, P., Bass, J. and Neugebauer, R. (2003) Group interpersonal psychotherapy for depression in rural Uganda: a randomized controlled trial. *Journal of the American Medical Association*, **289**, 3117–3124.
104. Layne, C.M., Saltzman, W.R. and Poppleton, L. (2008) Effectiveness of a school-based group psychotherapy program for war-exposed adolescents: a randomized controlled trial. *Journal of the American Academy of Child and Adolescent Psychiatry*, **47**, 1048–1062.
105. Dybdahl, R. *et al*. (2001) Children and mothers in war: an outcome study of a psychosocial intervention program. *Child Development*, **71**, 1214–1230.
106. Wallen, J. and Rubin, R.H. (1997) The role of the family in mediating the effects of community violence on children. *Aggression and Violent Behavior*, **2**, 33–41.

107. Otto, M.W. and Hinton, D.E. (2006) Modifying Exposure-Based CBT for Cambodian Refugees with Posttraumatic Stress Disorder. *Cognitive and Behavioral Practice*, **13**, 261–270.

108. Hinton, D.E. and Good, B.J. (eds) (2009) *Culture and Panic Disorder*, Stanford University Press, Stanford, CA.

109. Norris, F.H. and Kaniasty, K. (1996) Received and perceived social support in times of stress: a test of the social support deterioration deterrence model. *Journal of Personality and Social Psychology*, **71**, 498–511.

COMMENTARY

6.1 An Excellent Model for Low- and Middle-Income Countries

Dean Ajdukovic

Department of Psychology, University of Zagreb, Zagreb, Croatia

This chapter discusses the need and rationale for a public health approach to planning, providing, monitoring and evaluating mental health services in situations of organised violence and disaster. The disaster public mental health (DPMH) model is described in detail. This model is supported by extensive literature sources and the author's even more extensive first-hand experience in a number of countries in Africa and Asia.

The model is well grounded in systems theory and preventive science. It is generic but respects and accounts for social-contextual variables that are specific for given circumstances. Although the model can be useful for major incidents and disaster response in high-income countries, the emphasis of the whole chapter and most of the examples and social ramifications indicate that it is more targeted towards low- and middle-income countries. The reasons for this are provided by the author: it is in the poorer parts of the world that most of the casualties due to organised violence and natural disasters occur, where there is much less mental health provision and resources are severely limited. It is more likely therefore that the DPMH model will be implemented in these poorer parts – under the leadership of major international organisations that may already be involved in a particular country.

With this in mind, one sometimes has the feeling that the chapter was written primarily to be read by strong international players (who could take a lead in implementing this comprehensive model) and less for local governments, organisations or professional groups. Nevertheless, in some European countries with a more traditional approach to mental health services and severely

Post-traumatic Stress Disorder, First Edition. Edited by Dan Stein, Matthew Friedman, and Carlos Blanco.

limited resources this model should be welcome. Such countries include Kosovo, Albania, Moldova, Romania and Latvia, all of which have small numbers of trained mental health professionals, poor funding, a legacy of unquestionable professional authority, a traditional approach to mental disorders and treatment, a lack of training in psychological interventions and trauma treatment and a high stigma attached to mental health problems. To take the argument further, a considerable proportion of the displaced population after Hurricane Katrina (usually named internally displaced persons (IDPs), but not in the case of the USA) could have benefited from the proposed model. The author is quite right to point out that the gap between the mental health needs of the affected population and the services available is much larger in low- and middle-income countries (LAMICs) than in high-income countries, but that it still exists in both cases.

The values on which the model has been developed are very clear and commendable. They include: orientation toward the human rights of respect and protection, community development alongside emergency and post-emergency response, social justice and equality, participation and involvement of local people and communities, local ownership of programmes, social action and so on. The clear value orientation shows not only that the model fosters belief in the human capacity to deal with the aftermath of disaster, but also that it is deeply rooted in a humanistic perspective. This is clearly illustrated by highly relevant ethical considerations. The author is certainly very knowledgeable, with a wealth of insider's experience.

Consistent with these values is the author's notion that the best prevention of the mental health consequences of political violence is the prevention of conflict and war. This, of course, is a very true but rather idealistic position, and one that is dramatically undermined by the number of new and ongoing conflicts today.

The principles included in most important guidelines for mental health and psychosocial response after major incidents and disasters are embedded in the DPMH approach [1–4]. Without downplaying the importance of psychotropic medicine, the emphasis is on resources provided by the social (support) approach. The social approach is advocated as fundamental to protecting and promoting the well-being of affected populations. The seminal five intervention principles [5] are also integrated throughout the model. They are very appropriately supplemented with selective psychological and psychiatric interventions.

The chapter systematically presents a number of issues that are of paramount importance to both first and ongoing response by various stakeholders in the aftermath of massive political violence and traumatisation. They are very practical, whether they be related to assessment, intervention, management or evaluation. This feature of the text makes the chapter very user-friendly for any organisation that deals with mental health services. Another overarching message is that the public mental health approach requires a change of professional culture, and strong leadership in achieving such change. Resistance is likely because this approach can be seen as decreasing some of the benefits among the high-status professions. The model differs from day-to-day care in most countries, which might be perceived as a threat to the current power structures. On the other hand, the crisis brought about a disaster or the consequences of political violence might open up new ways forward, introducing new social structures and practices.

The essential role of the broader framework that needs to be accounted for when discussing mental health services in LAMICs is also appropriately emphasised. These issues include political, sociocultural and (un)safe circumstances which can obstruct planning and delivery of mental health services in countries with fragile governance and questionable rule of law.

The chapter describes three phases in the development of DPMH: assessment, criteria defining the priorities for mental health and psychosocial interventions, and the interventions themselves. The assessment paragraphs are very concrete and practical. The listing and description of the 10 criteria for setting the priorities is also very helpful.

However, I was less enthusiastic about Phase 3: Interventions. The primary prevention of mental health problems at the level of society-at-large really stretches the concept of 'eliminating the disorder before it can occur', entailing international involvement in preventing conflict (which conflict would inevitably lead to deterioration of mental health). I agree that prevention of organised violence (as any other violence) is a great contributor to good mental health and population well-being, but this form of prevention incorporates international relations and power struggles, international political and financial interests and so on under the banner 'mental health prevention'. I would suggest omission of such factors from the matrix and concentrating on the societal actions that can be more directly connected with mental health protection and interventions. As it stands now, the DPMH model matrix can be seen as a model for enforcing international peace!

The second objection to the matrix is that it focuses almost exclusively on post-conflict societies, while neglecting its applicability to post-natural disasters and post-manmade disasters (apart from war!). Though this reflects the author's bias towards the consequences of political violence, which we have seen in other parts of the chapter, it would be good if the matrix could present a better balanced list of possible interventions that would include specifics of the other types of disaster.

The DPMH model presented in this chapter is a highly relevant text which will provide readers with essential new knowledge and increase their cultural awareness of the manifold aspects of its introduction in a given setting. The author has skilfully used his enormous experience from many trouble spots around the world to highlight the issues that are essential in the planning and delivery of mental health services under severe constraints. The professional and human values that are built into the model clearly reflect the high ethical concern with international involvement in helping LAMICs deal with the mental health aftermath of political violence.

COMMENTARY

6.2 Disaster Mental Health and Public Health: An Integrative Approach to Recovery

Suresh Bada Math,[1] Channaveerachari Naveen Kumar[1] and Maria Christine Nirmala[2]

[1] *Department of Psychiatry, National Institute of Mental Health and Neurosciences (NIMHANS), Bangalore, India*

[2] *Lead Knowledge Management, Private Multinational Company, Bangalore, India*

INTRODUCTION

Dr Joop de Jong outlines in his chapter a series of issues related to disaster mental health management from a public health perspective by proposing a DPMH model. The proposed DPMH model uses a spectrum approach towards mental health and psychosocial issues. Careful analysis of the model reveals that though it is largely consistent with theory, it is silent about issues related to resilience. We certainly agree with the DPMH model regarding integrating public health principles into disaster mental health. However, the issue is, how can we integrate public health in the existing disaster mental health framework? To help address this question, we focus on the important paradigm shifts required to move from a curative to a preventive aspect of disaster mental health.

Contemporary disaster mental health is based on the principles of preventive medicine. This has necessitated a paradigm shift from relief-centred post-disaster management to a holistic, multidimensional integrated community approach incorporating disaster prevention, preparedness and mitigation. Community and individual reactions to disasters may follow a more or less predictable

Post-traumatic Stress Disorder, First Edition. Edited by Dan Stein, Matthew Friedman, and Carlos Blanco.

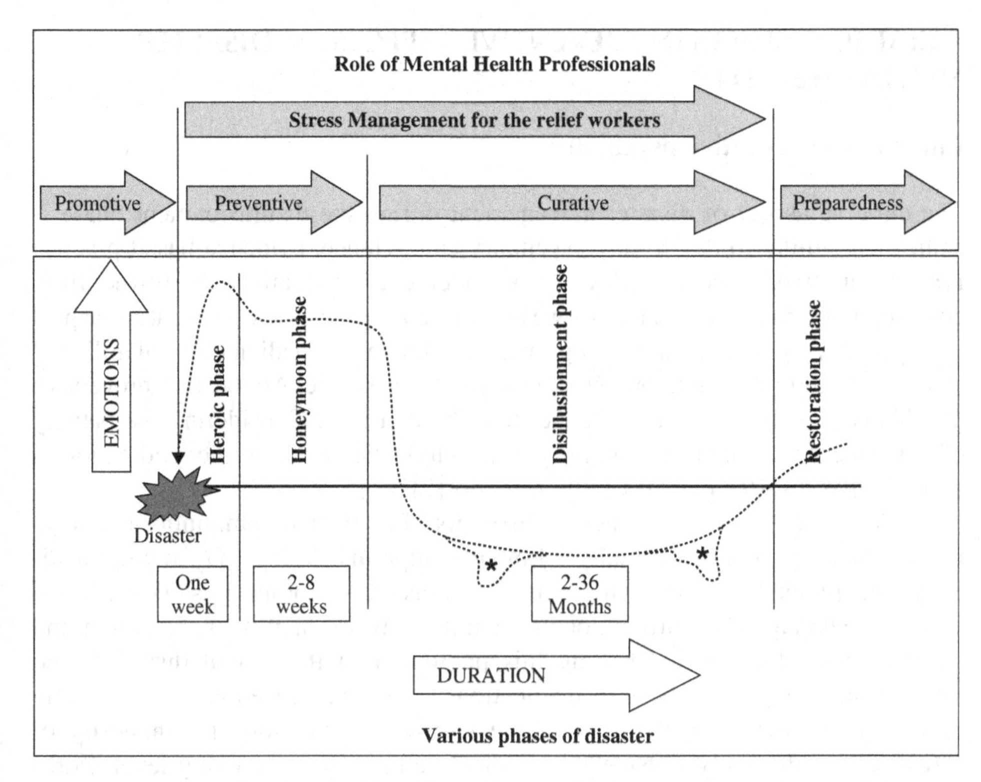

Figure 6.1 The role of mental health professionals during various phases of disaster. Immediately after the disaster, the heroic phase sets in. This is followed by the honeymoon phase. The disillusionment phase is the longest and the prevalence of mental health morbidity is high during this period. *, anniversary reactions.

pattern, involving the heroic phase, honeymoon phase, disillusionment phase and restoration phase [6, 7] (see Figure 6.1). Mental health disorders noted during the heroic and honeymoon phases are self-limiting and have low prevalence, whereas during the disillusionment phase the prevalence of mental disorders is high, necessitating assistance from mental health professionals. The window (heroic and honeymoon phases) immediately after the disaster calls for preventive measures in survivors. Identification of the high-risk group is essential in planning management so that preventive measures can be adopted to mitigate the suffering in survivors. This has ignited the paradigm shift from curative to preventive aspects of disaster management. The new paradigm can be understood on the basis of six 'R's: **R**eadiness (preparedness), **R**esponse (immediate action), **R**elief (sustained rescue work), **R**ehabilitation (long-term remedial measures using community resources), **R**ecovery (returning to normalcy) and **R**esilience (fostering).

PARADIGM SHIFTS IN PREVENTIVE ASPECTS OF DISASTER MENTAL HEALTH

Curative to preventive psychiatry

The curative aspect of disaster management during the disillusionment phase is somewhat similar to day-to-day psychiatry care. Hence, evidence-based practice for the curative aspects of disaster management care can be borrowed from contemporary psychiatry care. However, the challenge is the preventive aspect of psychiatry, which is similar to preventive and social medicine. Availability of evidence-based practice in preventive psychiatry is scarce. Advocating preventive psychiatry thus becomes a challenge in such situations. Considering the paucity of evidence it is difficult to recommend prophylactic psychotropic medication in a preventive disaster mental health scenario [8].

In addition to diagnosable mental disorders, the affected community may also harbour a large number of subsyndromal symptoms. Many may report medically unexplained somatic symptoms and unusual symptom clusters are often seen [9]. Mental health professionals should be aware of this phenomenon and restrain themselves from labelling this population with 'mental disorder' and treating them aggressively with medications [10]. Specialised care is generally only required for a small group of the survivor population. The majority of care occurs informally outside the medical setting by community-level workers. Training these community-level workers is an essential ingredient of disaster management. They must be able to identify severe cases and refer them to mental health professionals.

Demedicalisation

There is a need to demedicalise survivors' response to disaster, to deprofessionalise service delivery and focus on capacity building in the local community. By demedicalising, the stigma of mental illness can be decreased, and by deprofessionalising, there is an opportunity to train survivors, the lay-public, community leaders and significant others in providing care to the affected survivors. Demedicalisation need not threaten mental health professionals because they must still play a major role in disaster mental health, as shown in Table. 6.1.There is a need to recruit an army of trained, motivated grass-root workers to provide assistance during large-scale disasters.

Disaster assistance in the form of community empowerment

Assistance should be culturally appropriate and targeted towards empowering the affected community, in order to enhance their camaraderie and competence

Table 6.4 Role of mental health professionals in disaster [11, 12].

I. During pre-disaster period (preparedness)
  1. Public education – life-skills education, educating about disaster mental health
  2. Disaster response network – to develop collaboration with various existing agencies such as (non)governmental agencies and community health workers
  3. Disaster response training of trainers in:
     a. disaster mental health
     b. first aid (both medical and psychological)
     c. counselling skills
     d. stress management
     e. identifying common mental disorders and referral
     f. life-skills education
  4. Strengthening information, education and communication (IEC) activities

II. Immediately after the disaster (heroic and honeymoon phases)
  1. Being part of the multidisciplinary relief team
  2. Rapid assessment of:
     a. magnitude of the psychological impact
     b. available mental health resources in the affected community
     c. needs
     d. social, cultural and religious perspective of the community
  3. Providing health care:
     a. medical and psychological first aid
     b. treatment of preexisting mentally ill patients
     c. substance intoxication and withdrawal in survivors
     d. establishing the referral system
  4. Creating disaster psychiatry outreach teams to provide care
  5. Collaborating with administrative and funding agencies
  6. Dealing with victim and volunteer stress (stress management)
  7. Fostering mass grieving/mourning
  8. Mental health education – do's and do not's:
     a. educating administrative personnel, local leaders and the public
     b. utilising mass media to reach the survivors
  9. Initiating collaboration with local agencies for capacity building and outside agencies for support
  10. Planning research

III. During disillusionment phase
  1. Providing care for mentally ill patients
  2. Attending to referrals
  3. Continuing and expanding capacity-building activities (training of resourceful community members such as private physicians/doctors, primary health care staff, paramedical staffs, school teachers, grass-root workers, alternative complementary medicine personnels, religious leaders, spiritual leaders and faith healers
  4. Community-outreach camps
  5. Hand-holding of community health workers
  6. Assessment of the interventions and the feedback mechanism

to cope with future disasters [10]. Disaster management needs to follow the principle of democracy – 'of the people, by the people and for the people' – in order for the disaster assistance programme to be acceptable, accessible, adaptable and adoptable for long-term community participation and empowerment. This involves educating and training the local administration, community leaders, nongovernmental organisations, faith healers, community-level workers and survivors. The majority of disasters require not just temporary external aids but mainly permanent aid of community empowerment. Hence, the Sphere Project advocates humanitarian charter and identifies minimum standards for disaster assistance to promote accountability and share standards of good practice [13]. There is an urgent need to form a disaster policy or legislation at the international, regional and national levels for effective disaster management.

Changing focus from 'psychopathology' to 'resilience'

The concept of resilience has been applied to describe the adaptive capacities of individuals or communities in response to adversity or disaster. Majority of the research on disaster is on psychopathology rather than on resilience factors, which has led to a focus on services in curative rather than in preventive form. Hence, there is an urgent need to get disaster mental health services to focus on *fostering resilience factors*, which protect the people from developing mental health morbidity [14]. There are no systematic studies in this regard. However, preliminary research has yielded the following resilience factors: a cohesive community, adequate community resources, minimal displacement, absence of risk factors, good social support [15], preserved family system and support, altruistic behaviour of the community leaders, minimal materialistic needs, religious faith and spirituality. These were all noted in the native population of the Andaman and Nicobar Islands of India following the 2004 tsunami [10]. However, these resilience factors need to be studied systematically in a well-controlled disaster population.

Community-based interventions

Nonspecific community-based interventions play a major role in fostering the healing process. These interventions include: structuring of daily activities; avoiding displacement; fostering family, cultural and religious rituals; group discussions; validation of the emotions of the survivors' experience and survivors' guilt; providing factual information; educating parents and teachers; engaging children in various informal education methods using innovative ideas like drawing, sketching, singing, miming and so forth, utilising available community resources; engaging adult survivors in camp activities such as cooking, cleaning and assisting in relief work; setting up schools in the disaster-affected areas at the earliest possible date so that normalisation and structuring of daily activities occur in children; at the very least initiating informal education; teaching simple sleep hygiene techniques; educating survivors about the harmful effects of substance use; planning community-based group interventions such as art therapy (painting/drawing), group discussions, drama, storytelling, structuring the day, engaging in activities, prayers, yoga, relaxation and sports/games; stress management of relief workers; engaging willing survivors in spiritual activities; and involving survivors in rebuilding their community [16, 17].

CONCLUSION

Disaster mental health services needs to make the paradigm shift from curative to preventive aspects by including principles of public health. Nonspecific community-based group interventions are simple, easy to implement using local resources, effective in all groups, and provide important components of psychosocial rehabilitation such as normalising, stabilising, socialising, defusing emotions and feelings, and restoring a sense of identification with others and of safety and security, while allowing for the normal healing process and instilling hope for the future in survivors [18]. These interventions may help not only in the recovery of milder and subsyndromal symptoms, but also in the prevention of adverse mental health consequences. Such interventions, when feasible, should begin as early as possible.

COMMENTARY

6.3 Transcultural Aspects of Response to Disasters

Tarek A. Okasha
Department of Psychiatry, Institute of Psychiatry, Faculty of Medicine, Ain Shams University, Cairo, Egypt

Joop de Jong's chapter on '(Disaster) Public Mental Health' touches on many issues, but I would like to discuss just one: cultural sensitivity.

A report by the Red Cross has highlighted the differential impact of disasters in developing countries. In the period 1967–1991, an average of 17 million people living in developing countries were affected by disasters each year, as compared to about 700 000 in developed countries (a striking ratio of 166 to 1) [19]. These communities are particularly at risk in the face of disasters because they are already under strain and have few resources in reserve for use at times when rescue and protection are required. Their health systems tend to be rudimentary and to have little mental health capability. In Iraq at least 3 million people have been displaced by the war and another million are wounded or dead, 70% of them are women and children [20].

Social support is frequently mentioned as a critical factor that protects individuals following exposure to disasters [21]. The perception of social support is critically determined by the individual's personality. In a prospective study, personality characteristics such as neuroticism were an important determinant of the perception of social support [22]. Perceived social support also depends upon the belief about the availability of others to assist rather than the actual receipt of assistance. Solomon *et al.* [23] made the interesting observation that mid-range levels of support availability were associated with the most favourable outcomes for women. In contrast, women with high support availability did poorly. This study also found that women with excellent spouse support had worse outcomes than those with weaker spouse ties. In contrast, men tended to do better if they had a stronger spouse relationship. This suggests that there are

Post-traumatic Stress Disorder, First Edition. Edited by Dan Stein, Matthew Friedman, and Carlos Blanco.

gender differences, where the strength of attachment for women may be a burden rather than supportive at times of extreme stress.

Another important factor is resilience, which from a psychological perspective is defined as 'a person's capacity for adapting psychologically, emotionally and physically reasonably well and without lasting detriment to self, relationships or personal development in the face of adversity, threat or challenge' [24]. Usually children show a remarkable resilience to civilian disasters; it is surprising how often children and adolescents are reported to adapt to conditions of war and disaster with little evidence of manifest distress. The cognitive immaturity, plasticity and adaptive capacities of children have often veiled the effects of war [25].

Several factors affect resilience: (i) intelligence and temperament – there is research evidence showing that resilient children 'tend to possess an above average intelligence and a temperament that endears them to others'; (ii) family relationships and the level of support available from family – there is evidence that the role of family in the development of resilience is most important early in life and declines as children grow older; and (iii) external support from other persons and institutions – support of specific types for their families is a major discriminating factor in resilient urban children who have experienced life stresses. These positive social supports must actively include the children at risk and are best when whole families are supported [26].

In the warning phase of a disaster, there are often false alarms, which must be responded to rather than ignored. In the midst of the disaster, tolerance of a loss of control and the ability to function in the face of helplessness are attributes that facilitate adaptive behaviour. The individual must be able to move into an active stance when appropriate, rather than presuming that external help will resolve the situation or provide assistance. At a community and individual level, as the disaster further recedes into the past, an attitude that embodies optimism rather than demoralisation is critical to rebuilding a sense of a future world. Tolerance of distress in oneself and others and progression beyond post-disaster attachments are likely predictors of a positive outcome [27].

In the Gaza situation in Palestine the whole community, even the traditional sources of protection (e.g., parental authority) had been undermined. Gaza has a relatively large number of young individuals (age $< 20 = 60\%$): it is unknown what the long-term consequences are for the development of an individual when a whole generation has been traumatized.

Most children living in the Occupied Palestinian Territory (OPT) have directly experienced or witnessed physical or psychological violence. Curfews are considered as a collective punishment, turning every home into a prison; the result is the total breakdown of normal patterns of social and economic interactions. Curfews create frustration, and one of the main common responses to frustration is active aggression. If the stressful condition continues, and the individual is unable to cope with it, apathy may deepen into depression [28].

Palestinians have expressed serious concerns about the future consequences of these shattered parental bonds. There is a common belief that children who threw stones and fought against the occupation army may challenge their parents' authority [29].

A study in Gaza Community conducted by the Gaza Community Mental Health Program among children aged 10–9 years revealed that 32.7% suffered from PTSD symptoms requiring psychological intervention, 49.2% from moderate PTSD symptoms, 15.6% from mild PTSD symptoms, and only 2.5% had no symptoms [30].

After the tsunami disaster in Indonesia in 2004, it was found that many children who lost their parents had the resilience and coping behaviour not to develop post-traumatic stress disorder (PTSD). This was attributed to the power of religiosity and social support. The local population was a group of conservative Muslims who attributed the disaster to the wrath of God. The diagnosis of PTSD should be addressed with cultural sensitivity [20]. Traumatic events produce great damage not so much because of the immediate harm they cause but because of the lingering need to reevaluate one's view of oneself and the world [24, 31].

Advocates of 'cross-cultural universality' argue that syndromes hold true across cultures and tend to recommend full application of screening, assessment, diagnostic and intervention techniques that have been developed in Western approaches to mental health care. Proponents of 'cultural specificity' argue that the significance of experiences and symptoms should be understood in relations to the culture from which the affected individual comes. Delivery of mental health intervention in non-Western settings needs to incorporate prevailing cultural norms, including spiritual or religious involvement, basic ontological beliefs and related issues [32, 33].

In conclusion, it is essential to note that an understanding of vulnerability and protective factors is necessary in explaining the probability of developing post-disaster morbidity. PTSD and other trauma-related disorders represent the outcome of a complex biopsychosocial matrix of variables. These factors can operate along a variety of axes. The context in which the event occurs in the individual's life is the base from which the disorder emerges. The nature of the stressor, resilience, coping behaviour, cultural and religious factors, and the recovery environment involve a series of interactions that modify the ability of the individual to quench their immediate post-traumatic distress. It is in this post-disaster period that these vulnerability factors may play a critical role. On the other hand, it is important to emphasise that PTSD may emerge in previously healthy individuals whose modest vulnerability would otherwise have had little relevance.

COMMENTARY

6.4 Disaster Public Health: Health Needs, Psychological First Aid and Cultural Awareness

Robert J. Ursano,[1] Matthew N. Goldenberg,[2] Derrick Hamaoka[2] and David M. Benedek[1]

[1] *Department of Psychiatry and Neuroscience; Department of Psychiatry; Center for the Study of Traumatic Stress, Uniformed Services University of the Health Sciences, Bethesda, MD, USA*

[2] *Department of Psychiatry; Center for the Study of Traumatic Stress, Uniformed Services University of the Health Sciences, Bethesda, MD, USA*

Disasters are unfortunately common and span the globe. They include both natural events, such as earthquakes and hurricanes, and human-made disasters such as technological disaster and armed conflict, of which there are currently more than two dozen around the world [34–36]. Disasters result not only in bodily injury and death but also in mental health problems that can far outweigh the physical casualties in illness burden on the community. The costs of these often hidden injuries may be dramatic. Rarely is an adequate mental health response planned or funded. The mental health casualties of disaster disproportionately affect those who were disadvantaged prior to the disaster, including the poor and the previously ill. This disparity is the result of increased risk factors for individual distress (e.g. prior mental illness), the degree of community destruction (e.g. location in a flood plain) as well as the absence of recovery resources (e.g. post-disaster access to medical care, food, clean water).

As Dr de Jong points out in his chapter, planning for and responding to the mental health needs of a population following a disaster requires a public health approach rather than an individual treatment perspective [37]. Such an approach

Post-traumatic Stress Disorder, First Edition. Edited by Dan Stein, Matthew Friedman, and Carlos Blanco.

may be unfamiliar to many mental health providers, but sensitive and thoughtful public health practitioners can assist. Prior to a disaster, attention should be paid to developing and shoring up community emergency-response resources in the areas of public safety (police and fire), medical care, housing and communications. Public education campaigns must address the need for personal and family contingencies, including emergency supplies of food and water, and evacuation and reunification plans. During or immediately following a disaster, various interventions are called for. These include broadly administered interventions to mitigate widespread suffering and more targeted interventions aimed at those exhibiting significant distress, risky behaviours and/or mental illness.

Psychological first aid is a set of evidence-informed principles to guide early post-disaster interventions [38–40]. These include: (i) providing safety and care for injury; (ii) calming fears and worries; (iii) connecting people with loved ones and caring others for instrumental and emotional support; (iv) building confidence in the affected individual's own capabilities and enabling new skills; and (v) fostering hope. These principles, which can inform numerous interventions, are supported by empirical studies indicating that they enhance psychological recovery and health and sustain resilience.

Mental and behavioural health surveillance to identify those most in need of additional services is an important part of post-disaster response [37–39]. This includes identifying those whose behavioural health symptoms have emerged in the wake of the disaster as well as those with preexisting conditions that need care. Some people with preexisting illnesses may experience an exacerbation of their symptoms or become disconnected from prior support services as a result of disaster. Others may never have previously sought care but do so now because of its availability or changes in their social network patterns ('emergent mental health needs'). Even those without significant psychiatric history may develop concerning symptoms, behaviours and conditions, including distress, fear and anger, increased cigarette or alcohol use, and depression or PTSD.

Surveillance plans for schools, workplaces, hospitals, shelters and camps provides valuable information about the resource and care needs of the affected population. Screening, referral, provision of safety and other basic needs, keeping families and communities together, are important principles of post-disaster public mental health care [41–43].

Engagement with the disaster community is critical to the success of post-disaster interventions. Community leaders, from clergy to local healers and elected officials to teachers, are invaluable to disaster response and health care planning and delivery. Because they speak with and for their communities, local leaders provide vital information about their communities' culture, resources and needs. Culturally sensitive care and operations are the sine qua non of successful disaster mental health interventions, so it is critically important that response teams engage persons knowledgeable of local customs, structures, symbols and language. Alliance with community leadership provides disaster workers with the knowledge and credibility to work successfully with the community, to respond to disaster and to build the capacity for long-term recovery and care. The disaster worker is a visitor and his or her work must be both culturally sensitive and sustainable if it is to be effective.

Dr de Jong highlights sustainability as one of the three essential elements of an effective programme – along with political acceptability and ethical practice. Focusing on sustainability, beginning with the initial disaster response, increases the likelihood of long-term success. This must include planning for the rebuilding of the psychosocial support infrastructure and planning for the transition from surge support to reestablished local and more permanent resources. Political acceptance of an intervention is important. It can ensure both access to the population in need and resources for assistance. Finally, ethical practice – including the just treatment of all and respect for fundamental human rights – is indispensible.

In his comprehensive chapter, Dr de Jong emphasises that the mental health response begins before the event and extends long after. Disaster mental health care requires the desire to help; skills and knowledge of medical care and public health; and the ability to engage the affected community, manage the inevitable adversities and persist.

REFERENCES

1. Inter-Agency Standing Committee (IASC) (2007) *IASC Guidelines on Mental Health and Psychosocial Support in Emergency Settings*, IASC, Geneva.
2. NATO (2008) *Psychosocial Care for People Affected by Disasters and Major Incidents*, NATO, Bruxelles.
3. International Federation Reference Centre for Psychosocial Support (2009) Psychosocial Interventions – A Handbook, International Federation Reference Centre for Psychosocial Support, Copenhagen.
4. Bisson, J.I., Tavakoly, B., Witteveen, A.B., *et al*. (2010) TENTS guidelines: development of post-disaster psychosocial care guidelines through a Delphi Process. *The British Journal of Psychiatry*, **196**, 69–74.
5. Hobfoll, S.E., Watson, P., Bell, C.C. *et al*. (2007) Five essential elements of immediate and mid-term mass trauma intervention: empirical evidence. *Psychiatry*, **70**, 283–315.
6. Math, S.B., Girimaji, S.C., Benegal, V. *et al*. (2006) Tsunami: psychosocial aspects of Andaman and Nicobar islands. Assessments and intervention in the early phase. *International Review of Psychiatry*, **18**, 233–239.
7. Young, B.H., Ford, J.D., Ruzek, J.I. *et al*. (1998) Disaster Mental Health Services: A Guide for Clinicians and Administrators. National Center for Post-Traumatic Stress Disorder, Palo Alto, California.
8. Asher, S. and Jack, G. (2004) Psychopharmacological possibilities in the acute disaster setting. *The Psychiatric Clinics of North America*, **27** (3), 425–458.

9. North, C.S. (2002) Somatization in survivors of catastrophic trauma: a methodological review. *Environmental Health Perspectives*, **110**, 637–640.
10. Math, S.B., John, J.P., Girimaji, S.C. *et al*. (2008) Comparative study of psychiatric morbidity among the displaced and non-displaced populations in the Andaman and Nicobar Islands following the tsunami. *Prehospital and Disaster Medicine*, **23**, 29–34.
11. Math, S.B., Maria, C.N., Naveen, C.K. *et al*. Disaster Mental Health: A Paradigm Shift From Curative to Preventive Psychiatry. Submitted for publication in review process.
12. Math, S.B. and Chaturvedi, S.K. Disaster Psychiatry: Management and Disaster Preparedness. Submitted for publication in Asian Text Book of Psychiatry, in press.
13. The Sphere Project (2004) Humanitarian Charter and Minimum Standards in Disaster Response, WHO, Geneva: Sphere Project 2004. Available online http://www.sphereproject.org/component/option,com_docman/task,doc_download/gid,12/Itemid,26/lang,English/ (accessed 21 January 2010).
14. North, C.S., Hong, B.A., Suris, A. and Spitznagel, E.L. (2008) Distinguishing distress and psychopathology among survivors of the Oakland/Berkeley firestorm. *Psychiatry*, **71**, 35–45.
15. López-ibor, J.J., Christodoulou, G., Maj, M. *et al*. (eds) (2005) *Disasters and Mental Health*, John Wiley & Sons, Ltd, West Sussex, England.
16. Kar, N. (2009) Psychological impact of disasters on children: review of assessment and interventions. *World Journal of Pediatrics*, **5**, 5–11.
17. Math, S.B., Tandon, S., Girimaji, S.C. *et al*. (2008) Psychological impact of the tsunami on children and adolescents from the Andaman and Nicobar islands. *Primary Care Companion to the Journal of Clinical Psychiatry*, **10**, 31–37.
18. Suresh, S., Karim, M.E., Lourdes, L.-I. *et al*. (2008) Psychosocial responses to disaster. *An Asian Perspective. Asian Journal of Psychiatry*, **1** (1), 7–14.
19. International Federation of Red Cross and Red Crescent Societies (1993) World Disaster Report, 1993, Nijhoff, Dordrecht.
20. Okasha, A. (2010) Human rights is an investment for mental health. Plenary Lecture at the Annual Meeting of the Scandinavian Psychiatric Association, Sweden.
21. Norris, F. and Kaniasty, K. (1996) Received and perceived social support in times of stress: a test of the social support deterioration deterrence model. *Personality and Social Psychology*, **71**, 498–511.
22. Henderson, S., Byrne, G., Duncan-Jones, P. *et al*. (1980) Social relationships, adversity and neurosis: a study of associations in a general population sample. *British Journal of Psychiatry*, **136**, 574–583.
23. Solomon, Z., Mikulincer, M. and Hobfoll, S.E. (1987) Objective versus subjective measurement of stress and social support: combat-related reactions. *Consulting and Clinical Psychology*, **55**, 577–583.
24. Brett, R. and McCallin, M. (1998) Children: the Invisible Soldiers, Radda Barnen Swedish Save the Children.
25. Edwards, J.G. (1976) Psychiatric aspects of civilian disasters. *British Medical Journal*, **1** (6015), 944–947.

26. Condly, S.J. (2006) Resilience in children: a review of the literature with implications for education. *Urban Education*, **41**, 211–236.
27. McFarlin, A. (2005) Psychiatric morbidities following disasters: epidemiology, risk and protective factors, in *Disasters and Mental Health* (eds J.J. Lopez-Ibor, G. Christodoulou, M. Maj *et al.*), World Psychiatric Association, John Wiley & Sons, Inc., pp. 37–63.
28. Qouta, S. and El Sarraj, E. (1994) Palestinian Children under curfew. *Psychol Studies*, **4**, 1–12.
29. Garbarino, J., Kostelny, K. and Dubrow, N. (1991) What Children can tell us about living in danger? *American Psychologist*, **46**, 376–383.
30. Qouta, S. and El Sarraj, E. (2005) *Disaster and Mental Health: The Palestinian Experience*, *World Psychiatric Association*, Chapter 16, John Wiley & Sons, Ltd, pp. 229–237.
31. Yehuda, R. and Hyman, S.E. (2005) The impact of terrorism on brain, and behaviour: what we know and what we need to know. *Neuropsychopharmacology*, **30**, 1773–1780.
32. Williams, R. (2006) The psychosocial consequences for children and young people who are exposed to terrorism, war, conflict and natural disasters. *Current Opinion in Psychiatry*, **19** (4), 337–349.
33. Barenbaum, J., Ruchkin, V. and Schwab-Stone, M. (2004) *The psychosocial aspects of children exposed to war: practice and policy initiatives*. *Journal of Child Psychology and Psychiatry*, **45**, 41–62.
34. Benjamin, G., McGeary, M. and McCutchen, S. (eds), Committee on Medical Preparedness for a Terrorist Nuclear Event (2009) *Assessing Medical Preparedness to Respond to a Terrorist Nuclear Event: Workshop Report*, Institute of Medicine, Washington, DC.
35. Butler, A.S., Panzer, A.M. and Goldfrank, L.R. (eds) (2003) *Preparing the Psychological Consequences of Terrorism: A Public Health Strategy* (Committee on Responding to the Psychological Consequences of Terrorism Board on Neuroscience and Behavioral Health: Lewis R. Goldfrank, MD, Gerard A. Jacobs, PhD, Carol S. North, MD, M.P.E. Patricia Quinlisk, MD, MPH, Robert J. Ursano, MD, Nancy Wallace, CSW, Marlene Wong, LCSW, Andrew Pope, PhD, Adrienne Stith Butler, PhD), Institute of Medicine, The National Academies Press.
36. Fullerton, C.S., Reissman, D.B., Gray, C. *et al*. (2010) Earthquake response and psychosocial health outcomes: applying lessons from integrating systems of care and recovery to haiti. *Disaster Medicine and Public Health Preparedness*, **4** (1), 15–17.
37. Ursano, R.J., Fullerton, C.S., Raphael, B. and Weisaeth, L. (eds) (2007) *Textbook of Disaster Psychiatry*, Cambridge University Press, London.
38. Hamaoka, D., Benedek, D.M. and Ursano, R.J. (2008) Managing psychological consequences in disaster populations, in *Psychiatry*, 3rd edn, vol. 2 (eds A. Tasman, J. Kay and J. Lieberman), John Wiley & Sons, Ltd, Chichester, pp. 2465–2477.
39. Hamaoka, D., Benedek, D.M., Grieger, T. and Ursano, R.J. (2007) Crisis intervention, in *Encyclopedia of Stress*, 2nd edn (ed. G. Fink), Elsevier/Academic Press, London.

40. Hobfoll, S., Watson, P., Bell, C.C. *et al*. (2007) Five essential elements of immediate and mid-term mass trauma intervention: empirical evidence. *Psychiatry: Interpersonal and Biological Processes*, **70**(4), Winter, 283–315.
41. Benedek, D.M., Friedman, M.J., Zatzick, D. and Ursano, R.J. (2009) Guideline watch: practice guideline for the treatment of patients with acute stress disorder and posttraumatic stress disorder, *FOCUS*, **7**, 1–9.
42. Benedek, D.M. and Wynn, G.H. (2010) *Clinical Manual for Management of PTSD*, American Psychiatric Press, Washington, DC.
43. Blumenfield, M. and Ursano, R.J. (eds) (2008) *Early Intervention After Mass Violence*, Cambridge University Press, London.

Index

access to care 83–4
acute stress disorder (ASD) 1, 17–18
  cognitive behaviour therapy (CBT) 174
  early intervention 180–1
  epidemiology 66–7
adjustment disorders (ADs) 1, 19, 43
adrenocorticotrophic hormone (ACTH) 99
age as a risk factor for PTSD 62
agoraphobia, post-traumatic 187
alcohol abuse 64–5
allopregnanolone (ALLO) 98–9
allostatic stress hypothesis 120, 139–41, 143–4
γ-amino butyric acid (GABA) 94, 95
amygdala
  basolateral nucleus (BLA) 91–2, 94, 95–6
  central nucleus (CE) 91–2
  fear response 96–7
  monoaminergic modulation 94–5
  structural alterations in PTSD 107
  traumatic stimulus response 2
analgesia, stress-induced 2
anger 190
anterior cingulate cortex (ACC)
  connectivity 118
  structural abnormalities in PTSD 107–8, 117
anterior cingulate gyrus 2
anxiety disorders not otherwise specified (NOS) 6
archicortical system 105, 116, 119
avoidance behaviours 2
  external reminders (DSM-IV-TR Criterion C2) 13
  internal reminders (DSM-IV-TR Criterion C1) 13
avoidance, excessive 190

basolateral nucleus of the amygdala (BLA) 91–2, 94, 95–6
  fear response 96–7
BDNF gene 102, 103
brain imaging of PTSD
  functional 108–15
  structural 105–8

catastrophic thinking 190–1
central nucleus (CE) of the amygdala 91–2
Child Psychosocial Distress Screener (CPDS) 249
children
  cognitive processing therapy (CPT) 177
  individual and family therapy 252–3
  mental health and psychosocial support (MHPSS)
    classroom-based intervention (CBI) 251–2
    parental support 252
  peace education and conflict resolution at schools 246
  psychological interventions 203–4
    CBT 177
  classroom-based intervention (CBI) 251–2
clinical evaluation of PTSD 38–40, 41

Post-traumatic Stress Disorder, First Edition. Edited by Dan Stein, Matthew Friedman, and Carlos Blanco.

cognitive behaviour therapies (CBTs) 12–14, 172–3
  historical overview 171–2
  mechanisms 173–4
cognitive processing therapy (CPT) 173
  evidence
    adults 175–7
    children 177
combat exhaustion 49
communities in disasters 228
community-based rehabilitation (CBR) 223
community empowerment 244–5, 268–9
comorbidity
  complicated grief 186–7
  depression 185
  generalised anxiety disorder (GAD) 186
  mild traumatic brain injury (MTBI) 188–9
  post-traumatic agoraphobia and panic disorder 187
  psychiatric 64–5
  substance-use disorder 188
compensation 244, 249
complementary and alternative medicine (CAM) 233
complex PTSD 20–2
complicated grief 186–7
conditioned stress responses 97
  allopregnanolone/pregnanolone (ALLO) 98–9
  cortisol 100–1
  dehydroepiandrosterone (DHEA) 99–100
  neuropeptide Y (NPY) 97–8
conditioning 2
context of healing 217–18
contraindications for trauma-focused therapy 190–1
cortisol 100–1
counter-conditioning 172
course of PTSD 65–6
Critical Incident Stress Debriefing (CISD) 178
cultural aspects of public mental health interventions 237–8
cultural factors in PTSD 22–3
D-cycloserine (DCS) 165–6, 168
cytosine-guanine dinucleotide repeats (CpG) 102–3

Da Costa's syndrome 3
dehydroepiandrosterone (DHEA) 99–100
depression 185, 191
development and PTSD 23–4
dinucleotide methyltransferase (DNMT) 103
disaster public mental health (DPMH) model 221–3, 275–7
  Phase 1 – pre-programme and cyclical assessment 226–9
  Phase 2 – defining priorities 230
  Phase 3 – interventions 239–42
disasters 218–19
disorders of extreme stress not otherwise specified (DESNOS) 20–2
dissociative disorder not otherwise specified (DDNOS) 234
dissociative flashbacks (DSM-IV-TR Criterion B3) 12
dissociative identity disorder (DID) 234
dissociative subtype of PTSD 22
dopamine (DA) 92, 93, 94
dorsal striatum 2
DSM-III diagnostic criteria 35–6, 49–50
DSM-IV-TR diagnostic criteria 36–7
  Criterion A1 4, 5–10
  Criterion A2 8–10
  Criterion B 12–13
  Criterion C 13–14
  Criterion D 14–15
  Criterion E 15–16
  Criterion F 16
  factor structure 11
  summary 16–17
DSM-5 diagnostic criteria 37, 42–5

emotional arousal following reminders (DSM-IV-TR Criterion B4) 12
emotional numbing 2

emotional processing theory 2
Epidemiologic Catchment Area (ECA) 51
epidemiological research 75–6, 78
  challenges 76–7
  future horizons 77–8
epidemiology 49–50, 68
  acute stress disorder (ASD) 66–7
  course of PTSD 65–6
  gender-based 82, 84
    access to care 83–4
    prevalence of PTSD 82–3
    refugee status 83
  psychiatric comorbidity 64–5
  role in DPMH model 231–2
  sociodemographic risk factors 62
    age 62
    ethnicity 63
    gender 62
    marital status 63
    race 63
    socioeconomic education 64
    socioeconomic status 63–4
  trauma exposure in general population 50–1, 61
    Australia 55, 61
    Europe 53–5, 59–61
    Latin America 53, 58
    Lebanon 55, 61
    North America 51–8
epigenetic contributions to PTSD risk 102–3
  therapeutic aspects 103–4
ethnicity as a risk factor for PTSD 63
excessive avoidance 190
exposure therapy 171, 172, 211–12
extinction 95–6, 117
eye-movement desensitisation and reprocessing (EMDR) 174–5, 181–2

fear (DSM-IV-TR Criterion A2) 8–10
fear conditioning 2
fear conditioning and extinction 96–7, 142–4
  monoaminergic modulation
    amygdala 94–5
    prefrontal cortex (PFC) 93–4
  species-specific defence response (SSDR) 92–3
  unconditioned defence responses 91–2
fluoxetine 151
forensic evaluation of PTSD 40–1

gender as a risk factor for PTSD 62, 82, 84
  access to care 83–4
  prevalence 82–3
  refugee status 83
generalised anxiety disorder (GAD) 65, 186
genetic contributions to PTSD risk 101–2

helplessness (DSM-IV-TR Criterion A2) 8–10
hippocampus 2
  reduced volume in PTSD 105–7
historical perspective 3–4
horror (DSM-IV-TR Criterion A2) 8–10
humanitarian relief operations 243
hyperarousal 2
hyperarousal subtype of PTSD 22
hypervigilance 2
hypothalamic-pituitary-adrenal (HPA) axis 144
hypothalamus 2
hysteria 234

idiom of distress 233–4
Institute of Medicine (IOM) 152, 153, 167–8
insula 2
internally displaced persons (IDPs) 264
International Classification of Diseases (ICD) 50
interventions for public mental health 254
  nongovernmental organisations (NGOs) coordinating public mental health 239–42
  primary prevention 240
  primary prevention, community-focused 244–247
  primary prevention, family and individual 248–249

interventions for public mental health (*cont.*)
  primary prevention, societal 242
  secondary prevention 241
  secondary prevention, community-focused 274
  secondary prevention, family and individual 249–253
  secondary prevention, societal 243–244
  tertiary prevention 241, 254

key informant (KI) interviews 229
kindling hypothesis 120, 143

locus ceruleus (LC) 2, 92
low- and middle-income countries (LAMICs) 219
  suitability of MHPSS model 263–5
  treatment gaps in conflicts and disasters 220–1
  treatment needs and treatment gaps 219–20

major depressive disorder (MDD) 64
marital status as a risk factor for PTSD 63
medial prefrontal cortex 2
mental health and psychosocial support (MHPSS) 225, 226
  children 251–252
  integrative approach to recovery 266–271
  mental health 253
  psychosocial support
    counselling 250–1
    self-help groups 250
  suitability for LAMICs 263–5
N-methyl-D-aspartate (NMDA) 95
mild traumatic brain injury (MTBI) 188–9
mirtazepine 152
monoaminergic modulation
  amygdala 94–5
  prefrontal cortex (PFC) 93–4
motor-vehicle accident (MVA) survivors 67

National Institute for Clinical Excellence (NICE) 152–3
neurobiology 120–1
  background 89–90
    complexity and heterogeneity 90–1
  fear conditioning and extinction 91, 96–7
    conditioned stress 95–6
    monoaminergic modulation 93–5
    species-specific defence response (SSDR) 92–3
    unconditioned defence responses 91–2
  modulation of conditioned stress responses 97
    allopregnanolone/pregnanolone (ALLO) 98–9
    cortisol 100–1
    dehydroepiandrosterone (DHEA) 99–100
    neuropeptide Y (NPY) 97–8
  structural and functional neuroanatomy
    conceptual framework 104–5
    connectivity patterns 118–20
    functional brain imaging of PTSD 108–15
    structural brain imaging of PTSD 105–8
    synthesis of animal and human studies 116–18
neurocirculatory asthemia 3
neuropeptide Y (NPY) 97–8
  gene 101, 103
nongovernmental organisations (NGOs) coordinating public mental health 239–42
norepinephrine (NE; noradrenaline) 93, 94
nostalgia 3
nucleus accumbens (NA) 92
numbing symptom 11

ongoing stressors 191
orbitofrontal cortex 2

paleocortical system 105, 116
panic disorder 187

parahippocampal subdivision of the brain 104–5
parapiriform subdivision of the brain 104–5
partial PTSD 20
Pavlovian fear conditioning 2
pharmacotherapy 149, 158–9
  critical view 163
  development 149–52
  evidence 152–4
  key issues 154
    comparison with psychotherapy 157
    dose and duration 155
    optimal SSRI 154–5
    prophylaxis of PTSD 158
    PTSD subtypes and spectrum 155–7
    treatment-refractory PTSD 157–8
  need for new agents 167–8
  shortcomings 164–6
physiological arousal following reminders (DSM-IV-TR Criterion B5) 12
political violence 218–19
possession trance 234
post-traumatic agoraphobia 187
post-traumatic stress disorder (PTSD)
  complex 20–2
  cross-cultural factors 22–3
  developmental issues 23–4
  disorders of extreme stress not otherwise specified (DESNOS) 20–2
  features 1–2
  partial 20
  redefining for DSM-5 42–5
  subsyndromal 20
  subtypes 22
  treatment-refractory 157–8
prefrontal cortex (PFC) 92
  extinction 95–6
  fear response 96–7
  hypoactivation in PTSD 117
  monoaminergic modulation 93–4
pregnanolone (ALLO) 98–9
preventing mental ill-health following trauma 79–81, 239–242
prisoners of war 40–1
prophylaxis of PTSD 158
  early intervention for all trauma-exposed individuals 178–80
  early intervention for PTSD/ASD 180–1
  eye-movement desensitisation and reprocessing (EMDR) 181–2
prospective studies 144–5
psychiatric comorbidity 64–5
Psychological First Aid (PFA) 180
psychological interventions 171, 191–2
  children 203–4
  clinical guidelines 182–5
  comorbidity 185–189
  contraindications 190–191
  evidence 175
    CBT in adults 175–7
    CBT in children 177
    prophylactic approaches 177–82
  exposure therapy 211–12
  further evidence needed 208–10
  Hispanics 205–7
  historical overview 171–2
  major interventions
    cognitive behaviour therapy (CBT) 172–4
    eye-movement desensitisation and reprocessing (EMDR) 174–5
psychotherapy compared with pharmacotherapy 157
public mental health issues
  background 221
    political violence, war and disaster 218–19
    therapist, context and technique 217–18
    treatment gaps in LAMICs 220–1
    treatment needs and treatment gaps 219–20
  core concepts and definitions 225–6
  scope 221–3
    basic principles 224

quality of interventions 234, 243–4

race as a risk factor for PTSD 63
railway spine 3
raphe nuclei 92
recurrent intrusive recollections (DSM-IV-TR Criterion B1) 12
refugee status and PTSD 83
reparation 244, 249
repatriation, voluntary 244
reptilian brain 104–5
risk factors for PTSD 39–40
  sociodemographic 62
    age 62
    ethnicity 63
    gender 62
    marital status 63
    race 63
    socioeconomic education 64
    socioeconomic status 63–4

selective serotonin reuptake inhibitors (SSRIs) 150–1, 152–3
  dose and duration 155
  optimal for PTSD 154–5
serotonin 93
serotonin noradrenaline reuptake inhibitors (SNRIs) 154–5
severe depression 191
shell shock 3, 49
single nucleotide polymorphism (SNP) 102
socioeconomic education as a risk factor for PTSD 64
socioeconomic status as a risk factor for PTSD 63–4
soldier's heart 3, 49
species-specific defence response (SSDR) 92–3
stress-induced analgesia 2
stress-inoculation training 171
stressors and mental illness 1, 5–7
substance-use disorder 188
subsyndromal PTSD 20
subsystem clash hypothesis 120
suicide risk 191
systematic desensitisation 171, 172

technique selection 217–18
thalamus 2
therapist, importance of 217–18
timing of interventions 234
trauma-related borderline personality disorder 234
traumascape 226
traumatic exposure (DSM-IV-TR Criterion A1) 4–7, 9–10
  usefulness of 7–8
traumatic neurosis 3, 49
traumatic nightmares (DSM-IV-TR Criterion B2) 12
traumatic shock 49
truncated response hypothesis 120
two-factor theory 2

unconditioned stimuli (US) and the fear response 91–2

valproic acid 103
venlafaxine 151
ventral striatum 2
ventral tegmental area (VTA) 92
violence, political 218–19
volume of interventions 234

war 218–19
war psychoneurosis 49
World Health Organization (WHO) 50
  categories of violence 218

Printed in the United States
By Bookmasters